RHINOLOGY AND SINUSOLOGY
Diagnosis • Medical Management • Surgical Approaches

Series Editor

Howard L. Levine, M.D., F.A.C.S.
Director, The Mt. Sinai Nasal-Sinus Center
Chief, Section of Nasal-Sinus Surgery
The Mt. Sinai Medical Center
Cleveland, Ohio

Endoscopic Sinus Surgery

Howard L Levine, M.D., F.A.C.S.
Director, The Mt. Sinai Nasal-Sinus Center
Chief, Section of Nasal-Sinus Surgery
The Mt. Sinai Medical Center
Cleveland, Ohio

Mark May, M.D., F.A.C.S.
Director, Sinus Surgery Center
Shadyside Hospital

Clinical Professor
Department of Otolaryngology
University of Pittsburgh School of Medicine
Pittsburgh, Pennsylvania

Illustrated by Jon Coulter

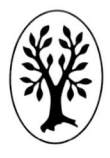

1993
THIEME MEDICAL PUBLISHERS, INC. New York
GEORG THIEME VERLAG Stuttgart · New York

Thieme Medical Publishers, Inc.
381 Park Avenue South
New York, New York 10016

ENDOSCOPIC SINUS SURGERY
Howard L. Levine
Mark May

Library of Congress Cataloging-in-Publication Data
Levine, Howard, 1944–
　　Endoscopic sinus surgery / Howard L. Levine, Mark May.
　　　　p.　　cm.—(Rhinology and sinusology)
　　Includes bibliographical references and index.
　　ISBN 0-86577-474-9 (TMP).—ISBN 3-13-794701-4 (GTV)
　　1. Paranasal sinuses—Endoscopic surgery.　I. May, Mark, 1936–
　　　II. Title.　III. Series.
　　[DNLM: 1. Endoscopy.　2. Paranasal Sinuses—surgery.　WV 340
L665e]
RF421.L48　1992
617.5′23—dc20
DNLM/DLC
for Library of Congress　　　　　　　　　　　　　　　　　　　　　　　　　92-49512
　　　　　　　　　　　　　　　　　　　　　　　　　　　　　　　　　　　　　　CIP

Copyright © 1993 by Thieme Medical Publishers, Inc. This book, including all parts thereof, is legally protected by copyright. Any use, exploitation or commercialization outside the narrow limits set by copyright legislation, without the publisher's consent, is illegal and liable to prosecution. This applies in particular to photostat reproduction, copying, mimeographing or duplication of any kind, translating, preparation of microfilms, and electronic data processing and storage.

Important note: Medicine is an ever-changing science. Research and clinical experience are continually broadening our knowledge, in particular our knowledge of proper treatment and drug therapy. Insofar as this book mentions any dosage or applications, readers may rest assured that the authors, editors, and publishers have made every effort to ensure that such references are strictly in accordance with the state of knowledge at the time of production of the book. Nevertheless, every user is requested to carefully examine the manufacturers' leaflets accompanying each drug to check on his own responsibility whether the dosage schedules recommended therein or the contraindications stated by the manufacturers differ from the statements made in the present book. Such examination is particularly important with drugs that are either rarely used or have been newly released on the market.

Some of the product names, patents, and registered designs referred to in this book are in fact registered trademarks or proprietary names even though specific reference to this fact is not always made in the text. Therefore, the appearance of a name without designation as proprietary is not to be construed as a representation by the publisher that it is in the public domain.

Printed in the United States of America.

5　4　3　2　1

TMP ISBN 0-86577-474-9
GTV ISBN 3-13-794701-4

In honor of my mother, Edith, and memory of my father, Samuel, whose hard work, encouragement, and life's commitment permitted me to become a physician.

To my wife, Susan, for her inspiration, support, and help in this textbook, my practice, and my life.

—*H.L.L.*

In memory of my parents, Paul and Pearl, who made personal sacrifices to provide me with my education. To my lifetime partner, companion, and mother to our seven children, Ida Ann. And finally to the thousands of sinus sufferers who gave me their confidence and allowed me to learn from them so that I might offer something better to those in the future.

—*M.M.*

Contents

Contributors xi

Preface xiii

Acknowledgments xv

1. **Complex Anatomy of the Lateral Nasal Wall: Simplified for the Endoscopic Sinus Surgeon** 1
   Howard L. Levine, M.D., F.A.C.S., Mark May, M.D., F.A.C.S., Michael Rontal, M.D., F.A.C.S., and Eugene Rontal, M.D., F.A.C.S.
   Anatomic Dissection of the Lateral Nasal Wall   2
      Turbinates   2
      Nasolacrimal and Sinus Drainage Sites   3
      Ostiomeatal Complex   4
      Structures Lateral to the Uncinate Process   6
      Maxillary Sinus   7
      Ethmoid Sinus   10
      Frontal Sinus   10
      Sphenoid Sinus   13
   Ethmoid Box and Surgical Zones   15
      Zone A   16
      Zone B   18
      Zone C   20
   Cross-Sectional Anatomy of the Paranasal Sinuses   22
   Summary   26

2. **Radiology of the Paranasal Sinuses** 29
   Section 1: Computed Tomography of the Paranasal Sinuses 29
   Gary G. Winzelberg, M.D., Kevin O'Hara, M.D., and Mark May, M.D., F.A.C.S.
   Computed Tomography Imaging Considerations   29
   Frontal Sinuses and Nasolacrimal Duct   30
      Frontal Sinus   30
      Nasolacrimal Duct   31
   Ethmoid Sinus   32
      Anatomy   32
      Variants   34

        Pathology   35
     Maxillary Sinus   38
        Anatomy and Variants   40
        Pathology   42
     Sphenoid Sinus   43
        Anatomy   44
        Pathology   44
     Adjacent Vital Structures   44
        Internal Carotid Artery   44
        Frontal Lobe   46
        Orbital Contents   47

Section 2: Advances in Paranasal Sinus Imaging: Screening Computed Tomography, 3-D Reconstruction, and Magnetic Resonance Imaging 49
    Charles F. Lanzieri, M.D., and Mae Urso, M.D.
    Screening Computed Tomography of Paranasal Sinuses   49
        Technique for Screening Computed Tomography   49
        Advantages of Screening Computed Tomography   51
    Surface-Rendered Three-Dimensional Reconstruction   51
    Magnetic Resonance Imaging   52
        Inflammatory Disease   53
        Neoplastic Disease   56
        Limitations of Magnetic Resonance Imaging   56
    Summary   59

3. Office Evaluation of Nasosinus Disorders: Patient Selection for Endoscopic Sinus Surgery 60
    Mark May, M.D., F.A.C.S., Sara J. Mester, R.T.(R), and Howard L. Levine, M.D., F.A.C.S.
    History   60
        Chief Complaint   61
        History of the Present Illness   62
        Past Medical and Surgical History   62
        Medications   62
        Symptom History   64
    Medical Management of Sinusitis   65
        Chronic Symptoms   65
        Allergy   65
        Acute Suppurative Sinusitis   65
        Treatment of Acute Suppurative Sinusitis   66
    Nasal Examination   68
        External Inspection   68
        Internal Examination   68
        Posterior Rhinoscopy   69
        Endoscopy   69
    Imaging of the Sinuses   85
        Plain Sinus Roentgenography   85

   Computed Tomography   85
  Case Selection for Surgery   87
   Informing the Patient   87
   Surgical Experience and Informed Consent   90
  Summary   90

4. Anesthesia for Endoscopic Sinus Surgery **91**
 Sawsan AlHuddud, M.D.
  Evaluation and Preparation for Anesthesia   91
   Anesthesia Evaluation   91
   Laboratory Tests   92
   Preoperative Medications   92
   Preparations in the Operating Room   93
  Local Anesthesia with Sedation   93
   Patient Oxygenation During Monitored Anesthesia Care   94
   Medications for Monitored Anesthesia Care   94
   Local Medications   95
   Complications During Monitored Anesthesia Care   96
  General Anesthesia   97
   Induction of Anesthesia   98
   Maintenance of Anesthesia   98
   Narcotic Anesthesia   99
   Complications of General Anesthesia   100
   Emergence from Anesthesia   100
  The Asthmatic Patient   101
  Postanesthesia Care   101
   Discharge Criteria   102
   Discharge Instructions   102
  Summary   102

5. Endoscopic Sinus Surgery **105**
 Mark May, M.D., F.A.C.S., Howard L. Levine, M.D., F.A.C.S.,
 Sara J. Mester, R.T.(R), and Marilyn Porta, R.N.
  Preparations for Surgery   106
   Special Preoperative Considerations   106
   On-Call to the Operating Room   107
  In the Operating Room   108
  Three Approaches to Sinus Surgery   108
   Video Endoscopic Sinus Surgery, Two-Handed
   Technique   108
   Two-Handed Endoscopic Versus Operating Microscope
   Technique   120
   The Wigand Technique   126
   Choice of Approach   126
  Anesthesia From the Surgeon's Point of View   126
   Choice of Anesthesia for Endoscopic Sinus Surgery   127
   Vasoconstriction and Local Anesthesia   128

Monitoring for Sinus Surgery 129
Endoscopic Sinus Surgery: Step-By-Step 129
   Nasal Septum 129
   Uncinate Process 130
   Maxillary Sinus Ostium 134
   Bulla Ethmoidalis 134
   Basal Lamella 134
   Roof of the Ethmoid Sinus 137
   Lamina Papyracea 141
   Sphenoidotomy 142
   Agger Nasi and Nasofrontal Recess 144
Special Surgical Situations 150
   Endoscopic Sinus Surgery 150
   Frontal Sinus Ostioplasty 157
   Maxillary Sinus Disease 164
   Traditional External Sinus Surgery 165
Prevention and Management of Bleeding 169
   Hemostasis 169
   Anterior Ethmoid Artery 169
   Sphenopalatine Artery 169
   Postoperative Dressings 170
Postoperative Care 170
   Outpatient Versus Inpatient Postoperative Care 170
   Routine Postoperative Orders 171
   Postoperative Medications 172
   Discharge Instructions to the Patient 173
   Postoperative Office Visits 173
Summary 174

6. Results of Surgery 176
Mark May, M.D., F.A.C.S., Howard L. Levine, M.D., F.A.C.S., Barry Schaitkin, M.D., and Sara J. Mester, R.T.(R)
Considerations for Systems to Report Results of Sinus Surgery 176
   Traditional Sinus Surgery 176
   Endoscopic Sinus Surgery 180
Sinus Surgery Results Reporting System of May and Levine 182
   Proposed Management of Nasosinus Disease by Endoscopic Sinus Surgery 184
   Results of Endoscopic Sinus Surgery in Levine and May Patient Series 185
Revision Endoscopic Sinus Surgery 188
   Reasons for Revision Surgery 189
   Treatment-Resistant Disease 190
Summary 191

7. **Complications of Endoscopic Sinus Surgery** 193
   Mark May, M.D., F.A.C.S., Howard L. Levine, M.D., F.A.C.S.,
   Barry Schaitkin, M.D., and Sara J. Mester, R.T.(R)
      System for Reporting Sinus Surgery Complications   193
         Classification   193
         Incidence   194
      Reported Complications of Traditional and Endoscopic Sinus Surgery   195
         Differences in Enumeration   195
         Surgeon's Learning Curve   198
         Type of Procedure   199
         Categorization of Complication   199
         Position of the Surgeon During Operation   200
         Complications for Traditional Versus Endoscopic Sinus Surgery   200
      Authors' Incidences of Endoscopic Sinus Surgery Complications   201
         Major Complications   202
         Minor Complications   203
      Prevention and Management of Complications   204
         Orbital Penetration   204
         Dural Complications of ESS   223
         Bleeding   229
         Lacrimal Complications   230
         Adhesions and Stenoses   230
         Asthma   237
         Other Complications   238
         Miscellaneous Complications   238
         Developing Surgical Skills to Avoid Complications   239
         Some Tips to Avoid Complications of Endoscopic Sinus Surgery   240
      Summary   242

8. **Endoscopic Sinus Surgery in Children** 244
   Rande H. Lazar, M.D., Ramzi T. Younis, M.D.,
   and Michael J. Gurucharri, M.D.
      Developmental Anatomy of the Paranasal Sinuses   244
         Ethmoid Sinus   245
         Maxillary Sinus   245
         Frontal Sinus   246
         Sphenoid Sinus   246
      Pathophysiology of Sinusitis in Children   246
         Ostial Obstruction   246
         Mucociliary Dysfunction   248
      Medical Management of Sinusitis in Children   248
         Antibiotic Medications   249

Other Medical Modalities **249**
Endoscopic Sinus Surgery in Children **251**
 Preoperative Evaluation **251**
 Endoscopic Sinus Surgery Technique in Children **251**
 Vasoconstriction **254**
 Procedure **254**
 Postoperative and Follow-up Care **255**
 Results of Endoscopic Sinus Surgery in Children **255**
Summary **255**

Appendix: Endoscopic Sinus Surgery Protocol 257
 Sinus Condition History **258**
 Symptom History **259**
 Nasal Endoscopic Findings **260**
 Computed Tomographic Scan Findings **261**
 Informed Consent **262**
 Findings at Surgery **263**
 Revision Surgery **264**

Index 265

Contributors

Sawsan AlHaddad, M.D.
Department of Anesthesiology
Cleveland Clinic Foundation
Cleveland, Ohio

Michael J. Gurucharri, M.D.
Chief of Surgery
Manatee Memorial Hospital
Bradenton, Florida

Charles F. Lanzieri, M.D.
Section of Neuroradiology
Cleveland Clinic Foundation
Cleveland, Ohio

Rande H. Lazar, M.D.
Director, Pediatric Otolaryngology
Director, Fellowship Training
LeBonheur Children's Medical Center
Memphis, Tennessee

Howard L. Levine, M.D., F.A.C.S.
Director, The Mt. Sinai Nasal-Sinus Center
Chief, Section of Nasal-Sinus Surgery
The Mt. Sinai Medical Center
Cleveland, Ohio

Mark May, M.D., F.A.C.S.
Director, Sinus Surgery Center
Shadyside Hospital

Clinical Professor
Department of Otolaryngology
University of Pittsburgh School of Medicine
Pittsburgh, Pennsylvania

Sara J. Mester, R.T.(R)
Research Assistant
Sinus Surgery Center
Shadyside Hospital
Pittsburgh, Pennsylvania

Kevin O'Hara, M.D.
Chief, Ultrasound
Department of Radiological Sciences and
    Diagnostic Imaging
Shadyside Hospital
Pittsburgh, Pennsylvania

Marilyn Porta, R.N.
Staff Development Coordinator
Shadyside Hospital
Pittsburgh, Pennsylvania

Eugene Rontal, M.D., F.A.C.S.
Clinical Associate Professor
Department of Otolaryngology–Head and
    Neck Surgery
University of Michigan
School of Medicine
Ann Arbor, Michigan

Michael Rontal, M.D., F.A.C.S.
Clinical Associate Professor
Department of Otolaryngology–Head and
    Neck Surgery
University of Michigan
School of Medicine
Ann Arbor, Michigan

Barry Schaitkin, M.D.
Sinus Surgery Center
Shadyside Hospital
Pittsburgh, Pennsylvania

Mae Urso, M.D.
Fellow, Section of Neuroradiology
Cleveland Clinic Foundation
Cleveland, Ohio

Gary G. Winzelberg, M.D.
Vice Chairman, Department of Radiological
   Sciences and Diagnostic Imaging
Shadyside Hospital
Pittsburgh, Pennsylvania

Ramzi T. Younis, M.D.
Staff Otolaryngologist
LeBonheur Children's Medical Center
Memphis, Tennessee

Preface

Otolaryngologists have always taken great interest in the evaluation and management of nasal and sinus disorders. The evaluation of the patient has involved careful history, physical examination, and imaging. Management has been both medical and surgical. In the past, the examination was performed with head mirror and nasal speculum and imaging with plain sinus roentgenography. Medical management involved nasal douche, fluid displacement, sinus irrigation, and antibiotics. Surgical management involved drainage with trephination, traditional Caldwell-Luc procedure, and sphenoethmoidectomy.

Recently, there has been a preoccupation by otolaryngologists with nasal and sinus disorders because of a major change in the manner in which nasal and sinus disorders have been detected and cared for. Much of this interest has been stimulated by the development of nasal and sinus endoscopy by European investigators and of computed tomographic imaging. This has created an increasing pursuit in the understanding of the pathophysiology of nasal and sinus disease.

Because of these new developments, there has been great exhilaration in otolaryngology. This excitement has been translated into countless teaching courses, research articles, national and international programs, and textbooks. For many practicing otolaryngologists, it has totally changed the manner in which they approach nasal and sinus disease.

The evaluation of the patient with nasal or sinus symptoms now includes nasal endoscopy, which has permitted the practitioner the ability to determine more thoroughly and reliably the cause of the symptoms. Computed tomographic scanning has shown the components of the anatomy of the ostiomeatal complex and contributed to the understanding of disease. Nasal endoscopes have allowed a meticulous, delicate removal of disease while preserving normal mucosa and structures. As results begin to be accumulated, there is even more enthusiasm for endoscopic sinus surgery as a functional, conserving approach.

With this excitement, there has been a demand for as much knowledge as possible within the field of rhinology and sinusology. As a result, this series, *Rhinology and Sinusology*, has been inaugurated.

This volume, *Endoscopic Sinus Surgery*, seems a most fitting topic source, and to a great extent it has been the basis for the enthusiasm. In this volume, there is an attempt to deal completely with nasal endoscopic diagnosis and management. Evaluation is discussed in chapters on office technique, patient selection, and radiographic imaging. Management of the adult and pediatric patient is included in chapters on surgical anatomy, anesthesia, and nasal endoscopic surgery and its complications. Most importantly, there is a discussion of results.

Many of the concepts described in this volume are not unique, but are the result of student and faculty discussion at teaching courses given by the authors at Shadyside Hospital in Pittsburgh, Pennsylvania, the First International Symposium in Contemporary Sinus Surgery (November 4–6, 1990), and countless visits by professionals to the offices and operating rooms at Shadyside Hospital, the Cleveland Clinic Foundation, and the Mt. Sinai Medical Center in Cleveland, Ohio.

Subsequent volumes in *Rhinology and Sinusology* will cover current, specific topics within this discipline. Although a book manuscript must someday go to the publisher and be considered "finished," the subject of nasal and sinus disease, as with all topics in medicine, is ongoing, and therefore the need exists for a continuing series. It is anticipated that this series will continue to provide ongoing, current topics of interest to the practicing otolaryngologist.

Howard L. Levine, M.D., F.A.C.S.
Mark May, M.D., F.A.C.S.

Acknowledgments

We would like to thank the many people who were involved in the creation of this book—the many residents who we had the privilege to teach and who along the way taught us what we did not know.

We are also grateful to Jon Coulter for his superb illustrations, Diana Mathis for copyediting and helping to revise the manuscript, and Roselle Solomon and Romayne Bodnar for typing and helping with the book's organization.

We acknowledge with gratitude the granting of permission to reproduce, either in their original or in modified form, illustrations published in the *Archives of Otolaryngology—Head and Neck Surgery*, *Laryngoscope*, and *Operative Techniques in Otolaryngology—Head and Neck Surgery* (Chapters 1 and 5). In addition, we would like to thank Xomed, Inc., who kindly supplied the photography of the Xomed-Treace MPS2000 Micro-Craft drill with Micro-Slim handpiece, which is shown in Chapter 5, as well as Karl Storz Instrument for providing photographs of instruments noted in Chapter 5.

Howard L. Levine, M.D., F.A.C.S.
Mark May, M.D., F.A.C.S.

1
Complex Anatomy of the Lateral Nasal Wall: Simplified for the Endoscopic Sinus Surgeon

HOWARD L. LEVINE, M.D., F.A.C.S.
MARK MAY, M.D., F.A.C.S.
MICHAEL RONTAL, M.D., F.A.C.S.
EUGENE RONTAL, M.D., F.A.C.S.

The growing popularity of endonasal endoscopic sinus surgery has led to a resurgence of interest in the anatomy of the nose and paranasal sinuses. In an effort to understand nasal and sinus anatomy and pathophysiology better, modern sinus surgeons have returned to the writings of anatomists and otolaryngologists who decades ago described the recesses, spaces, and bony structures of this region. Paranasal anatomy is complex, however, and traditional descriptions are not always useful for physicians planning and executing endoscopic surgical management of sinus disease.

The way we present the complex anatomy of the lateral nasal wall in this chapter should simplify the process by which endonasal endoscopic sinus surgeons gain an understanding of pertinent surgical anatomy. First, we describe the anatomy of the lateral nasal wall as it would be revealed by medial-to-lateral dissection. Then, we describe the ethmoid sinus as a box divided into distinct surgical zones. Finally, we describe the cross-sectional anatomy of the paranasal sinuses. The goal of this presentation is to help the sinus surgeon visualize the anatomy of the lateral nasal wall in three dimensions, a necessary prerequisite to operating in this region.

ANATOMIC DISSECTION OF THE LATERAL NASAL WALL

In dissecting the lateral nasal wall from medial to lateral, the first structure encountered is the medial wall of the nose or nasal septum. The nasal septum is a relatively simple structure that has an impact on sinus disease only when the septum is deviated significantly (Fig. 1–1).

Turbinates

In contrast, the lateral wall of the nose, which is the next structure encountered when the nasal septum has been removed, is a complex structure that is frequently involved in sinus disease. The most prominent features of the lateral wall of the nose (Fig. 1–2) are the turbinates. These are usually three, or possibly four, in number, and they appear as delicate scrolls of bone, covered by ciliated columnar mucous epithelium, that project from the lateral nasal wall. Inferior, middle, and superior turbinates are present in nearly all patients; occasionally, a very small supreme turbinate may be present as well.

Often, a prominence may be seen at the anterior attachment of the middle turbinate. This prominence appears variably as a slight elevation in some patients to a definite rounding in others, depending on the degree of pneumatization of the anterior portion of the ethmoid sinus. The prominence overlies the agger nasi (Fig. 1–2), anterior to the nasofrontal recess, and is thought to be a remnant of an additional turbinate found in animals. The agger

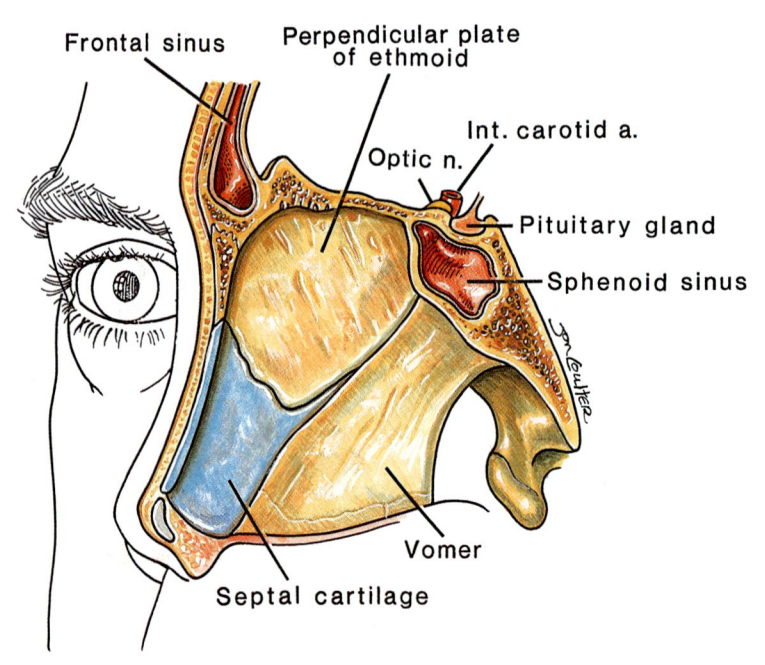

Figure 1–1. Oblique view of right nasal septum. a.: artery; Int.: internal; n.: nerve.

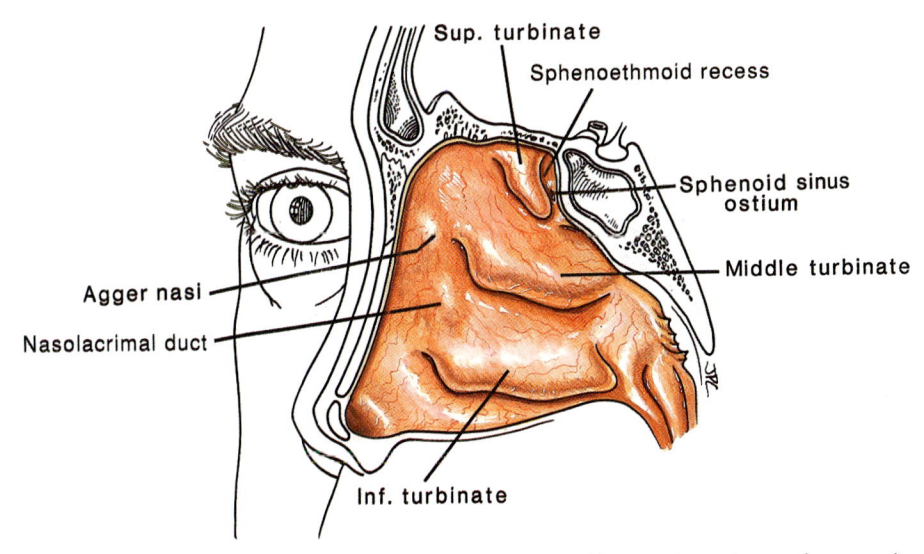

Figure 1–2. Oblique view of lateral nasal wall demonstrates the turbinates and prominence of agger nasi and lacrimal duct. Inf.: inferior; Sup.: superior.

nasi cells themselves overlie the lacrimal sac and are separated from this sac by a thin layer of bone.

Nasolacrimal and Sinus Drainage Sites

When the anterior attachment of the inferior and middle turbinates has been removed, lacrimal and sinus drainage system elements may be seen (Fig. 1–3). The nasal opening of the *nasolacrimal duct* is visible in the anterior third of the inferior meatus. The course of this duct, from the lacrimal sac under the agger nasi to its opening under the anterior end of the inferior turbinate, may be noted as a prominence in the lateral nasal wall.

The anterior sinus drainage system (frontal, maxillary, and anterior ethmoid) lies in the middle third of the lateral nasal wall, under the middle turbinate (the middle meatus) (Fig. 1–4A).[1] The *uncinate process* (the first lamella), a structure shaped like a wing or boomerang, forms the anterior border of this system. The uncinate process attaches anteriorly to the posterior edge of the lacrimal bone and inferiorly to the superior edge of the inferior turbinate. Superiorly, the uncinate process may attach to the lamina papyracea, roof of the ethmoid sinus, or middle turbinate.

The drainage of the anterior system is into a channel, the *infundibulum*. The infundibulum is bordered anteriorly by the uncinate process, posteriorly by the *face of the bulla ethmoidalis* (the second lamella), and laterally by the lamina papyracea. The infundibulum is open on its medial side, which is referred to as the hiatus semilunaris (Fig. 1–4A).[1] Secretions from the frontal, maxillary, and anterior ethmoid sinuses are swept by

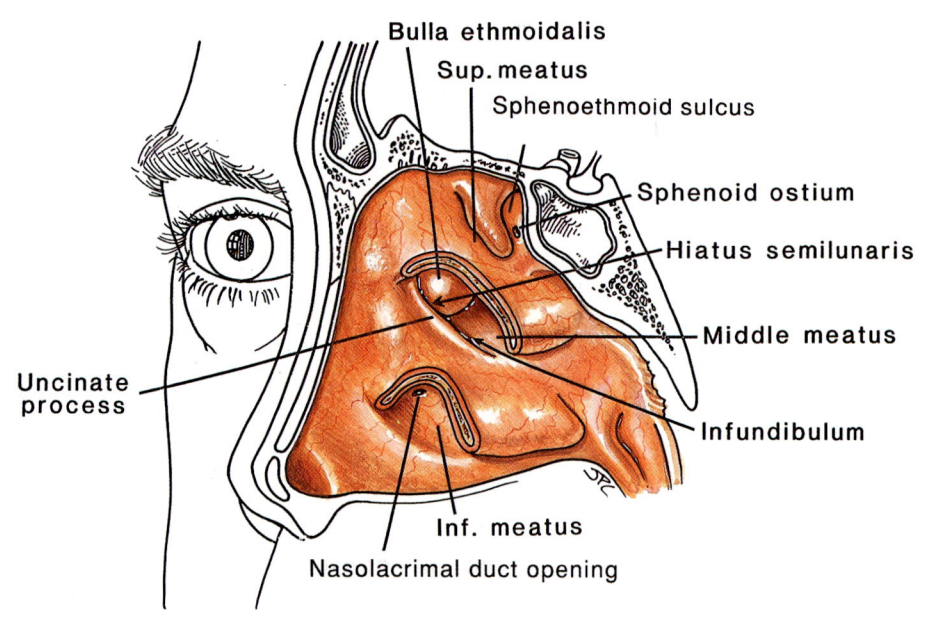

Figure 1–3. Oblique view of right lateral nasal wall with the anterior portions of the middle and inferior turbinate removed. Major structures of the lateral nasal wall that appear after this dissection are the nasolacrimal duct opening, uncinate process, hiatus semilunaris, and bulla ethmoidalis. The sphenoid sinus ostium may also be seen posterior to the superior turbinate. Inf.: inferior; Sup.: superior.

mucociliary flow toward the nasopharynx over the sulcus formed by the superior boundary of the inferior turbinate and under the prominence of the torus tubarius (Fig. 1–4B).

The *basal lamella* (the third lamella, also called the ground lamella because it appears transparent or the grand lamella because it is an important surgical landmark) forms the boundary between this anterior sinus drainage system and more posterior systems. Thus, posterior ethmoid cells drain under the superior turbinate into the superior meatal sulcus. The sphenoid sinus drains into the sphenoethmoid recess through the sphenoid sinus ostium. Both the posterior ethmoid cells and sphenoid sinus drain over the upper surface of the torus tubarius (Fig. 1–4B).

Ostiomeatal Complex

Endoscopic sinus surgeons use the term "ostiomeatal complex" (OMC) to refer to the area bounded by the middle turbinate medially, the lamina papyracea laterally, and the basal lamella superiorly and posteriorly. The inferior and anterior borders of the OMC are open. This space contains the agger nasi, nasofrontal recess, infundibulum, bulla ethmoidalis, and anterior ethmoid cells (Fig. 1–4A).[1]

One of us (H. L.) suggests that this area, now referred to as the OMC, be called the *anterior OMC* and the space behind the basal lamella containing the posterior ethmoid cells be referred to as the *posterior OMC*. This new terminology further recognizes the basal

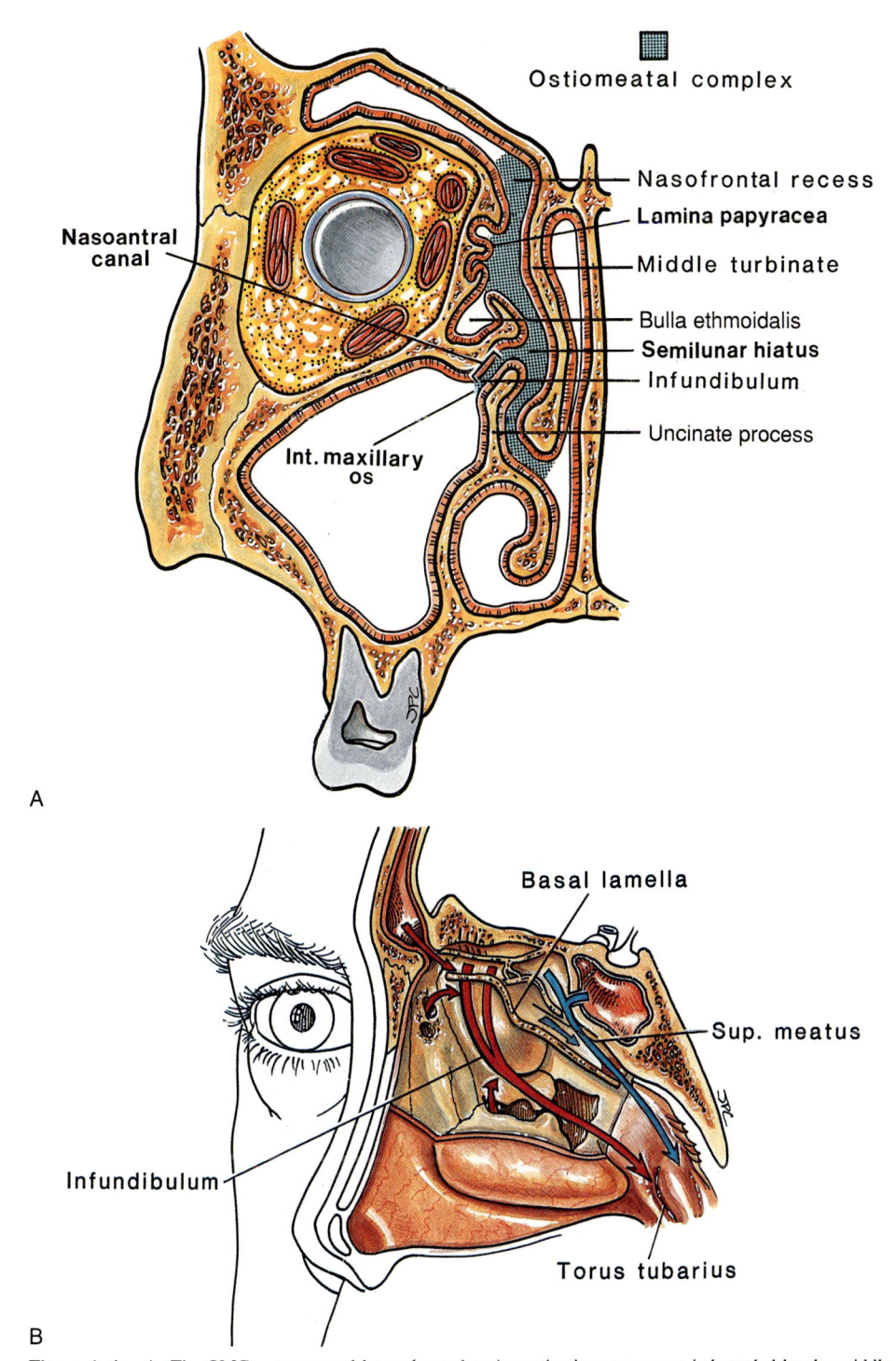

Figure 1–4. **A**: The OMC, a term used by endonasal endoscopic sinus surgeons, is bounded by the middle turbinate, lamina papyracea, and basal lamella. Int.: internal; os: ostium. (Modified from Kennedy et al.[1]) **B**: The basal lamella divides the OMC into anterior and posterior compartments that drain mucociliary flow anteriorly or posteriorly (as suggested by H. L.). Sup.: superior.

lamella as an important anatomic landmark that separates the anterior from the posterior sinus drainage systems (Fig. 1–4B). These separate drainage pathways are important in the pathophysiology of sinus disease and also to its surgical treatment. Thus, when disease is limited to the anterior compartment of the OMC, ethmoid cells are opened and diseased tissue removed as far as the basal lamella; not disturbing the basal lamella in such cases avoids the risk of penetrating the roof of the ethmoid sinus and possibly causing a cerebrospinal fluid leak or worse injury to intracranial structures.

Structures Lateral to the Uncinate Process

The ethmoid infundibulum, which lies lateral to the uncinate process, may be seen more clearly when the uncinate process has been removed (Fig. 1–5). When this infundibulum extends anteriorly and superiorly to the nasofrontal recess, it may be considered the frontal infundibulum. If it ends blindly, as it may when the frontal sinus drains between the middle turbinate and the uncinate process, this pocket may be referred to as a *sinus terminalis*.

The bulla ethmoidalis forms the posterior aspect of the ethmoid infundibulum. This bulla, the most prominent of the anterior ethmoid air cells, is pneumatized in 60 to 70% of cases.[2] Superior and posterior to the bulla ethmoidalis, a small depression, the sinus lateralis (Fig. 1–5), is present in some individuals. The sinus lateralis separates the bulla ethmoidalis and the basal lamella.

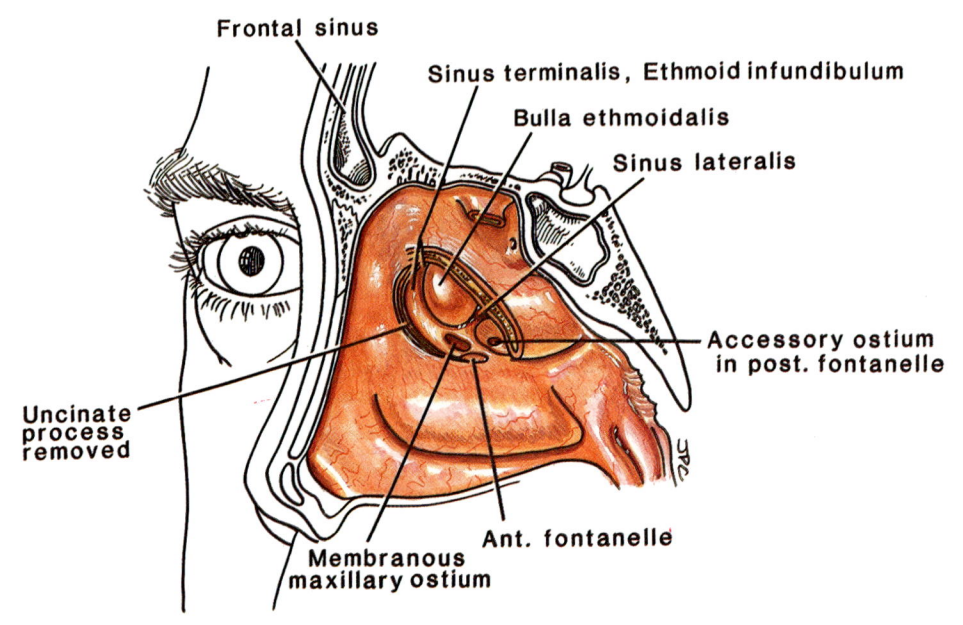

Figure 1–5. Oblique view of right lateral nasal wall with the uncinate process removed. Note relationship of the membranous maxillary sinus ostium to the bulla ethmoidalis. Ant.: anterior; post.: posterior.

Maxillary Sinus

The membranous *maxillary sinus ostium* is formed by the confluence of the maxillary sinus mucosa and the mucosal lining of the nasal infundibulum (Fig. 1–4A). This ostium, normally hidden from view by an intact uncinate process, is usually found at the junction of the anterosuperior and posteroinferior aspects of the infundibulum.

Based on a study of 163 specimens, Van Alyea[3] found the most common site for the maxillary ostium to be in the posterior third of the infundibular groove (72%). The ostium was located in the anterior third in only 6% of specimens; in 12% of specimens the ostium was at the extreme posterior tip of the groove.

The location and configuration of the maxillary sinus ostium and the relationship of the ostium to the orbit are of practical significance to the endoscopic sinus surgeon. Of particular relevance is the ostium's configuration as seen through the 0° endoscope and its location with respect to the orbit, uncinate process, bulla ethmoidalis, and any accessory ostia. When the internal maxillary ostium is viewed directly in the dissection laboratory, this opening on the maxillary sinus side appears shaped like an ellipse, teardrop, or hourglass, with its long axis oriented horizontally or obliquely. This ostium was consistently found (within 2 to 3 mm) just below the junction of the medial wall of the maxillary sinus with the orbital plate of the maxilla (orbital floor) roughly halfway between the anterior and posterior walls (Fig. 1–6A).[4]

The image of this ostium obtained through a wide-angled endoscopic lens appears to be an optical illusion and can be disorienting: the ostium is the same shape, but its long axis appears to have been rotated 45° counterclockwise (Fig. 1–6B)[4]; the transcanine endoscopic image of the ostium on the left side would appear rotated 45° clockwise.

This change in appearance of the maxillary sinus ostium has practical implications for the surgeon working through the endoscope in the antrum, particularly when widening the ostium or forming a communication between it and the accessory ostium. The change in appearance of the ostium and loss of depth of field can easily lead the surgeon to mistake the orbital floor for the posterior wall of the antrum. The floor of the orbit will appear more vertically oriented through the endoscope and may appear behind, rather than above, the ostium. The surgeon must keep these effects of the endoscopic view in mind and must have a thorough knowledge of the relevant anatomic relationships to avoid injuring the orbit when opening the natural ostium.

The endoscopic sinus surgeon must also distinguish the natural maxillary sinus ostium from the accessory ostium. These ostia differ in location and configuration, with the accessory ostium usually being located within the posterior fontanelle and being more rounded than the natural ostium. In addition, mucociliary flow is not directed toward the accessory ostium, but rather around it toward the natural ostium. Endoscopically, the accessory ostium generally appears inferior to the natural ostium because of the optical illusory effect described earlier, although it is actually located posterior to the natural ostium.

When surgeons begin to perform endoscopic sinus surgery, they may experience a higher incidence of orbital complications than average. This is because identification of the natural ostium of the maxillary sinus from the nasal side during surgery may be more difficult than identification in the dissection laboratory. To decrease the risk of orbital complications, surgeons should avoid blind probing or nibbling with the forceps in this region.

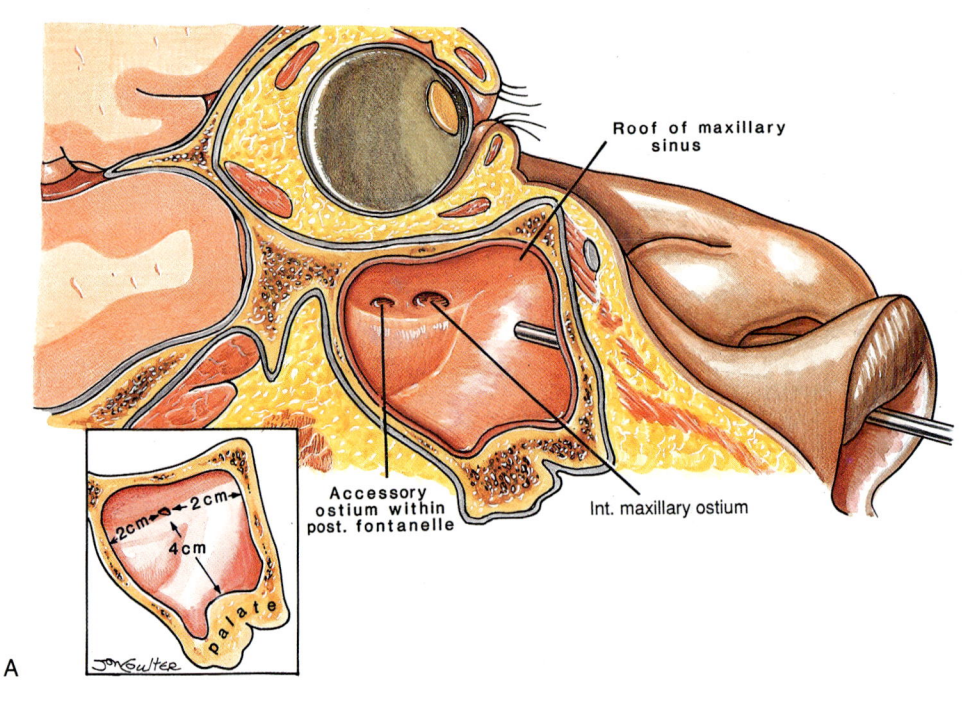

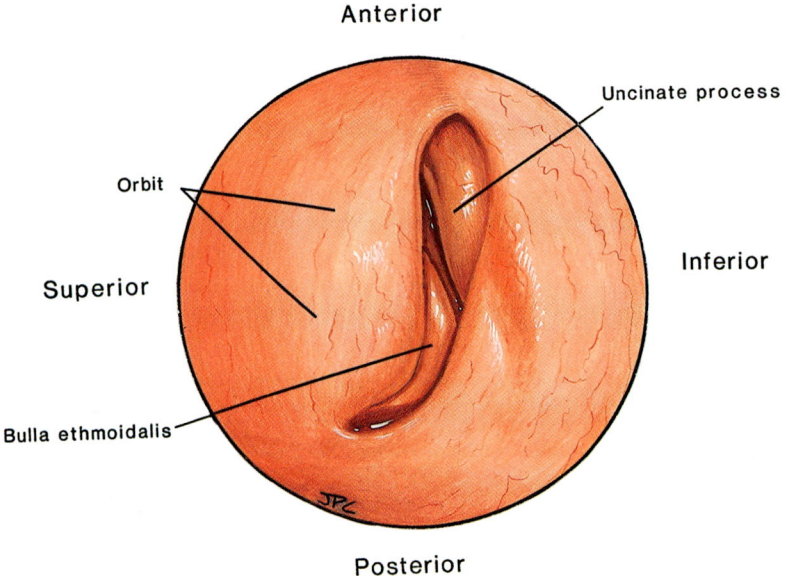

Figure 1–6. Right transcanine fossa approach to the maxillary sinus. **A**: Right sagittal section through orbit and maxillary sinus shows internal maxillary ostium located just beneath the floor of the orbit and accessory ostium located posterior to it in the posterior fontanelle. *Inset*: Average distance of the internal maxillary ostium from the anterior and posterior maxillary wall and floor of maxillary sinus (palate). Int.: internal; post.: posterior. **B**: Endoscopic view through right canine fossa of internal maxillary ostium. Note that anterior is at the top and posterior is at the bottom. This rotation is due to the optical distortion associated with the endoscope. (Modified with permission from May et al.[4]).

Fontanelle

Just posterior to the maxillary sinus ostium and inferior to the lamina papyracea is the membranous wall or *fontanelle* that separates the maxillary sinus from the nasal cavity. This fontanelle is bounded inferiorly by the superior border of the inferior turbinate and posteriorly by the ascending process of the palatine bone (Figs. 1–5 and 1–7). The fontanelle may be divided into anterior and posterior segments by the uncinate process. The smaller anterior fontanelle is the portion covering the bony dehiscence between the inferior edge of the uncinate and its attachment to the inferior turbinate. The posterior fontanelle lies above the posterosuperior edge of the uncinate process.

Accessory Ostium

According to a number of studies, an *accessory ostium* is present in the posterior part of the fontanelle in some 10 to 50% of specimens.[3] It is not known whether such ostia are congenital or occur secondarily. A possible mechanism for secondary formation of accessory ostia is obstruction of the natural ostium by maxillary sinus infection followed by rupture of infectious material through a weak area of the fontanelle. The surgeon should be careful to distinguish an accessory ostium from the maxillary sinus ostium because mucociliary flow and normal sinus drainage are through the natural ostium and not through the accessory ostium.[4]

The lateral boundary of the ethmoid complex and of the bulla ethmoidalis is formed by the lamina papyracea (orbital wall), which is wider anteriorly and narrows posteriorly (Fig. 1–7). When the middle turbinate has been removed, its lateral attachment to the lamina papyracea, the basal lamella, can be visualized (Fig. 1–7). This view demonstrates the basal lamella as the structure that divides the anterior and posterior drainage systems (Fig. 1–4B).

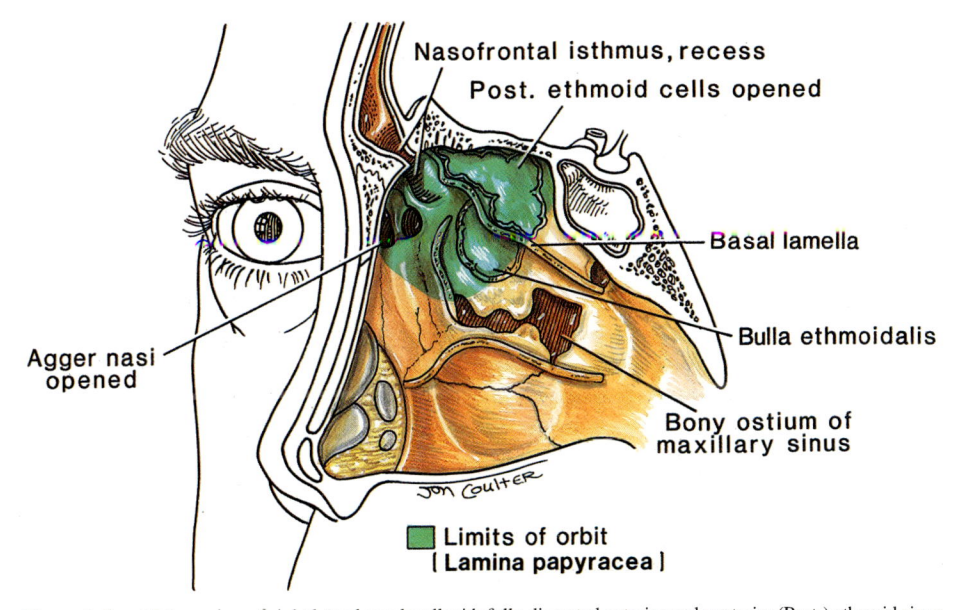

Figure 1–7. Oblique view of right lateral nasal wall with fully dissected anterior and posterior (Post.) ethmoid sinus. The medial aspect of the orbit (lamina papyracea) on the lateral nasal wall is the cone-shaped area colored green.

Ethmoid Sinus

The ethmoid sinus is a cavity made up of a honeycomb network of small cells that vary in number from one individual to the next. This cavity, or space, is contained within a box with sides of varying dimensions. The box is narrow (approximately 0.5 cm across) anteriorly and widens (to approximately 1.5 cm) as it extends posteriorly to the front face of the sphenoid sinus. The box is wider along its roof than its inferior aspect. It is approximately 4 to 5 cm long and 2.5 to 3 cm high.

The roof of the ethmoid sinus is relatively smooth, as is the lamina papyracea, which forms the lateral wall of the ethmoid sinus. The medial wall of the ethmoid sinus, formed by the middle turbinate, is less smooth.

Frontal Sinus

The frontal sinus, nasofrontal isthmus, and nasofrontal recess are shaped something like the upper portion, waist, and lower portion of an hourglass (Fig. 1–8).

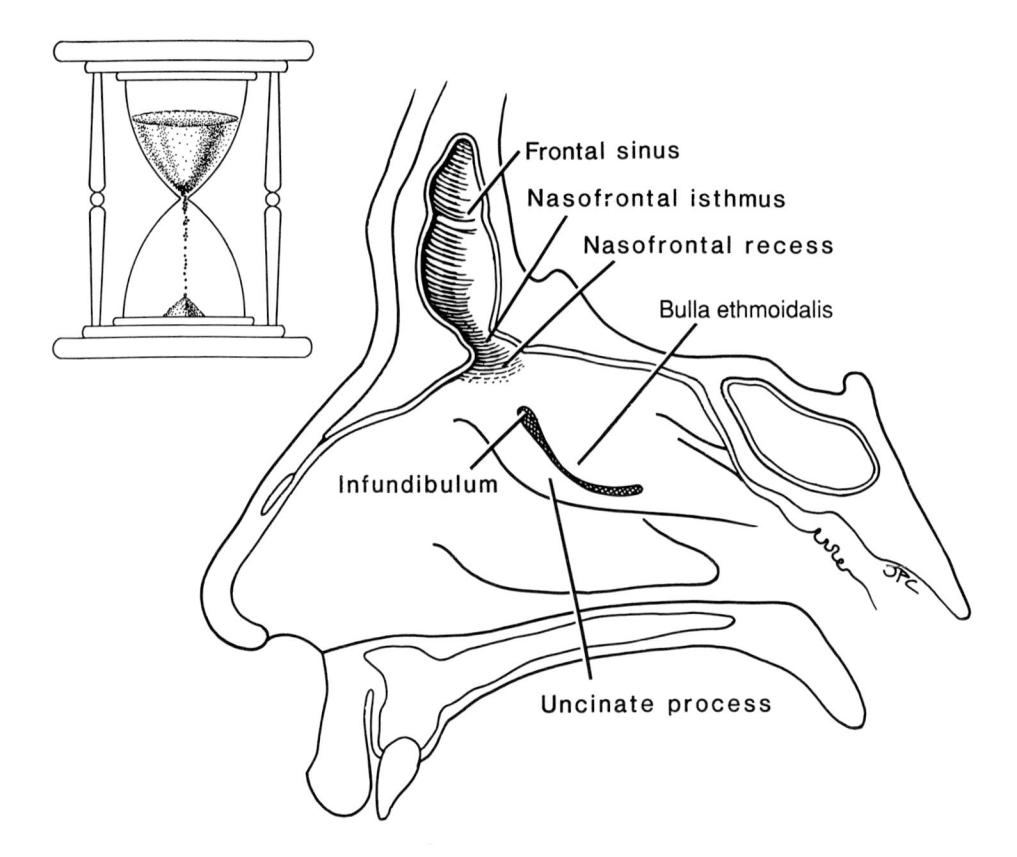

Figure 1–8. Lateral view of right paranasal structures showing relationship of the frontal sinus to the nasofrontal recess. *Insert*: The complex of frontal sinus, isthmus, and nasofrontal recess is shaped like an hourglass.

Several different patterns of *frontal sinus drainage* have been described. Van Alyea[5] described two major types of frontal drainage, depending on whether the sinus drains directly into the infundibulum or not. Van Alyea found that in 86% of patients the frontal sinus drains anterior to (Fig. 1–9A), superior to (Fig. 1–9B), or posterior to (Fig. 1–9C) the infundibulum. When the frontal sinus drains medial to the infundibulum, the uncinate process is usually attached to the orbit and the infundibulum ends superiorly, against the lamina papyracea, as a sinus terminalis (Fig. 1–9D). In such cases the nasofrontal recess drains into the space between the uncinate and the lateral wall of the middle turbinate.[6]

Van Alyea[5] found that in the other 14% of cases the frontal sinus drains directly into the infundibulum (Fig. 1–10A). The uncinate process in these cases is attached to the roof of the ethmoid (Fig. 1–10B) or the superior lateral attachment of the middle turbinate (Fig. 1–10C).[6]

Kasper,[7] however, reported different findings regarding drainage of the frontal sinus. In 34% of the cadavers that Kasper dissected, the frontal sinus arose from and drained into the ethmoid infundibulum. In another 4% of the cadavers the frontal sinus was in direct anatomic continuity with the ethmoid infundibulum.[7]

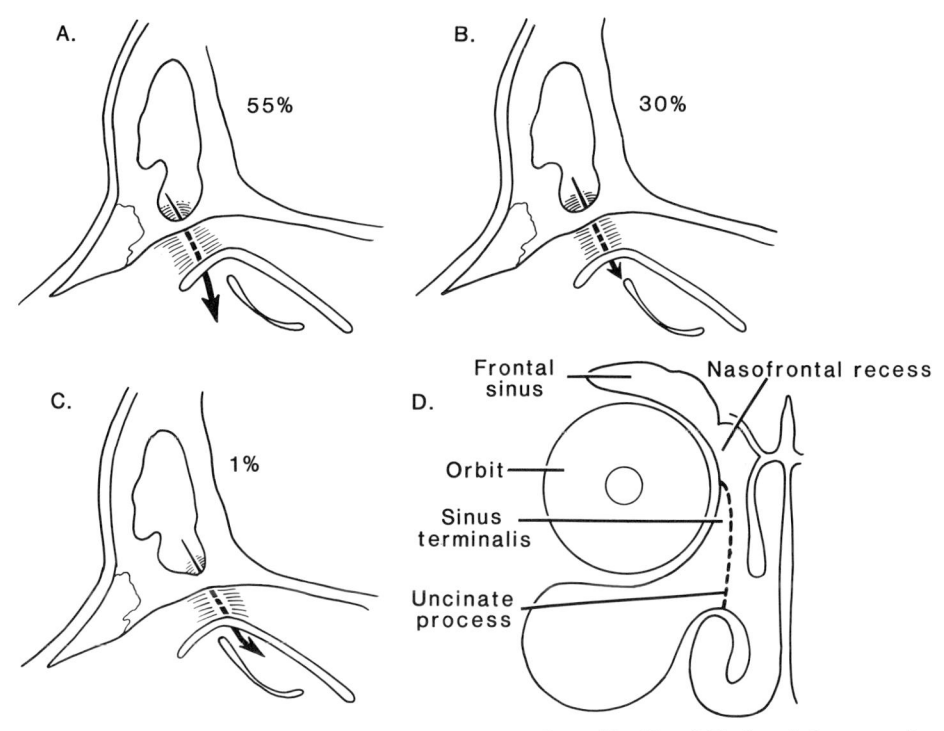

Figure 1–9. Right lateral view of frontal sinus drainage according to Van Alyea.[5] The frontal sinus most often drains between the middle turbinate and uncinate either anterior to the infundibulum (**A**), above the infundibulum (**B**), or posterior to the infundibulum (**C**). **D**: When the uncinate process is attached to the lamina papyracea, the nasofrontal recess drains between the uncinate and middle turbinate. In these cases the infundibulum ends blindly to form a sinus terminalis.[6]

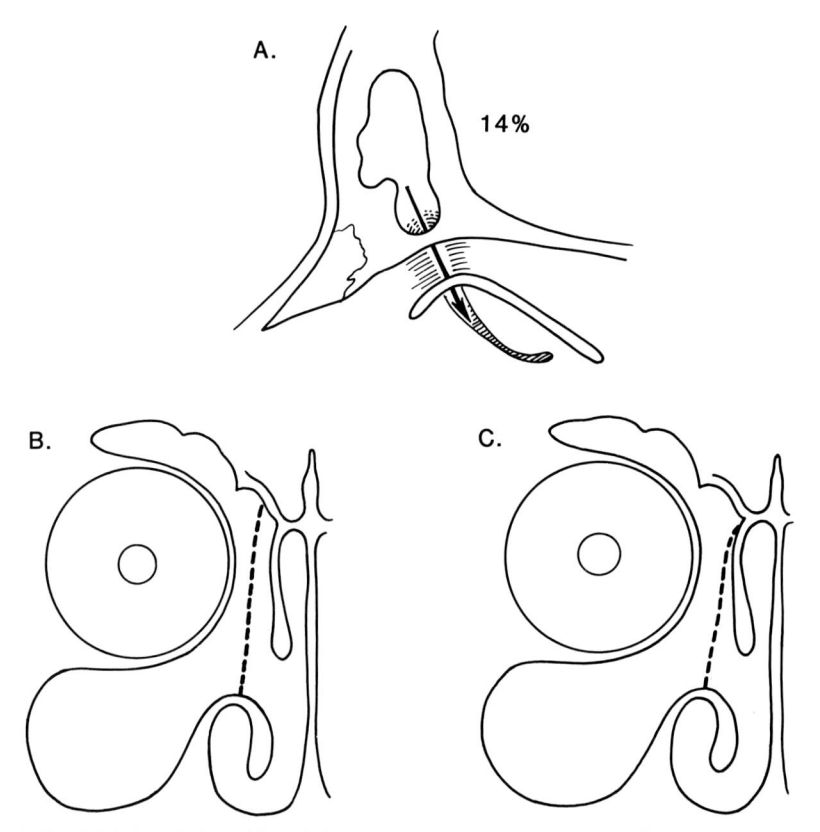

Figure 1–10. Right lateral view of frontal sinus drainage according to Van Alyea.[5] **A**: The frontal sinus drains into the infundibulum when the uncinate attaches to the roof of the ethmoid (**B**) or the anterior superior attachment of the middle turbinate (**C**).[6]

When viewed from the frontal sinus in the axial plane (Fig. 1–11),[8] the nasofrontal isthmus appears surrounded medially and anteriorly by agger nasi air cells. The nasolacrimal sac lies about 1 to 2 mm anterior to the isthmus.

The *anterior ethmoid artery*, a branch of the ophthalmic artery, lies in the roof of the ethmoid sinus just posterior to the nasofrontal recess. This artery is in the same coronal plane as the anterior aspect of the ethmoid bulla, and, after it leaves the orbit through the anterior ethmoid foramen, it passes between the ethmoid air cells and enters the olfactory groove. It then passes through a slit by the side of the crista galli and returns through the cribriform plate to enter the nasal cavity.

The *agger nasi cells* lie in approximately the same coronal plane as the nasofrontal recess and nasolacrimal duct (Fig. 1–12).[8] The relationship of the agger nasi cells to the frontal sinus is variable and may affect frontal sinus drainage. The nasofrontal recess is bounded by agger nasi cells anteriorly and by the anterosuperior face of the bulla ethmoidalis posteriorly (Fig. 1–13A). Van Alyea[5] found that in 50% of cases the agger nasi cells impinge on the frontal sinus, and in one third of these cases the region of the

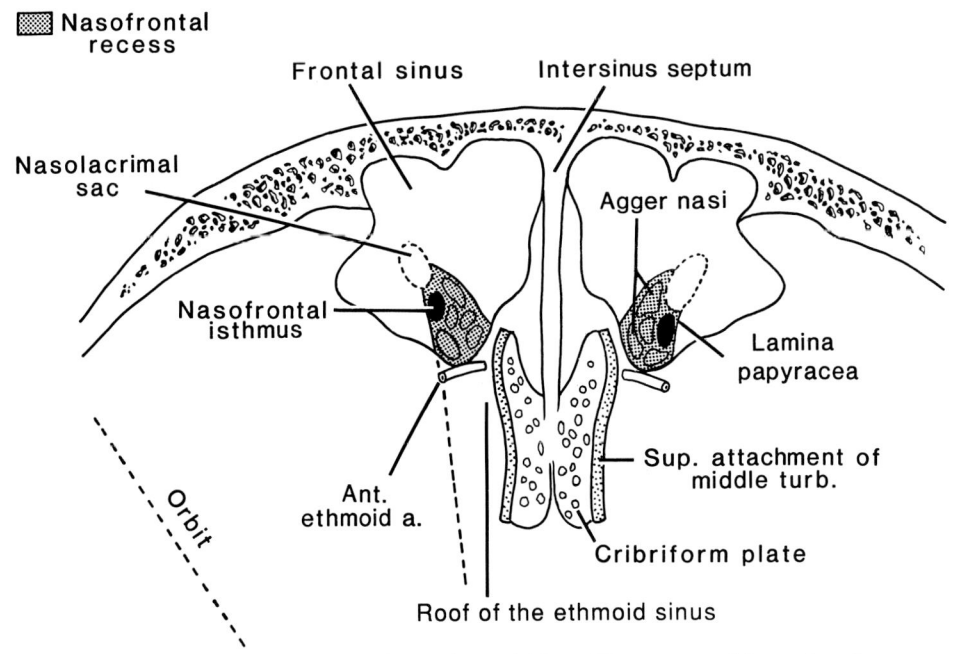

Figure 1–11. Superior axial view through the anterior cranial fossa. The structures of the nasofrontal recess are presented as though the bone over the nasofrontal recess were transparent. In this way, the frontal sinus, superior (Sup.) attachment of the middle turbinate (turb.), and cribriform plate can be seen at the same time as the structures related to the nasofrontal recess. Note that the nasofrontal isthmus is lateral to the anterosuperior attachment of the middle turbinate and lies against the lamina papyracea (orbit) in the anterior aspect of the nasofrontal recess. Ant.: anterior; a.: artery. (Modified with permission from May.[8])

nasofrontal isthmus is affected. He believed that these configurations would cause frontal sinus obstruction and thus sinusitis.

One type of obstruction to frontal sinus outflow is a *frontal sinus bulla*, which occurs when agger nasi cells push superiorly into the floor of the frontal sinus (Fig. 1–13B). A frontal sinus bulla may also occur as a result of the contralateral frontal sinus impinging on the sinus. Alternatively, obstruction to frontal sinus outflow may be caused by a middle turbinate that is enlarged or convex laterally rather than medially so that it obstructs the nasofrontal recess.

Sphenoid Sinus

The sphenoid sinus has been called the most variable bilateral cavity in the human body.[9] This sinus is usually contained entirely within the body of the sphenoid bone, although it may extend into the greater wing of the sphenoid bone or into the pterygoid process.[9,10] Its size varies widely, from 0.5 to 30 cc (average, 7.5 cc).[11] Because the opening of the sphenoid sinus into the sphenoethmoid recess, which lies superior and posterior to the superior turbinate, is about 1.5 cm above the sinus floor, mucus must be moved out of the sphenoid sinus by active mucociliary flow (Fig. 1–4B).

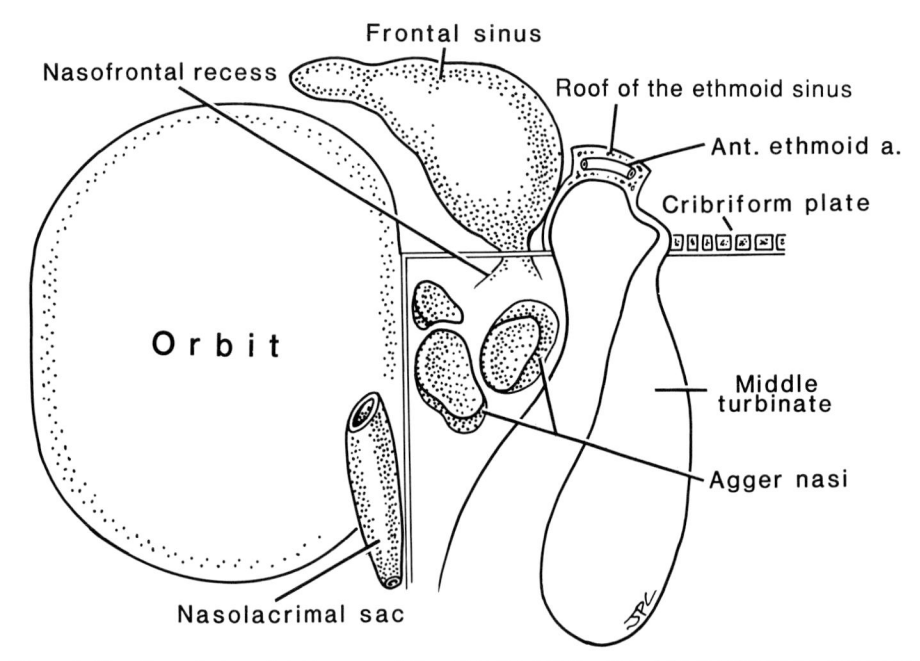

Figure 1–12. Coronal view of right paranasal structures through the area of the nasofrontal isthmus showing relationships of anterior (Ant.) ethmoid artery (a.), orbit, nasolacrimal sac, and cribriform plate to frontal sinus, agger nasi cells, and middle turbinate. (Reprinted with permission from May.[8])

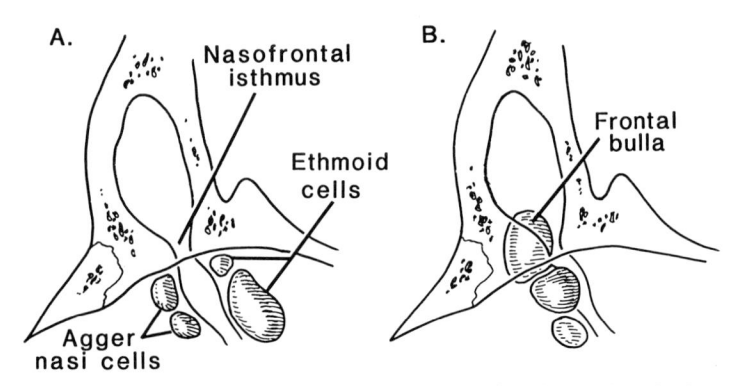

Figure 1–13. Right lateral views of nasofrontal complex show nasofrontal recess bounded by agger nasi cells anteriorly and ethmoid cells posteriorly (**A**) and encroachment of agger nasi cells into the nasofrontal complex (**B**). Such encroachment is referred to as a frontal bulla and can obstruct nasofrontal drainage.

Structures and spaces contiguous to the sphenoid sinus are of great importance to the endoscopic sinus surgeon. These structures include the pituitary gland superior to this sinus and the optic nerve and carotid artery laterally. The roof of the sphenoid sinus is usually level with the roof of the ethmoid sinus.

When the sphenoid sinus is well-pneumatized, many structures contiguous with this sinus can deform the sinus walls (Fig. 1–1). For example, if the sphenoid sinus has pneumatized into the anterior and posterior clinoid processes, the sella turcica can project into the roof of the sinus. The internal carotid artery has been found to project into the posterolateral aspect of the sphenoid sinus in 65% of cases,[12] and in 8 to 25% of specimens the wall of the sphenoid sinus may be dehiscent over this artery.[13,14] In other cases (7 to 78%)[9,12,13] the optic canal may project into the sphenoid sinus. In a study by Fujii et al,[13] the optic nerve sheath in 4% of specimens was separated from the sphenoid sinus by only sinus mucosa. Finally, the maxillary division of the fifth cranial nerve may indent the lateral wall of this sinus.[9,10,13]

ETHMOID BOX AND SURGICAL ZONES

Earlier in this chapter the ethmoid complex was described as a space contained in a box with sides of variable dimensions. To help the endoscopic sinus surgeon visualize the anatomy of this region in three dimensions, it may be useful to review the boundaries and contents of this box for their surgical significance. The sides of the box are open anteriorly and inferiorly (Fig. 1–14).[15] The roof of the box is the roof of the ethmoid sinus, the lateral wall

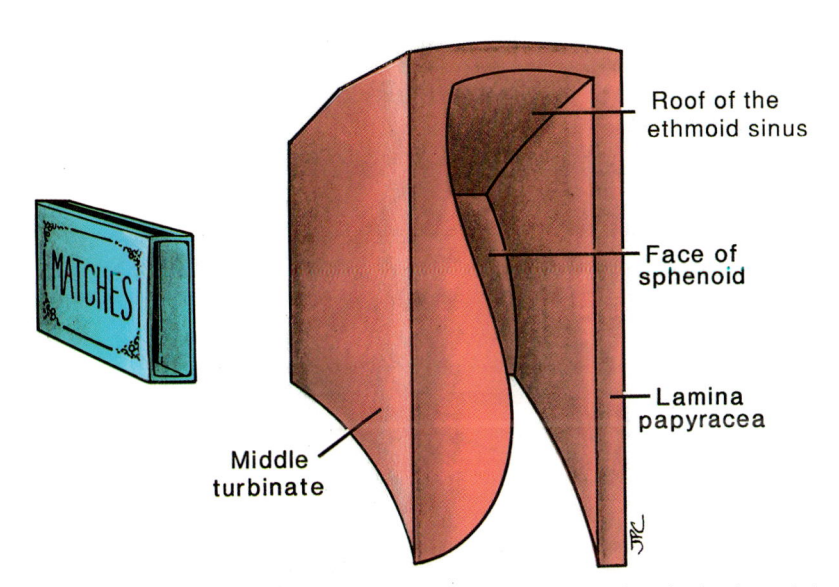

Figure 1–14. Left lateral view of ethmoid complex. The complex, approximately the size and shape of a matchbox, is 0.5 cm wide, 1.5 cm high, and 5 cm deep. It has four bony sides—a roof, lateral wall (the lamina papyracea), medial wall (the middle turbinate), and posterior wall (face of the sphenoid)—and is open on two sides. (Reprinted with permission from May.[15])

is the lamina papyracea, the medial wall is the middle turbinate, and the posterior wall is the face of the sphenoid sinus.

The ethmoid box may be divided into three zones (Fig. 1–15)[15]: A, (the anterior OMC) from the anterosuperior attachment of the middle turbinate to the posterolateral attachment of the middle turbinate; B, (the posterior OMC) from the posterolateral attachment of the middle turbinate to the face of the sphenoid bone; and C, (the sphenoid) from the face of the sphenoid sinus to include the sphenoid sinus and its neighboring structures.

Zone A

Within zone A (the anterior OMC) are the nasofrontal recess, agger nasi cells, anterior ethmoid artery, lamina papyracea, uncinate process, infundibulum, natural ostium of the maxillary sinus, and bulla ethmoidalis (Fig. 1–16A and B). Zone A is narrowest and its walls thinnest in its most anterior extent.

The roof of zone A is the roof of the ethmoid sinus. This plate of bone separates the ethmoid cavity from the anterior cranial fossa, and, at its anterosuperior and medial aspect, it is paper thin. The bone in this vicinity of the ethmoid sulcus is up to 10 times thinner than

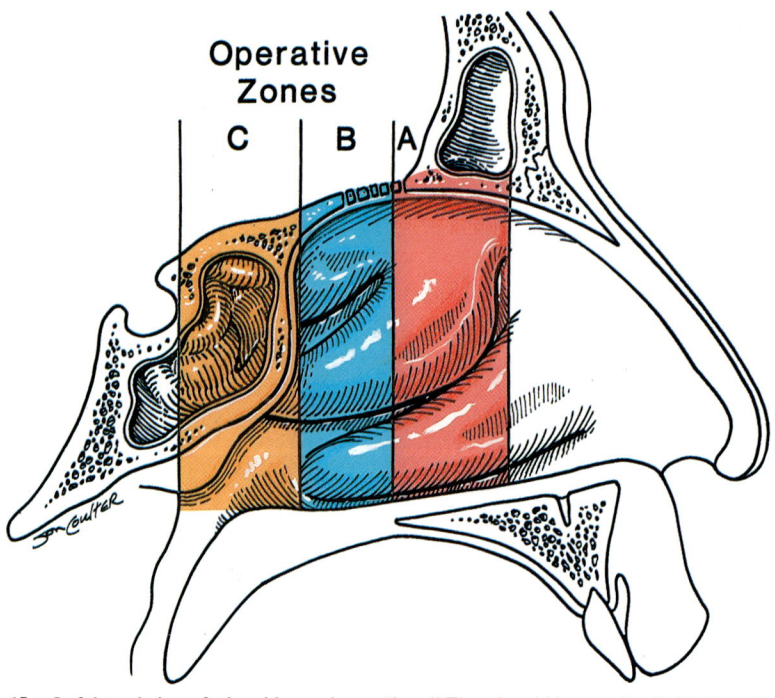

Figure 1–15. Left lateral view of ethmoid complex or "box." The ethmoid box can be divided into three zones: A (anterior OMC): anterior to the anterior superior attachment of the middle turbinate; B (posterior OMC): from this attachment to the posterior lateral attachment of the middle turbinate; and C: (sphenoid) from the face of the sphenoid to include the sphenoid sinus and its neighboring structures. (Reprinted with permission from May.[15])

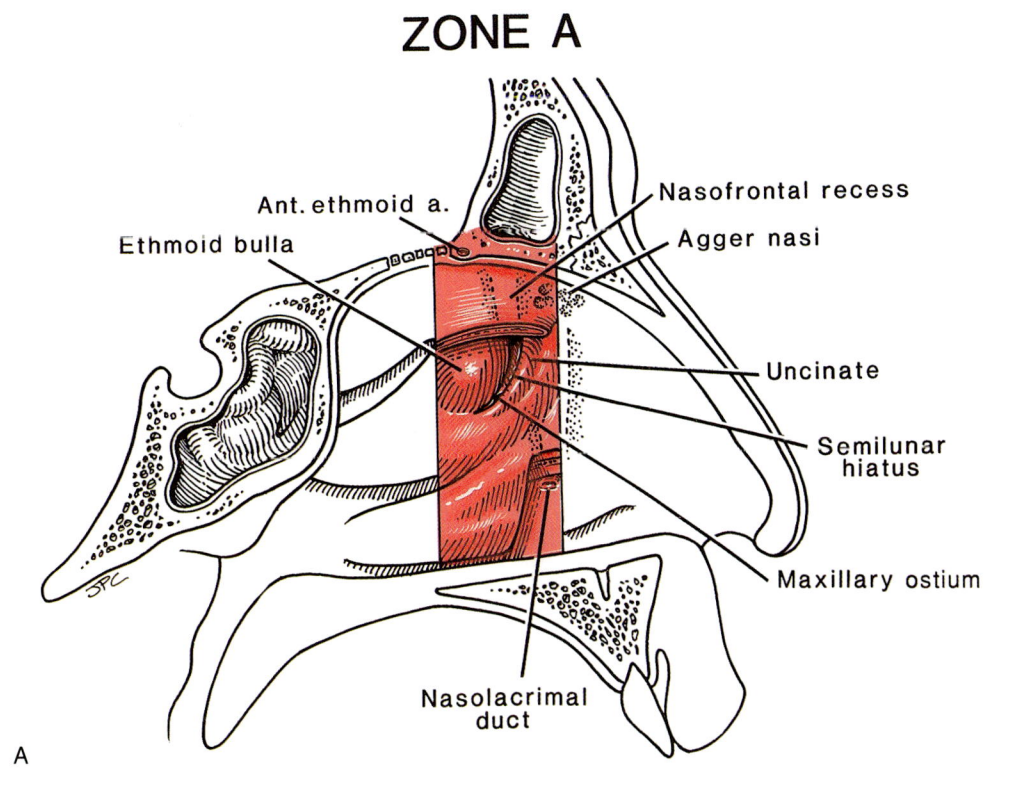

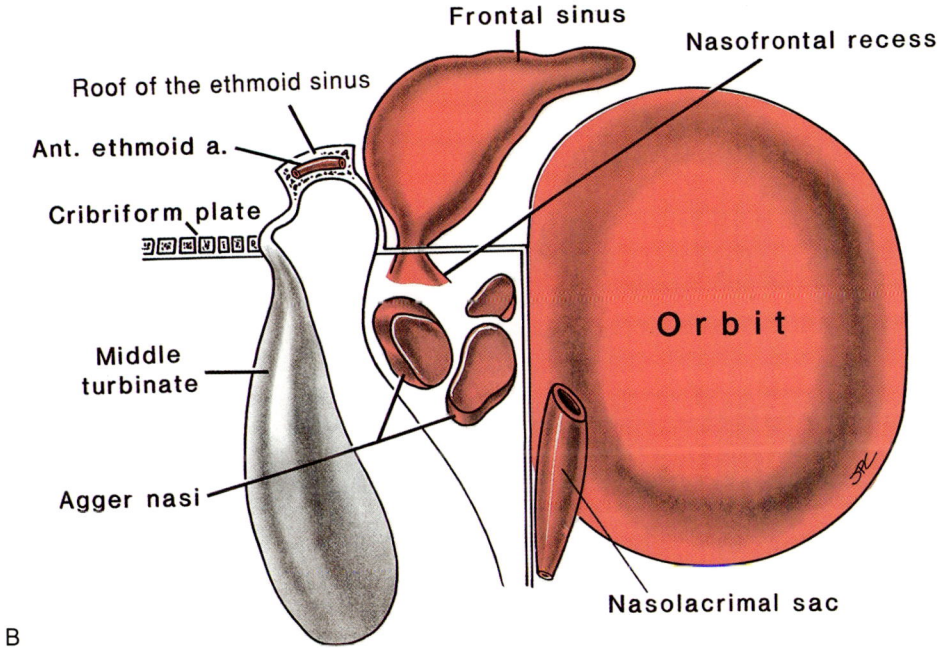

Figure 1–16. Lateral view (**A**) and coronal view (**B**) of zone A of left ethmoid box. Ant.: anterior; a.: artery. (Reprinted with permission from May.[15])

the neighboring roof of the ethmoid sinus.[16] As a result, the anterior cranial fossa in this area is vulnerable to penetration during sinus surgery.

Another risk factor for penetration of the anterior cranial fossa is the steepness of the slope between the roof of the ethmoid sinus and the floor of the cribriform plate (Fig. 1–17A and B). The distance between these structures may vary between 3 and 16 mm.[16]

Structures that lie lateral to the ethmoid in zone A, the orbit and the nasolacrimal duct, are also vulnerable.

Zone B

Zone B (the posterior OMC) begins at the horizontal-oblique attachment of the middle turbinate, just posterior to the bulla ethmoidalis and sinus lateralis (Fig. 1–18A and B).[15] An important landmark in zone B is the basal lamella, which separates the anterior from the posterior ethmoid air cells and must be penetrated during operations to manage disease in the posterior ethmoid sinus.

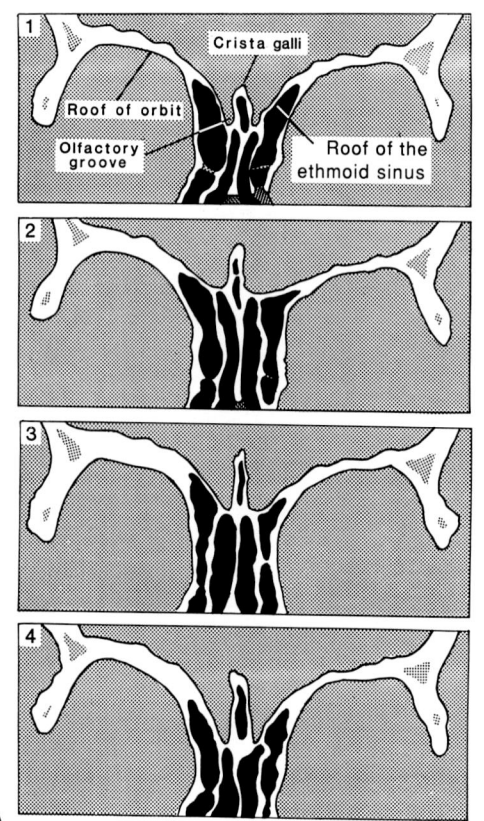

Figure 1–17. **A**: The variable (1, 2, 3, 4) steepness of the slope between the roof of the ethmoid sinus and the floor of the cribriform plate. (Figure continued on next page).

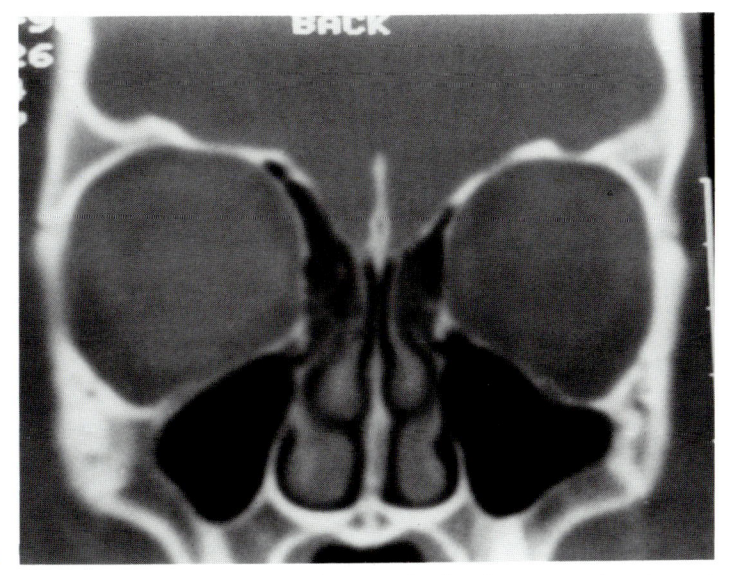

Figure 1–17. (*Continued*). **B**: Coronal computed tomography view demonstrates the extreme steepness of the roof of the ethmoid sinus. The endoscopic sinus surgeon should note this anatomic situation because it poses increased risk of penetrating the anterior cranial fossa.

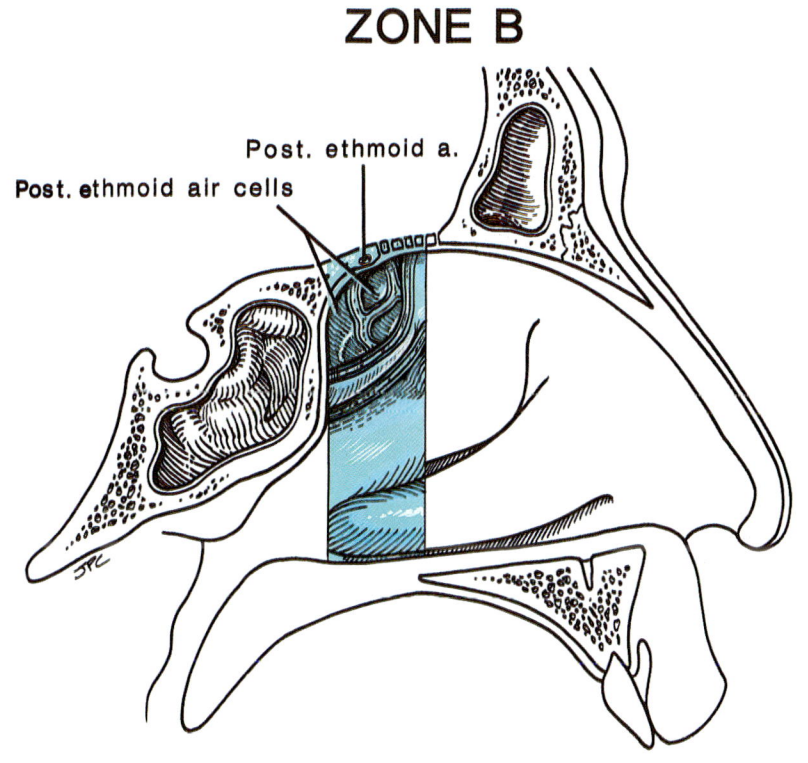

Figure 1–18. **A**: Lateral view of zone B of left ethmoid box. Post.: posterior; a.: artery. (Reprinted with permission from May.[15]) (Figure continued on next page.)

ZONE B

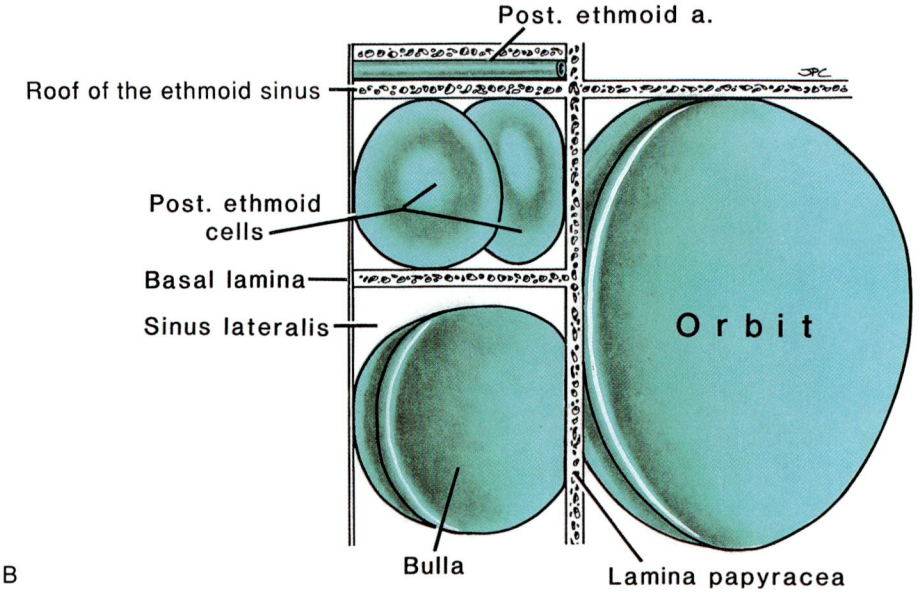

Figure 1–18. *(Continued).* **B**: Coronal view of zone B of left ethmoid box. (Reprinted with permission from May.[15]) Post.: posterior; a.: artery.

The roof of the ethmoid sinus may be confused at surgery with the basal lamella, and penetration of the roof of the ethmoid sinus will result in a cerebrospinal fluid leak. Thus, the surgeon must make every attempt to identify the basal lamella positively before penetrating a bony wall in this region. The basal lamella is attached anteriorly to the lamina papyracea close to the roof of the ethmoid sinus, but as the basal lamella extends obliquely posteriorly, the distance between the basal lamella and roof of the ethmoid sinus becomes greater (Fig. 1–7). Penetrating the basal lamella posteriorly thus provides the safest approach to the posterior ethmoid cells.

Zone C

Because zone C (the sphenoid) contains the optic nerve and carotid artery, violation of sphenoid sinus walls in this zone may lead to loss of the patient's sight or massive hemorrhaging and possibly death (Fig. 1–19A and B).[15] Extreme caution must thus be exercised when operating in this zone. The anterior boundary of zone C is the front face of the sphenoid sinus, which lies 6 to 7 cm from the anterior nasal spine and at an angle of 25° to 35° from the plane of the floor of the nose.

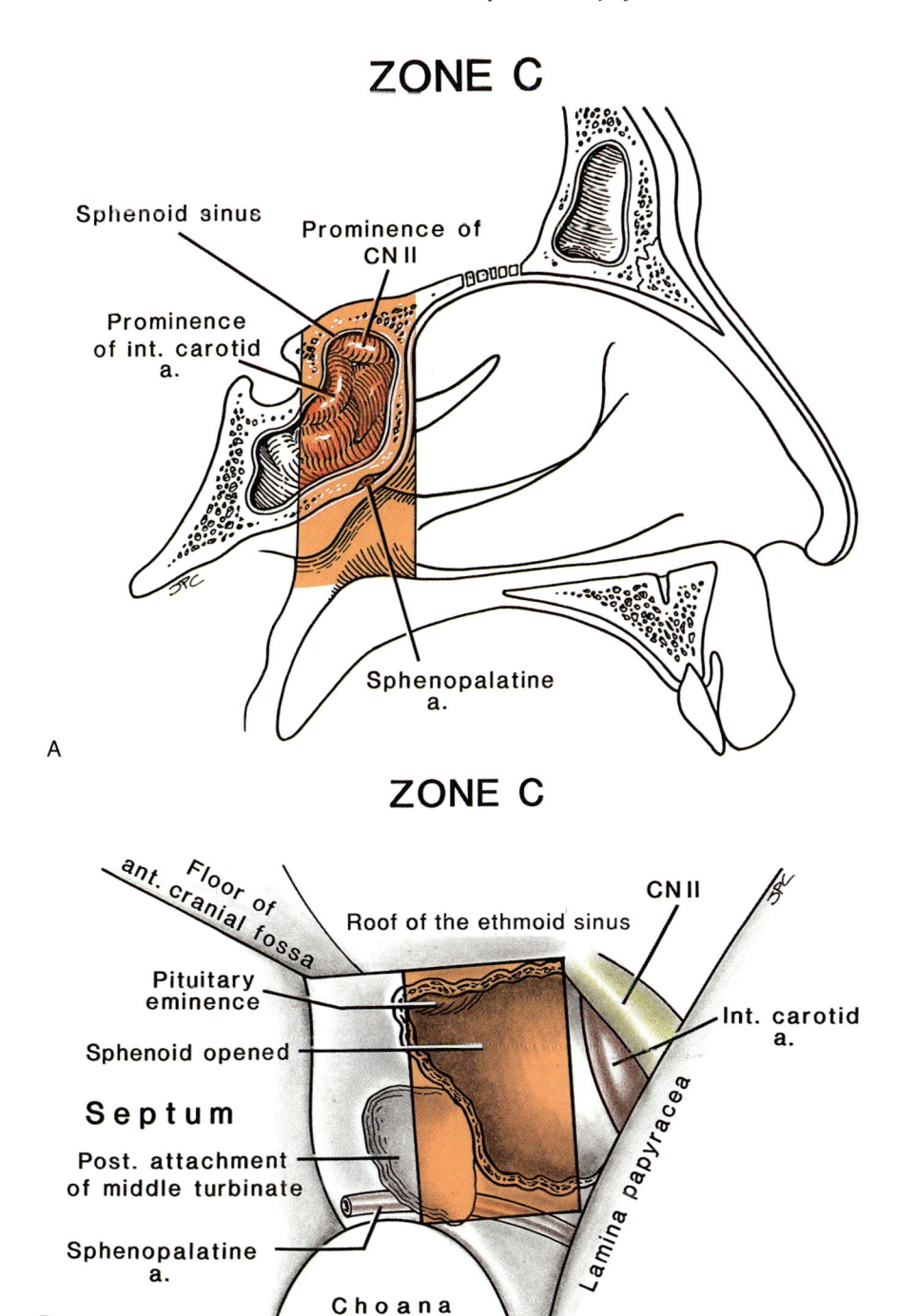

Figure 1–19. Lateral view (**A**) and coronal view (**B**) of zone C of left ethmoid box. Note that the safe way to approach the sphenoid sinus is above the posterior choana, near the nasal septum and the posterior attachment of the middle turbinate. a.: artery; ant.: anterior; CNII: cranial nerve II; int.: internal; post.: posterior. (Reprinted with permission from May.[15])

CROSS-SECTIONAL ANATOMY OF THE PARANASAL SINUSES

The endoscopic sinus surgeon can combine a knowledge of gross anatomy, information gained by computed tomography, and an examination of coronal, axial, and sagittal sections through the paranasal sinuses to visualize this region in three dimensions. The following presentation of coronal, axial, and parasagittal sections through the sinuses is designed to aid the surgeon in this task.

The relationship of the lacrimal duct, middle turbinate, and uncinate process may be understood by examining a coronal section through the anterior portion (corresponding to *zone A*) of the paranasal sinus block (Fig. 1–20).[17] At this point, the nasolacrimal duct, which may be seen at the lower end of the uncinate process and also anterior and deep to the most anterior attachment of the middle turbinate, may be surrounded by relatively thin bone and thus be vulnerable to injury. The duct forms a prominence in the very anterior aspect of the medial wall of the maxillary sinus, and it opens into the inferior meatus.

The uncinate process varies in shape from quite thick (Fig. 1–20)[17] to quite thin (Figs. 1–21 and 1–22).[17]

Figure 1–21,[17] a coronal section anterior to the maxillary sinus ostium, shows *orbital structures* important to the sinus surgeon. The medial wall of the orbit (lamina papyracea) is very thin and thus may easily be penetrated, especially with removal of the thick-walled ethmoid cells that lie along it. However, orbital fat fills the area between the medial orbital wall and the globe and surrounds the globe's suspensory ligaments and the medial rectus muscle. This fat, and the lack of any significant blood vessels in the region of the globe in zone A, make it unlikely that any significant bleeding will occur if the lamina papyracea is breached in this area.[18]

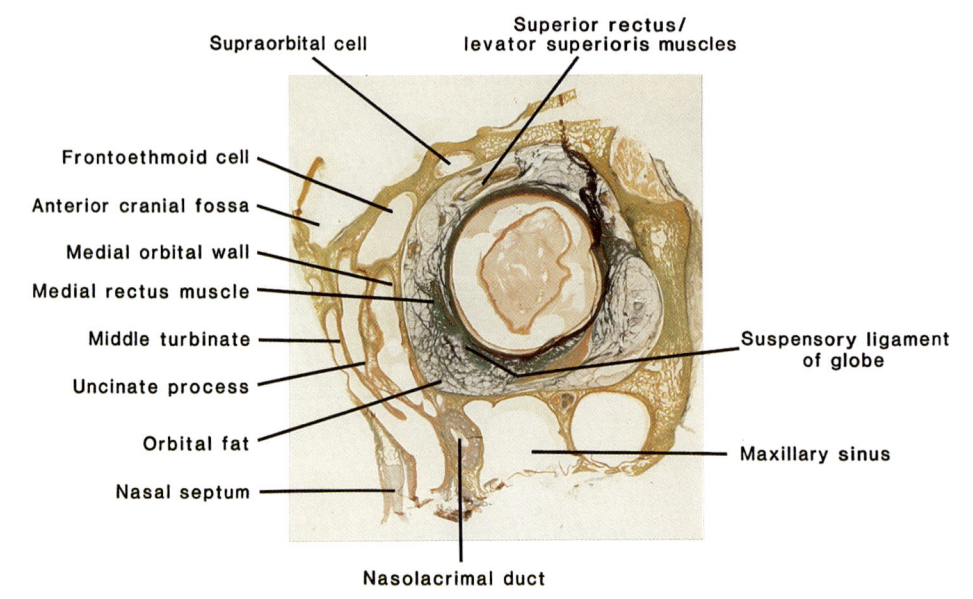

Figure 1–20. Very anterior coronal section through left globe and paranasal sinus structures. Note relationship of nasolacrimal duct, middle turbinate, and uncinate process. (Modified from Rontal and Rontal.[17])

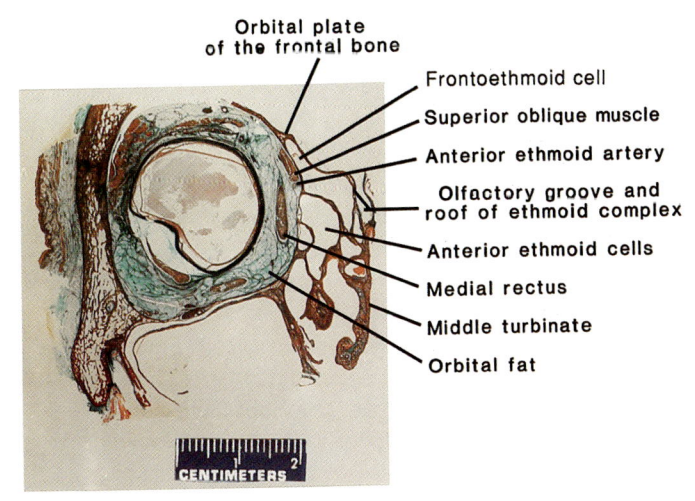

Figure 1–21. Coronal section through right globe anterior to maxillary ostium. Note how thin the medial wall of the orbit (lamina papyracea) can be relative to the anterior ethmoid cells. The wall of the orbit is so thin at this location that it is transparent and appears yellow because of the orbital fat showing through. Also note relationship between the superior oblique muscle and medial wall of the orbit; this muscle could be injured during dissection of a frontoethmoid cell. (Modified from Rontal and Rontal.[17])

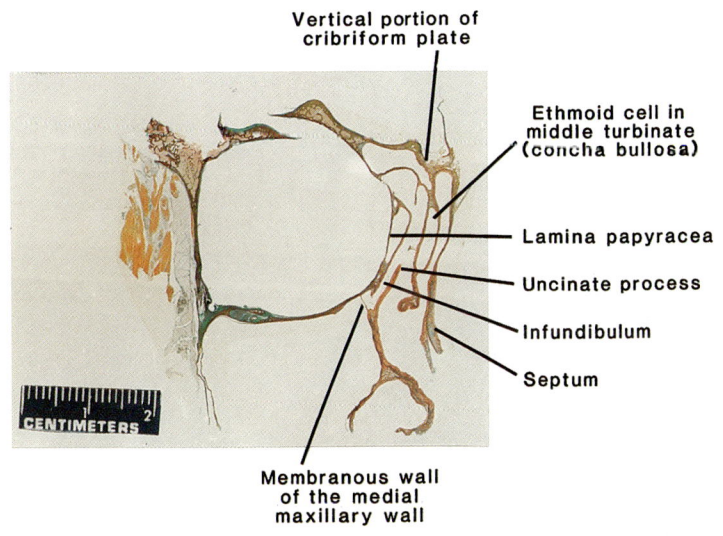

Figure 1–22. Coronal section through right globe just anterior to maxillary ostium. (Modified from Rontal and Rontal.[17])

24 *Endoscopic Sinus Surgery*

The anterior medial aspect of the *roof of the ethmoid* is also thin, and if it is penetrated cerebrospinal fluid leakage could occur. Twisting or attempting to fracture the middle turbinate could also result in fracturing the thin roof of the ethmoid and a cerebrospinal fluid leak.

Figure 1–22[17] shows a *concha bullosa*, a pneumatized middle turbinate. This figure also shows the thin lamina papyracea.

The ostium of the maxillary sinus is located just at the inferior border of the globe (Fig. 1–23).[17] The uncinate process and bulla ethmoidalis are also seen at this level.

A coronal section through the posterior orbital cone (Fig. 1–24)[17] shows the relationships among paranasal sinus structures at the level of the posterior ethmoid artery. A laterally pneumatized *posterior ethmoid cell* (also called an Onodi cell) may be quite large and extend as far posterior as the orbital apex. Particularly when the Onodi cell extends posteriorly and laterally, it may be mistaken for the sphenoid sinus; if this mistake occurs and the surgeon then penetrates the posterior wall of the Onodi cell, the optic nerve and muscles, which are not protected by fat at this level, can be damaged.

The relationships of paranasal sinus structures to the *cavernous sinus* are shown in Figure 1–25.[17] As the optic nerve, surrounded by the third, fourth, and sixth cranial nerves, leaves the orbit at its apex, these nerves and the origins of the extraocular muscles lie close to the sphenoid sinus. Because of this confluence, disease in the sphenoid sinus could involve any or all of these structures. Such involvement has been termed "orbital apex syndrome."

An axial section through the roof of the ethmoid sinus shows the relationship of the anterior and posterior ethmoid arteries to each other and to other structures in the region (Fig. 1–26).[17] Both ethmoid arteries are surrounded by bone. The *anterior ethmoid artery* is seen on coronal sections (including computed tomography scans) at the posterior aspect of the globe. This artery marks the anterosuperior extent of the bulla ethmoidalis, the anterior

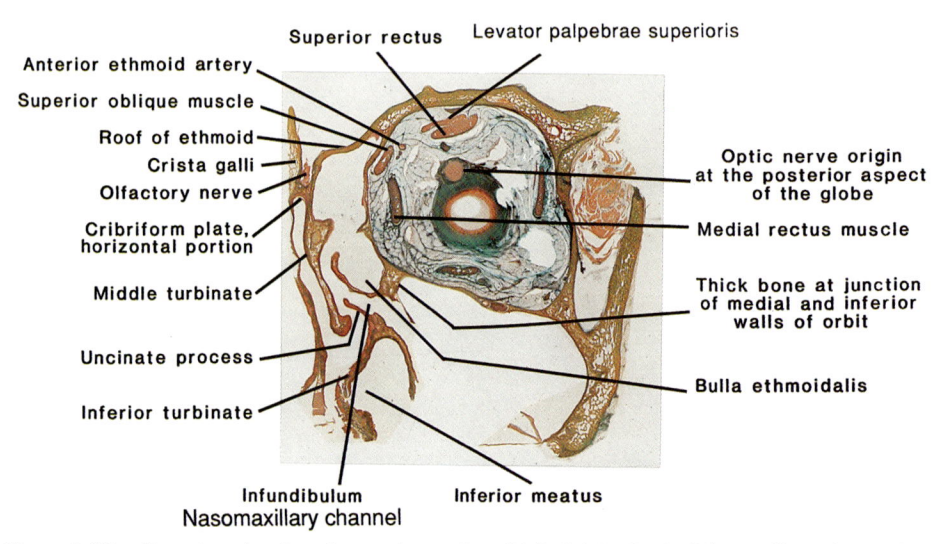

Figure 1–23. Coronal section through posterior portion of left globe at level of the maxillary sinus ostium showing its relationship to the uncinate process, bulla ethmoidalis, and inferior turbinate. (Modified from Rontal and Rontal.[17])

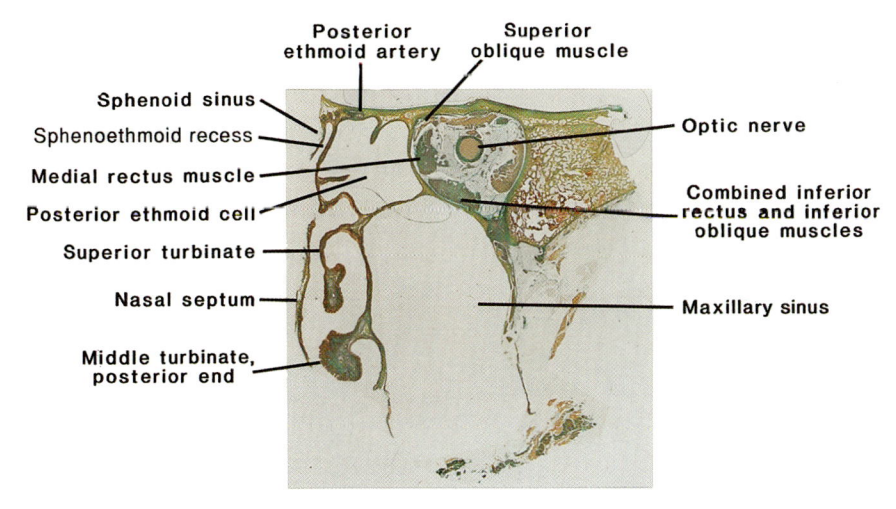

Figure 1–24. Coronal section through left posterior orbital cone and posterior ethmoid artery at level of the sphenoethmoid junction. (Modified from Rontal and Rontal.[17])

extent of the cribriform plate, and the division between the anterior and posterior ethmoid cell groups.

Although the anterior ethmoid artery is well-protected in the orbit as it passes between the medial rectus and superior oblique muscles, it may be injured during surgery in the ethmoid sinus. Bleeding from this artery can usually be controlled by application of pressure and a hemostatic agent such as oxymetazoline (Afrin); if a bleeding anterior ethmoid artery retracts into the orbit, however, an intraorbital expanding hematoma may result.

The *posterior ethmoid artery* is found in the region of the sphenoethmoid junction and at the posterior extent of the cribriform plate.

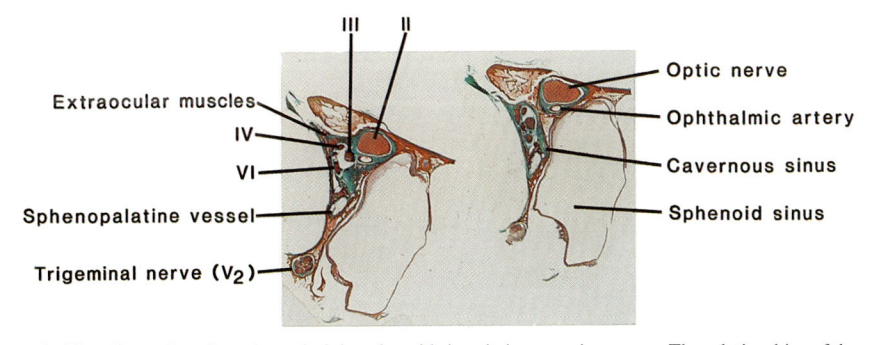

Figure 1–25. Coronal sections through right sphenoid sinus in its posterior aspect. The relationships of the optic nerve and structures within the cavernous sinus are demonstrated. (Modified from Rontal and Rontal.[17])

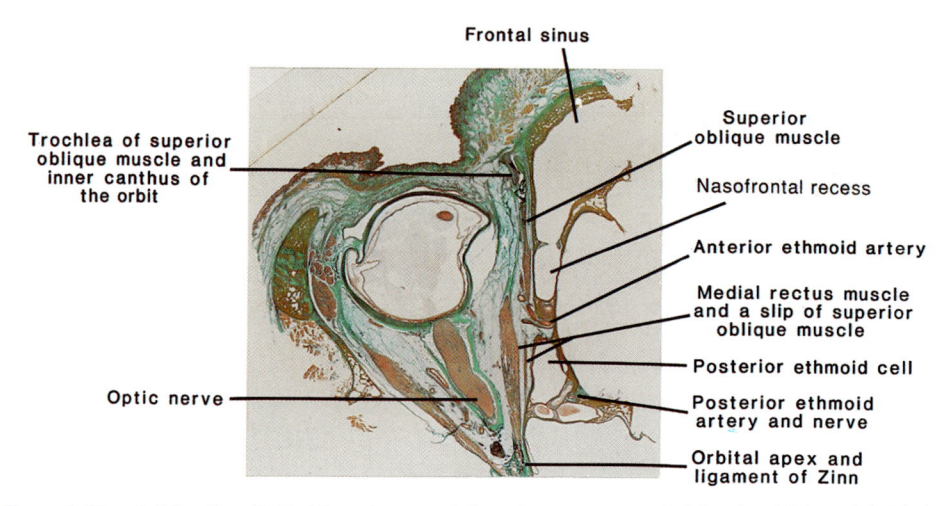

Figure 1-26. Axial section of left globe and paranasal sinus structures near roof of the ethmoid sinus. (Modified from Rontal and Rontal.[17])

Figure 1-27, a section through the orbital apex high on the lateral ethmoid wall, shows a posterior ethmoid (Onodi) cell enveloping the optic nerve.[17] The bone enveloping the optic nerve is usually thick, but, on occasion, as in this case, the posterior ethmoid cells expand into this bone and leave the optic nerve quite vulnerable.

A parasagittal section through the infundibulum (Fig. 1-28)[17] shows how the uncinate process, anterior ethmoid cell, anterior ethmoid artery, and frontal sinus relate to one another. Note that the basal lamella is at the level of the anterior ethmoid artery in this section. As has been discussed, the basal lamella separates the anterior ethmoid cells and their drainage into the infundibulum from the posterior ethmoid cells and their drainage into the superior meatus or sphenoethmoid recess.

A parasagittal section through the orbital apex (Fig. 1-29) shows the maxillary sinus roof sloping upward at an angle of 30° to 45° from anterior to posterior. Branches of the *sphenopalatine artery* cross the anterior face of the sphenoid sinus just posterior to the middle turbinate and just superior to the posterior choana. If brisk bleeding is encountered when the posterior end of the middle turbinate is removed or when working in the inferior aspect of the face of the sphenoid sinus, the bleeding is most likely from one of these sphenopalatine artery branches.

SUMMARY

By studying paranasal sinus anatomy by cadaver dissections, schematic reconstructions, and histologic sections obtained in different planes through this area, surgeons can gain a three-dimensional understanding of anatomy in this region. Such an understanding forms the foundation for safe and effective endonasal endoscopic sinus surgery.

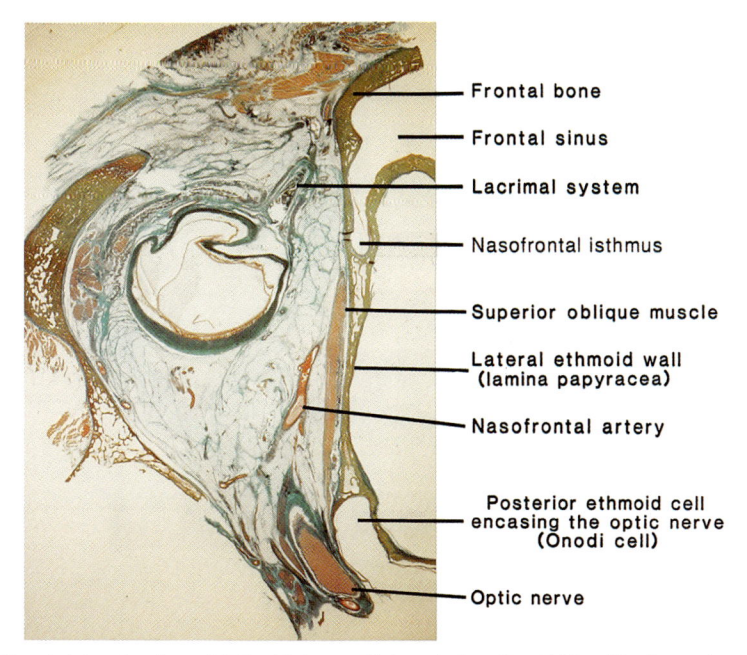

Figure 1–27. Axial section through left orbital apex. Note posterior ethmoid (Onodi) cell encasing optic nerve. (Modified from Rontal and Rontal.[17])

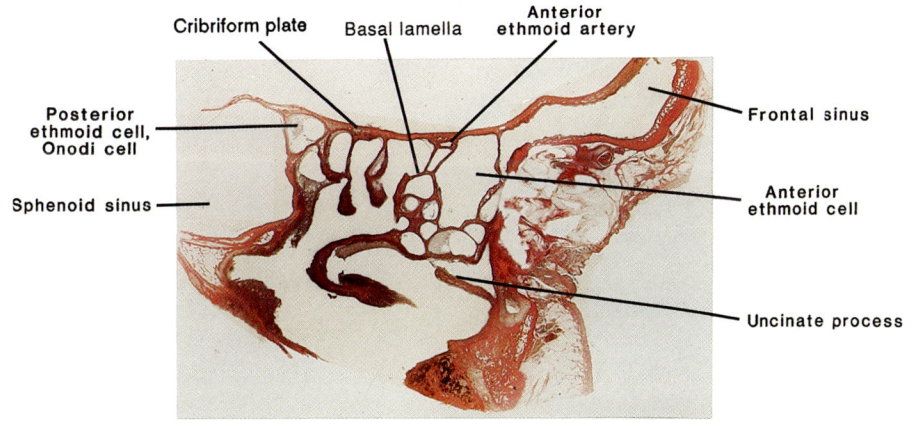

Figure 1–28. Parasagittal section through left infundibulum. (Modified from Rontal and Rontal.[17])

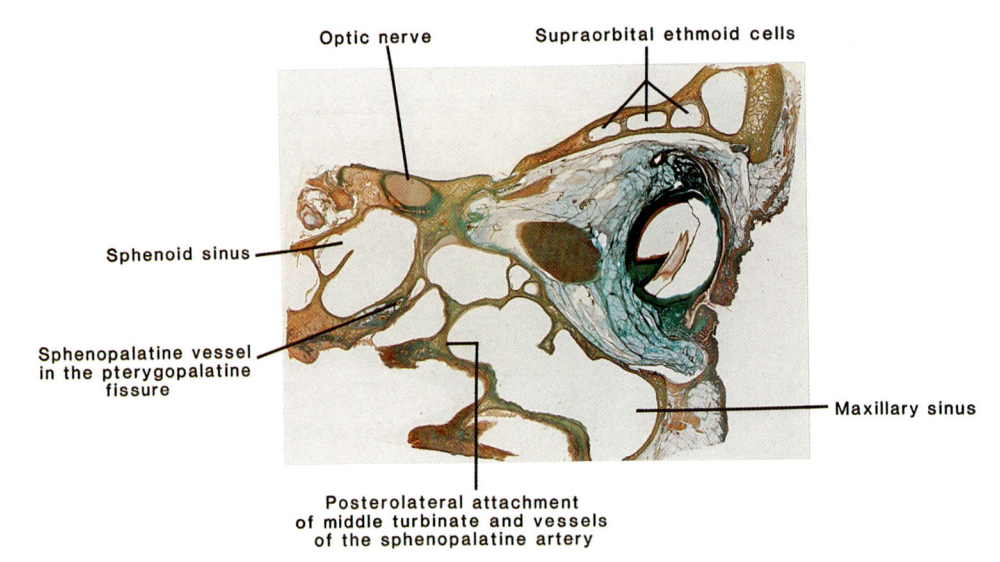

Figure 1–29. Parasagittal section through left orbital apex. (Modified with permission from Rontal and Rontal.[17])

REFERENCES

1. Kennedy DW, Zinreich SJ, Rosenbaum AE, Johns ME: Functional endoscopic surgery. Theory and diagnostic evaluation. Arch Otolaryngol Head Neck Surg 111:576-582, 1985.
2. Lang J: Clinical Anatomy of the Nose, Nasal Cavity and Paranasal Sinus. New York: Thieme Medical Publishers, 1989, p 58.
3. Van Alyea OE: The ostium maxillare: Anatomic study of its surgical accessibility. Arch Otolaryngol 24:553-569, 1936.
4. May M, Sobol SM, Korzec K: The location of the maxillary os and its importance to the endoscopic sinus surgeon. Laryngoscope 100:1037-1042, 1990.
5. Van Alyea OE: Frontal sinus drainage. Ann Otol Rhinol Laryngol 55:267, 1946.
6. Stammberger H: Functional Endoscopic Sinus Surgery. Philadelphia: BC Decker, 1991, pp 80-81.
7. Kasper KA: Nasofrontal connections, a study based upon one hundred consecutive cadaver dissections. Arch Otolaryngol 23:322, 1936.
8. May M: Frontal sinus surgery: Endonasal endoscopic ostioplasty rather than external osteoplasty. Op Tech Otolaryngol Head Neck Surg 2:247-256, 1991.
9. Peele JC: Unusual anatomical variations of the sphenoid sinuses. Laryngoscope 67:208-231, 1957.
10. Van Alyea OE: Sphenoid sinus. Anatomic study with consideration of the clinical significance of the structural characteristics of the sphenoid sinus. Arch Otolaryngol 34:225-253, 1941.
11. Hollingshead WH: Anatomy for Surgeons. Vol. 1: Head and Neck, ed 3. Philadelphia: Harper & Row, 1961 p 267.
12. Dixon FW: A comparative study of the sphenoid sinus. A study of 1600 skulls. Ann Otol Rhinol Laryngol 46:687, 1937.
13. Fujii K, Chambers SM, Rhoton AL: Neurovascular relationships of the sphenoid sinus: A microsurgical study. J Neurosurg 50:31-39, 1979.
14. Kennedy D, Zinreich S, Hassab M: The internal carotid artery as it relates to endonasal sphenoethmoidectomy. Am J Rhinol 4:7-12, 1990.
15. May M: Complex paranasal anatomy simplified for the surgeon. Op Tech Otolaryngol Head Neck Surg 2:214-217, 1991.
16. Kaintz J, Stammberger H: The roof of the anterior ethmoid: The place of least resistance in the skull base. Am J Rhinol 3:191-199, 1989.
17. Rontal M, Rontal E: Studying whole-mounted sections of the paranasal sinuses to understand the complications of endoscopic sinus surgery. Laryngoscope 101:351-366, 1991.
18. Stankiewicz J: Blindness and intranasal endoscopic ethmoidectomy: Prevention and management. Otolaryngol Head Neck Surg 101:320-329, 1989.

2
Radiology of the Paranasal Sinuses

SECTION 1: COMPUTED TOMOGRAPHY OF THE PARANASAL SINUSES

Gary G. Winzelberg, M.D., Kevin O'Hara, M.D., and Mark May, M.D., F.A.C.S.

For some four decades physicians have used radiographic techniques to help in the assessment of suspected paranasal sinus disease. When plain films show partial or complete opacification of one or more sinuses, the physician should suspect that sinus disease is present. Routine sinus films do not allow the physician to ascertain details of bone or soft tissue structure, however. In fact, the only sinus disease that correlates well with plain film findings is acute sinusitis, which is indicated by an air-fluid level in a sinus.

Accurate assessment of bone and soft tissues of the paranasal sinuses has become possible recently with increased availability of high-resolution computed tomography (CT).[1] This technique is indeed optimally suited for assessment of these structures. To help the sinus surgeon use such images to best advantage, this first portion of the chapter reviews some considerations for CT scanning of the paranasal sinuses and adjacent vital structures and presents—from anterior to posterior—normal anatomy, anatomic variants, and pathologic changes of the sinuses as they appear on CT images.

COMPUTED TOMOGRAPHY IMAGING CONSIDERATIONS

The *primary objectives* of CT in patients suspected of having sinus disease are to help the physician identify normal anatomic landmarks and variant anatomy,[2] to aid in the diagnosis of pathologic changes, and to provide the operating surgeon with a road map for surgery. To fulfill these objectives, CT images must clearly show not only the paranasal sinuses, but also vital structures near these sinuses such as the roof of the ethmoid sinus, cribriform plate, lamina papyracea, lacrimal duct, carotid artery, and optic nerve.

Technical considerations for obtaining the most helpful images include the plane of imaging (coronal or axial) and equipment settings.

The ostiomeatal complex (OMC), ethmoid sinus, and sphenoid sinus are best visualized when CT scanning is performed in the coronal plane (direct coronal CT scanning), and usually a complete coronal CT examination is all that is necessary. Sophisticated software is available for the most modern CT equipment to allow for reconstruction of axial or sagittal views from thin-section coronal images. The resolution of such images, however, may not be as good as the resolution of axial images obtained directly. For this reason, direct axial CT scanning may be performed in specific cases, particularly to help the physician evaluate the position of other vital structures, such as the carotid artery and optic nerve.[1]

For direct coronal CT scanning, the patient is placed prone with the neck extended, and the scanning beam is directed perpendicular to the infraorbital-meatal line. Section thickness is usually set at 4 mm, and contiguous 3-mm sections are obtained through the paranasal sinuses.[1] The CT images should be photographed on "bone" (average, 2000H window) settings because images obtained with bone settings are best to show fine details of the OMC, uncinate process, and ethmoid and sphenoid sinuses. Evidence of bone expansion or bone erosion are also best seen on images obtained with bone settings. Images obtained with soft tissue settings (average, 250H window), however, help the physician to evaluate any associated orbital or intracranial pathologic changes. For example, images are obtained with soft tissue settings for patients with opaque sinuses because these are suspicious of fungal sinusitis. If there is suspicion that a neoplasm or vascular abnormality may be present, a contrast agent should be given intravenously, before CT scanning, to enhance the delineation of soft tissues.

FRONTAL SINUSES AND NASOLACRIMAL DUCT

The frontal sinuses and the nasolacrimal duct are the first paranasal structures notable on anterior-to-posterior coronal CT images of the head.

Frontal Sinus

The frontal sinus first becomes apparent on roentgenograms of the skull at about 8 years. Most individuals have a right and a left frontal sinus, but in some cases one or both of the frontal sinuses may be missing.

The CT appearance of *obstructive sinusitis* on a CT image varies, depending on the duration of the sinusitis and its severity. In mild cases only membrane thickening may be noted, in other cases the sinus may be completely opacified, and in acute cases (Fig. 2–1) an air-fluid level may be visible on the CT image. Evidence of bone sclerosis suggests a chronic condition.

The frontal sinuses are also a common location for *mucoceles*.[3] Mucoceles appear on CT scans as opacification and expansion of the sinus; if they are not treated early, mucoceles may erode frontal sinus bone and extend into the orbit or anterior cranial fossa. The frontal sinuses may also be involved by *fibrous dysplasia* (Fig. 2–2) or *osteomas*.

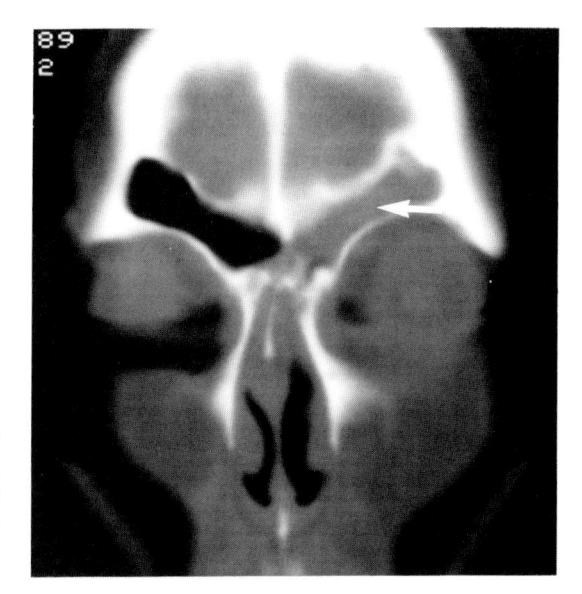

Figure 2–1. Coronal CT of a 42-year-old man with headaches related to acute bacterial sinusitis involving the left frontal sinus. This sinus is opacified (arrow) with intact cortical margins and no apparent expansion or sclerosis. The right frontal sinus is well pneumatized and is not opacified.

Nasolacrimal Duct

The nasolacrimal duct may be seen on the most anterior coronal CT images. It appears as a vertically oriented tubular structure with well-defined cortical margins filled by soft tissue, but it may be air-filled[4]; it extends from the lacrimal fossa inferomedially to the level of the inferior turbinate. Remembering that the nasolacrimal duct appears just anterior to the uncinate process (Fig. 2–3) will help avoid confusing the nasolacrimal duct with anterior structures in the OMC.

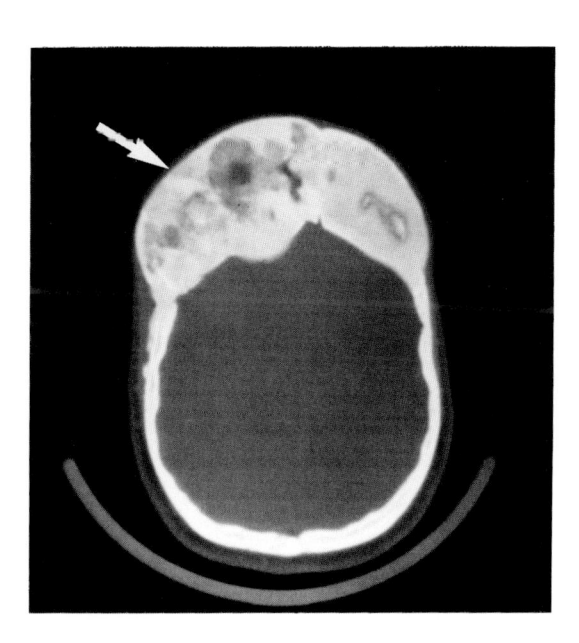

Figure 2–2. Axial CT at the level of the frontal sinus in a 22-year-old woman with fibrous dysplasia of the calvarium (arrow) involving the frontal bones. Frontal sinuses are totally opacified and nonpneumatized; sinuses and frontal bones are enlarged and sclerotic, with decreased attenuation in some central areas related to abnormal bone matrix.

32 Endoscopic Sinus Surgery

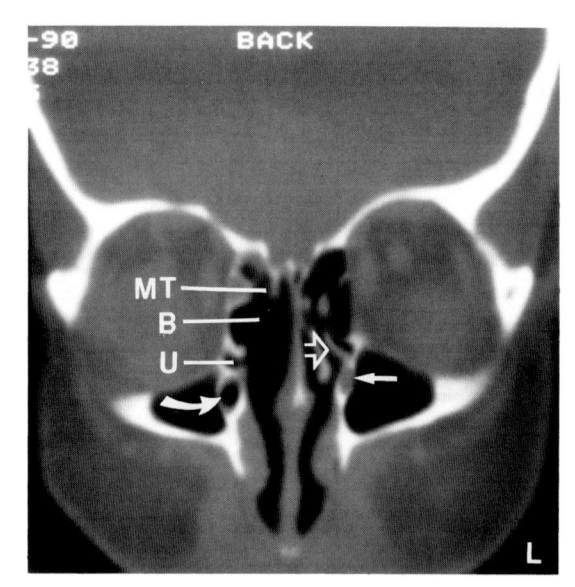

Figure 2–3. Coronal CT shows close relationship of the uncinate process to the lacrimal fossa. The nasolacrimal duct (solid arrow) is visible just inferior to the left uncinate process (open arrow). Because the image was obtained at a slightly oblique angle, the duct on the right side (curved arrow) appears at a slightly different level than that on the left. Remnant of the right middle turbinate (MT) and lack of medial wall of the bulla ethmoidalis (B) and the uncinate process (U) on the right side are results of previous surgery.

ETHMOID SINUS

The ethmoid sinus is the most common location for sinus infection. The anatomy of this sinus is complex, and many normal variants have been identified.[5]

Anatomy

The ethmoid sinus is comprised of vertically oriented air cells, up to 15 in number, that are septated so that they form a honeycomb of mucosa-lined spaces that drain into each other.[6] The *bulla ethmoidalis* is variable in size and bordered anteroinferiorly by the infundibulum and hiatus semilunaris, laterally by the lamina papyracea, and superoposteriorly by the sinus lateralis (Fig. 2–4). The bulla ethmoidalis communicates with the nasal cavity via an ostium that is variable in position but most often lies posteriorly.

Three *turbinates*—thin plates of bone covered with ciliated respiratory mucosa—are usually present on each lateral nasal wall. The superior turbinate, usually the smallest, is anchored superiorly to the cribriform plate (Fig. 2–5).

The middle turbinate is one of the principal structures in the ethmoid sinus. Anteriorly, the middle turbinate attaches to the ethmoid roof at the lateral lamella of the cribriform plate (Fig. 2–4). Posteriorly, the middle turbinate inserts laterally into the lamina papyracea via the *basal lamella* (Fig. 2–4), a bony structure oriented from anterosuperior to posteroinferior and lying superior and posterior to the bulla ethmoidalis.

The space between the posterior wall of the bulla ethmoidalis and the basal lamella (if present) is the *sinus lateralis* (Fig. 2–4).

The inferior turbinate is usually the largest and forms the superior border of the inferior meatus. The *uncinate process*, a slender mucosa-covered bony plate that projects from the

Radiology of the Paranasal Sinuses   33

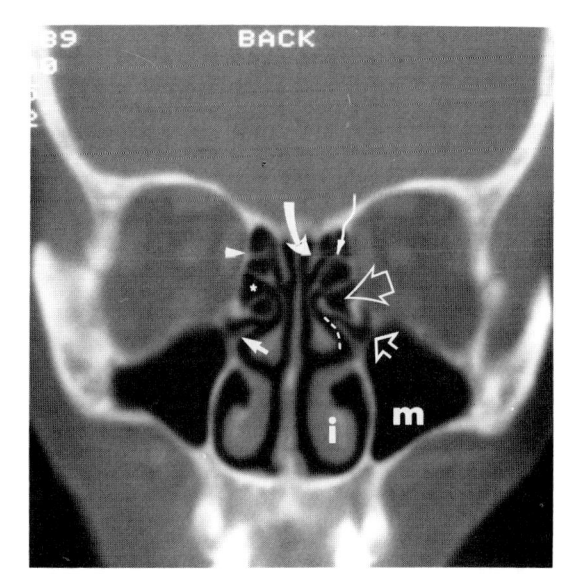

Figure 2–4. Coronal CT shows normal anatomy. Beginning at 12 o'clock and moving clockwise, the following are indicated: superior turbinate (curved arrow), basal lamella and attachment of middle turbinate to lamina papyracea (wavy arrow), bulla ethmoidalis (large open arrow), middle meatus (dotted line), maxillary ostium (small open arrow), maxillary sinus (m), inferior turbinate (i), uncinate process (small straight arrow), sinus lateralis (*), and lamina papyracea (arrowhead).

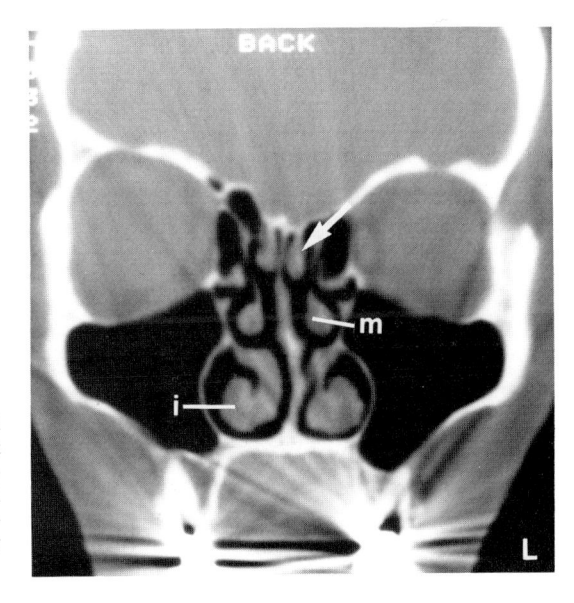

Figure 2–5. Coronal CT of a 46-year-old woman with nasal septal deviation to the left of midline. Inferior (i) and middle (m) turbinates can be seen clearly, as can bilateral superior turbinates (arrow) attached to cribriform plate. The right and left maxillary antra are well pneumatized.

inferior turbinate, forms the medial boundary of the infundibulum. The uncinate process extends from the posterior edge of the lacrimal bone (Fig. 2–3).

Variants

Many variations to normal anatomy may be seen in the ethmoid sinus.[7] A *concha bullosa* (pneumatization of the middle turbinate) is present in up to 30% of patients; the middle turbinate may be pneumatized unilaterally or bilaterally[8] (Figs. 2–6 and 2–7A and B), and most often the concha bullosa drains into the frontal recess. A unilateral concha bullosa is often seen with a deviated nasal septum and underdeveloped contralateral middle turbinate (Fig. 2–8). A concha bullosa may be completely opacified (Fig. 2–9) as a result of obstruction, inflammation, osteitis, or even retention of secretions with fungal debris. Such an opacified middle turbinate may be the cause of "sinus" pain, fullness, and pressure, which may be cured by removing the turbinate.

A *paradoxical turbinate* is convex laterally instead of the normal configuration—convex medially. This variant may occur bilaterally (Fig. 2–10) or unilaterally (Fig. 2–11) and may be associated with a laterally deviated nasal septum.

Agger nasi cells, pneumatized cells that form the most anterior portion of the anterior ethmoid labyrinth (Fig. 2–11), are anterior to the uncinate process and may be large enough to obstruct the OMC. The OMC may also be obstructed by *Haller cells*, ethmoid air cell extensions anteriorly near the orbit. Haller cells can obstruct the OMC by their close proximity to the uncinate process (Fig. 2–12).

Nasal septal deviation and obstruction of the middle meatus can also occur in association with congenital deformities of the palate (Fig. 2–13).

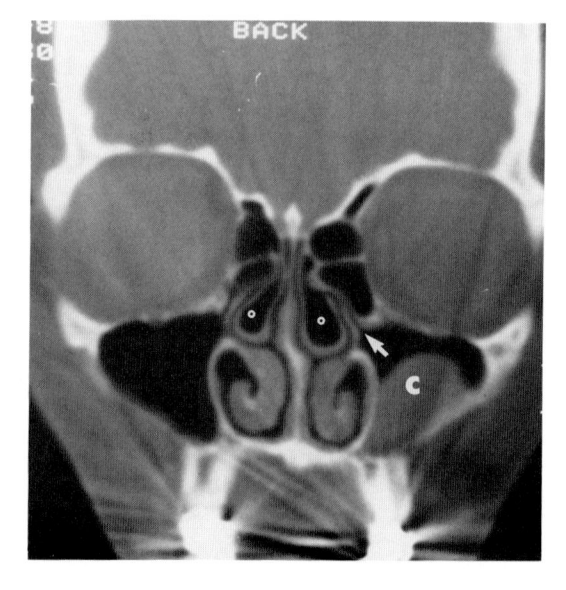

Figure 2–6. Coronal CT of a 37-year-old woman with headaches. Bilateral middle turbinate conchae bullosae (open white circles), a mucous retention cyst in the left maxillary antrum (c), and narrowing of the infundibulum (arrow) bilaterally are noted.

Radiology of the Paranasal Sinuses 35

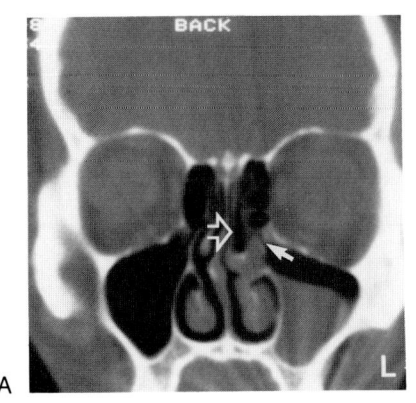

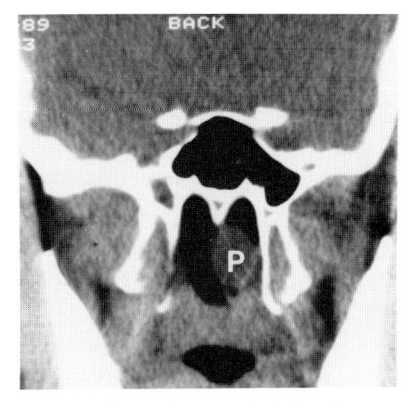

Figure 2–7. Coronal CT images of a 41-year-old man with nasal stuffiness. **A**: A concha bullosa is present on the left (open arrow) with narrowing of the middle meatus. The left infundibulum is narrowed (solid arrow) and the left maxillary antrum opacified. **B**: On a more posterior section, a polypoid mass (p) is visible on the left side; this proved to be an antral choanal polyp.

Pathology

The ethmoid sinuses are a common site of pathologic changes.[9] *Inflammation* of the ethmoid sinuses is often associated with narrowing of the ostiomeatal unit, which in turn may be related to thickening of inflamed mucosal surfaces (Figs. 2–14A and B, 2–15, and 2–16). The OMC may also be obstructed by polyps, a displaced uncinate process, or extrinsic masses such as a concha bullosa, Haller cells, or agger nasi cells. Most often,

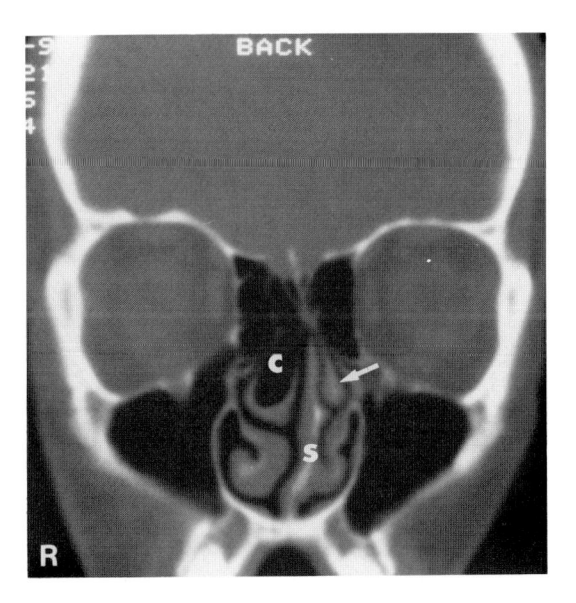

Figure 2–8. Coronal CT of a 25-year-old man with nasal septum (s) deviated to the left of midline. A middle turbinate concha bullosa (c) is present on the right; on the left the middle turbinate is small (arrow) and the middle meatus is narrowed.

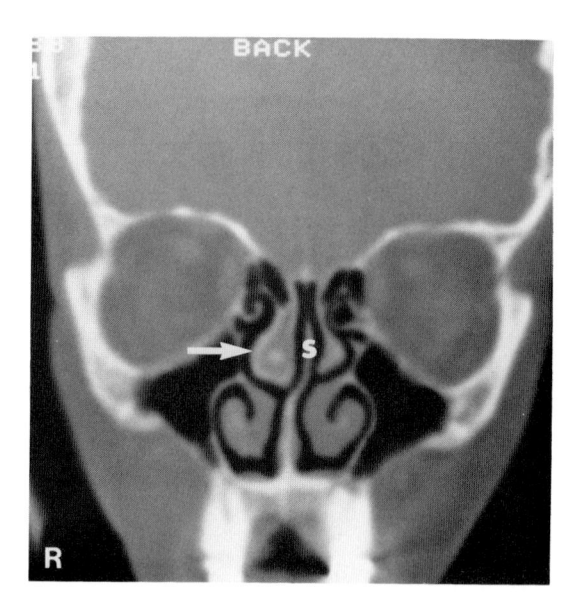

Figure 2–9. Coronal CT of a 57-year-old man with nasal stuffiness and right-sided nasofacial pain relieved following right middle turbinectomy. An opacified concha bullosa (middle turbinate) is visible on the right (arrow). The nasal septum (s) is slightly deviated to the left of the midline. Right and left maxillary antra are well pneumatized.

sinusitis appears on CT images as opacification of the sinus or thickening of the sinus mucosa. When inflammation is chronic, bone thickening or sclerosis can occur.

Mucoceles of the ethmoid sinuses occur most often in the anterior ethmoid air cells and may be suspected on clinical examination by the presence of proptosis or lateral displacement of the eye.[3] On CT images, anterior ethmoid sinuses that contain mucoceles appear opacified and expanded (Fig. 2–17A, B, and C). Mucoceles occur less often in the posterior than in the anterior ethmoid cells; on presentation, posterior ethmoid mucoceles may appear to be in the sphenoid sinus because they impinge on the apex of the orbit and cause symptoms of visual or optic nerve disturbance.

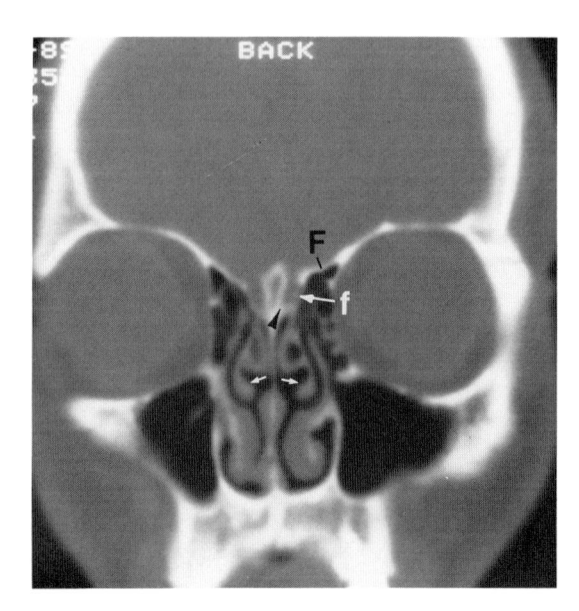

Figure 2–10. Coronal CT of a 30-year-old man with bilateral paradoxical middle turbinates (small arrows). Note difference in thickness between the anterior roof of the ethmoid sinus (F) and thin medial wall (vertical plate of the olfactory groove) (f) that separates the roof of the ethmoid sinus from the anterior cranial fossa. This is an area of potential surgical penetration into the anterior cranial fossa. The cribriform plate (black arrowhead) is separated from the medial wall of the ethmoid by the anterior superior attachment of the middle turbinate.

Radiology of the Paranasal Sinuses 37

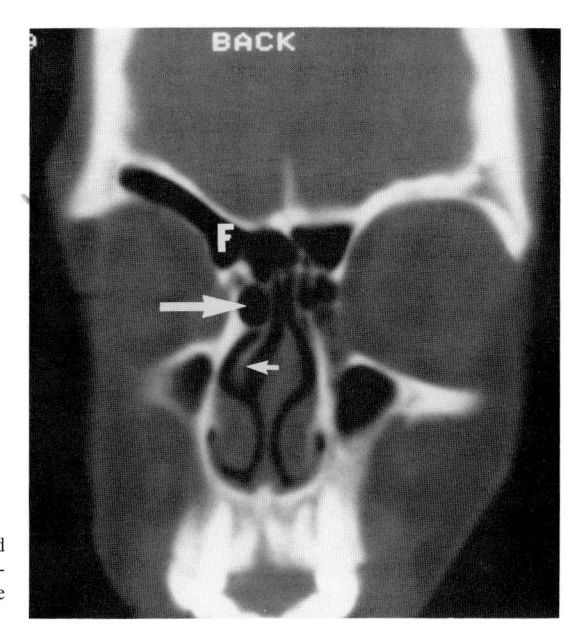

Figure 2–11. Coronal CT of a 24-year-old man. Agger nasi cell (large arrow) and paradoxical middle turbinate (small arrow) are present on the right side. F, frontal sinus.

Slow-growing masses, whether benign (including polyps) or malignant, appear similarly on CT images as sinus opacification and expansion, with preservation of the lamina papyracea but destruction of the ethmoid septa. Some benign tumors, such as inverted papillomas, have no characteristic appearance on CT images.

Rapidly growing malignancies in the ethmoid sinuses cause bone destruction without remodeling. This condition may appear on CT images as opacification of the sinuses, which

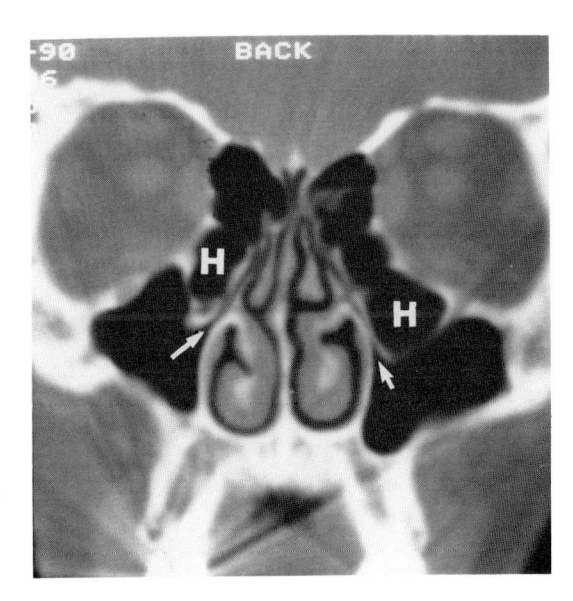

Figure 2–12. Coronal CT of a 41-year-old man with nasal stuffiness. Bilateral Haller cells (H) have narrowed the ostiomeatal complex bilaterally (arrows).

38 *Endoscopic Sinus Surgery*

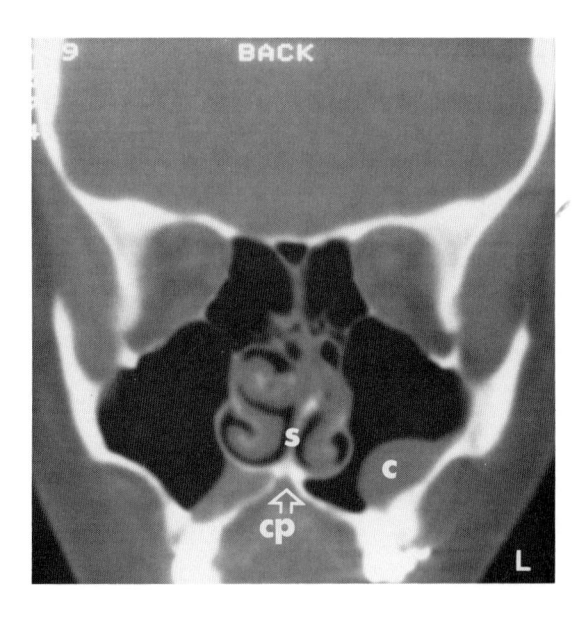

Figure 2–13. Coronal CT of a 15-year-old boy with cleft palate (arrow, cp). The nasal septum (s) is deviated to the left of midline and a mucous retention cyst (c) is present in the left maxillary antrum.

can be enhanced with contrast. Abnormalities that can produce these findings include adenocarcinomas, sarcomas, metastatic disease, and squamous cell cancers.

MAXILLARY SINUS

The maxillary sinus is linked to the nasal cavity by the maxillary sinus ostium, which opens into the infundibulum.[1] The infundibulum is bound laterally by the orbit, posteriorly by the bulla ethmoidalis, and medially by the uncinate process (Fig. 2–18A and B).

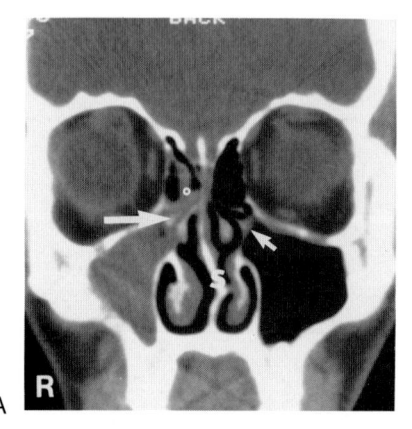

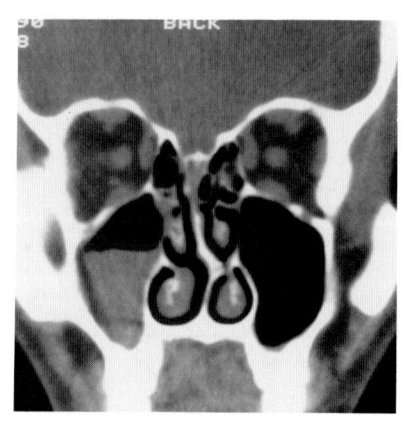

Figure 2–14. Coronal CT of a 29-year-old man with acute bacterial sinusitis. **A**: On the right the maxillary antrum, ostiomeatal complex (long arrow), middle meatus, and anterior ethmoid sinuses (white circle) are opacified. The nasal septum (s) is deviated to the left of the midline. On the left mucoperiosteal narrowing of the ostium to the maxillary antrum is visible (short arrow). **B**: More posteriorly, an air-fluid level can be identified in the right maxillary antrum, as can opacification of both ethmoid air cells. The lamina papyracea is intact bilaterally.

Radiology of the Paranasal Sinuses   **39**

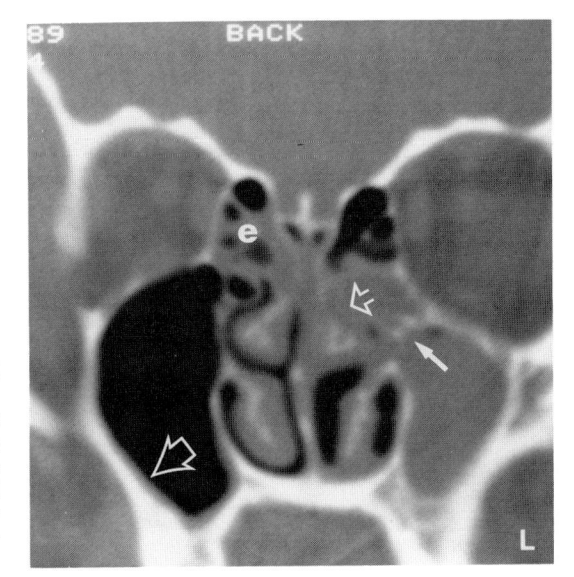

Figure 2–15. Coronal CT of a 20-year-old woman with acute left maxillary sinusitis. The left maxillary antrum and infundibulum (arrow) are opacified, as is the middle meatus (open arrow). The nasal septum is deviated to the right of the midline, mucoperiosteal thickening is notable in the right maxillary antrum (large open arrow), and the right anterior ethmoid sinus (e) is opacified.

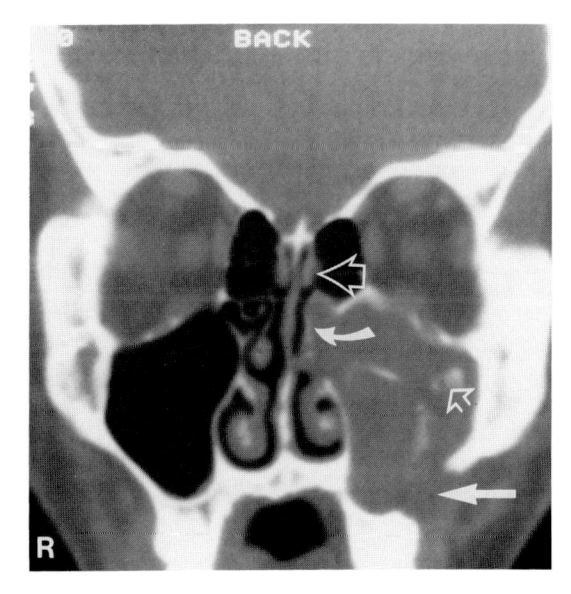

Figure 2–16. Coronal CT of a 23-year-old man with recurrent left maxillary sinusitis after a left-sided Caldwell-Luc procedure (straight arrow). The bony density in the left maxillary antrum (inferior open arrow) is related to an odontogenic cyst. The left middle meatus is totally opacified (curved solid arrow). On the right side, inferior and middle turbinates are present. Superior turbinates (large open arrow) are present bilaterally.

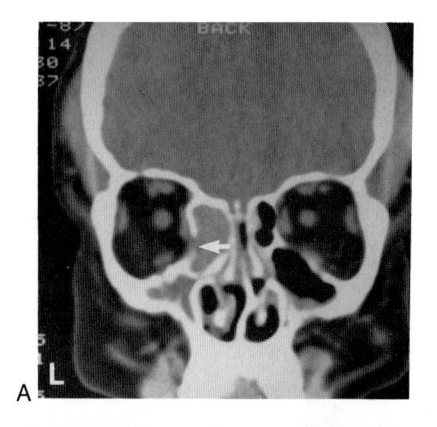

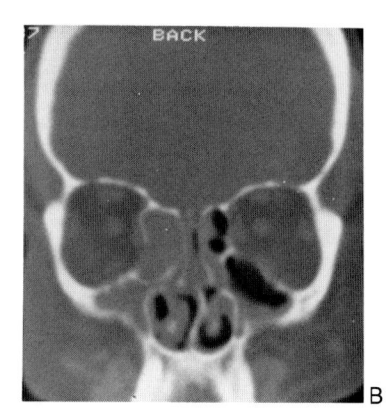

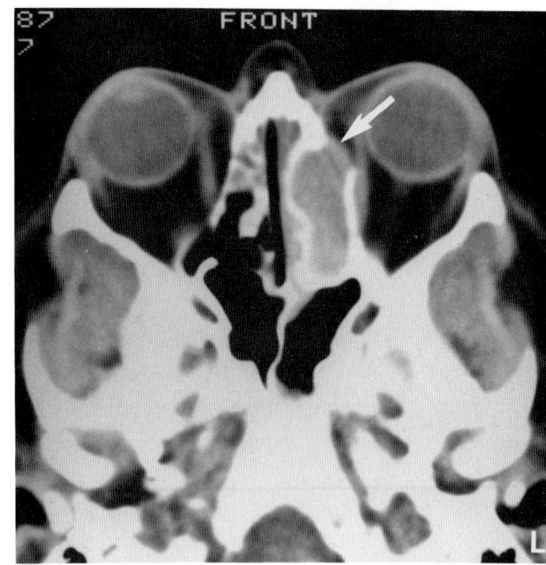

Figure 2–17. CT of a 47-year-old woman with a mucocele involving the left ethmoid sinus. The patient's left side is on the left in images obtained in the coronal plane. **A:** Coronal CT shows opacification of left ethmoid air cells and erosion of the lamina papyracea (arrow). The right maxillary antrum is also opacified. **B:** Coronal CT on soft tissue setting shows soft tissue opacification and erosion of bone. **C:** Axial CT shows opacification of left ethmoid sinus with erosion of anterior lamina papyracea (arrow).

Anatomy and Variants

The maxillary sinuses are usually bilaterally symmetrical in size, although occasionally one or both maxillary sinuses are *hypoplastic*[10–12] (Fig. 2–19). Such sinuses appear opacified on routine sinus roentgenograms,[13] but their decreased volume is apparent on CT images.

Bolger et al[11] found the prevalence of congenital maxillary sinus hypoplasia to be 10.4%. They also found this variant to be associated in many cases with anomalies of the uncinate process, and so they classified hypoplasia of the maxillary sinus as follows: type I when the uncinate process was normal, type II when the uncinate process was hypoplastic, or type III when the uncinate process was absent. If these anomalies are not recognized, the surgeon might inadvertently cause damage to the orbit.

Asymmetry of the maxillary sinuses due to unilateral acquired atelectasis was reported

Radiology of the Paranasal Sinuses 41

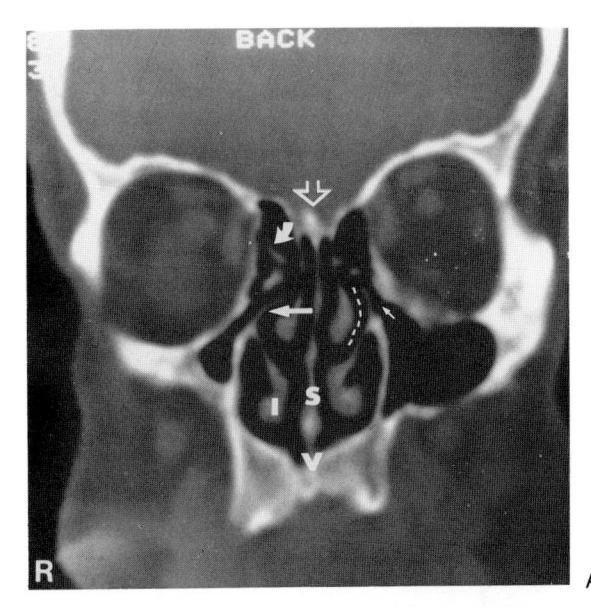

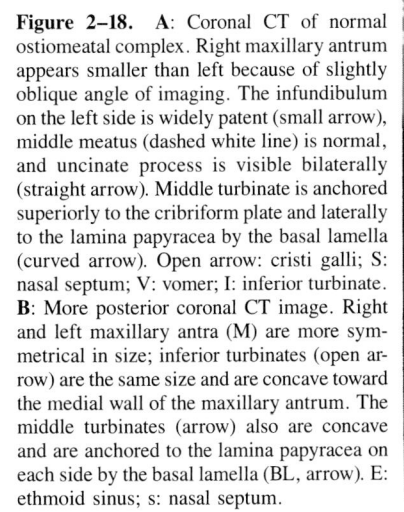

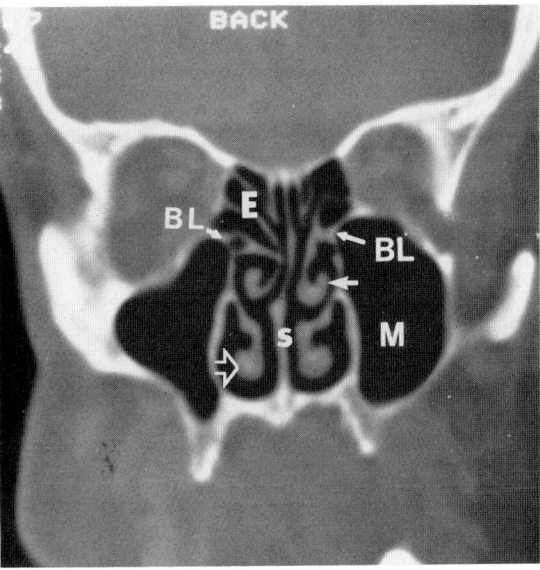

Figure 2–18. **A**: Coronal CT of normal ostiomeatal complex. Right maxillary antrum appears smaller than left because of slightly oblique angle of imaging. The infundibulum on the left side is widely patent (small arrow), middle meatus (dashed white line) is normal, and uncinate process is visible bilaterally (straight arrow). Middle turbinate is anchored superiorly to the cribriform plate and laterally to the lamina papyracea by the basal lamella (curved arrow). Open arrow: cristi galli; S: nasal septum; V: vomer; I: inferior turbinate. **B**: More posterior coronal CT image. Right and left maxillary antra (M) are more symmetrical in size; inferior turbinates (open arrow) are the same size and are concave toward the medial wall of the maxillary antrum. The middle turbinates (arrow) also are concave and are anchored to the lamina papyracea on each side by the basal lamella (BL, arrow). E: ethmoid sinus; s: nasal septum.

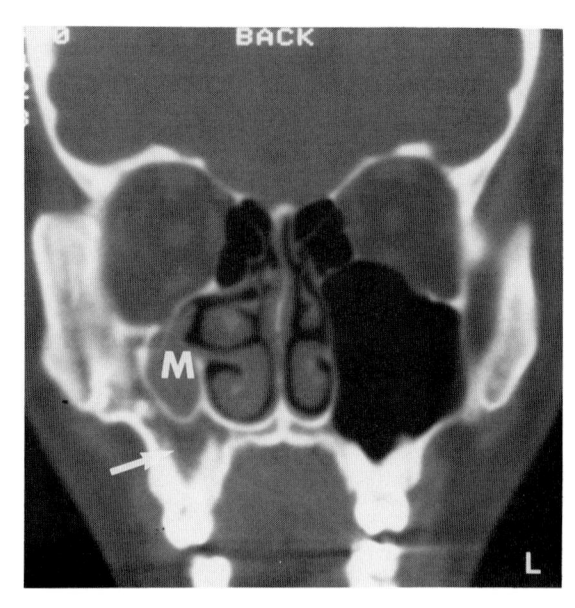

Figure 2–19. Coronal CT of a 29-year-old man with congenitally hypoplastic right maxillary antrum. The bone of the right maxilla is markedly thickened (arrow) and the right maxillary antrum (M) is opacified.

by Furin et al[12] as a distinct anatomic variant. The uncinate process is not affected by such acquired hypoplasia of a maxillary sinus. The atelectatic maxillary sinus is characterized by the posterior fontanelle being displaced laterally. The acquired hypoplastic maxillary sinus is usually secondary to chronic infection or previous Caldwell-Luc surgery.

Pathology

Maxillary *sinusitis* most often occurs secondarily as a result of obstruction of the natural maxillary sinus ostium by disease involving the infundibulum or anterior OMC (Figs. 2–14A and B, 2–15, and 2–16). Maxillary sinusitis appears on CT images as membrane thickening and opacification of the sinuses with an air-fluid level but no destruction of bony structures.

Stammberger et al[14] and later Zinreich et al[15] reported on the appearance of fungal sinusitis on images of the maxillary sinus. This condition can be suspected when CT images show increased soft tissue densities or calcifications within an opacified sinus cavity (the calcifications represent metal ions and calcium salts concentrated within necrotic areas of fungal mycelium) (Fig. 2–20). Conditions to be considered in the differential diagnosis include inspissated mucus, thick pus, a thrombus, and a space-occupying lesion (carcinoma, sarcoma, meningosarcoma, ossifying esthesioneuroblastoma, osteoblastoma, and osteoma surrounded by an inflammatory soft tissue mass).[15]

A *mucous retention cyst* appears on CT images as a well-demarcated soft tissue density, often with a convex margin (Figs. 2–21 and 2–22). One or more *polyps* in the paranasal sinuses can appear as a focal soft tissue mass, but more often they appear as diffuse opacification of one or more sinuses (Fig. 2–22). Bone remodeling can also occur when polyps are present. *Mucoceles* that involve the maxillary antrum may expand the cavity.[16]

Radiology of the Paranasal Sinuses 43

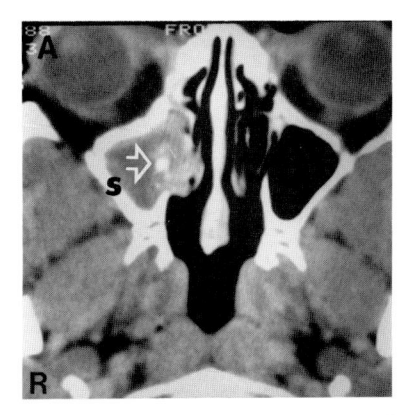

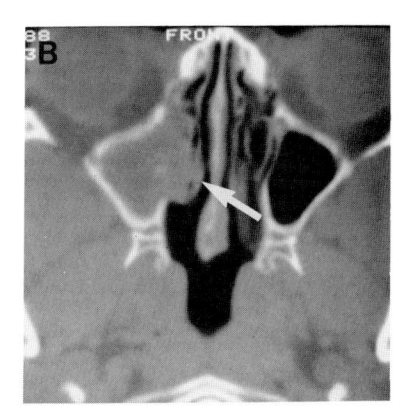

Figure 2–20. Axial CT of a 48-year-old woman. Opacification and sclerosis (s) of right maxillary antrum are evident on both bone (A) and soft tissue (B) settings. **A:** The area of increased attenuation in the right maxillary antrum (open arrow) is characteristic of fungal sinusitis. This patient's sinus cultures grew *Aspergillus*. **B:** Right maxillary antrum has been destroyed medially (arrow), allowing a soft tissue mass to protrude into the middle meatus.

Inverted papillomas (Fig. 2–23) and malignant *neoplasms* such as adenocystic carcinomas, plasmocytomas, melanomas, and lymphomas (Fig. 2–24) can also involve the maxillary antrum. Such neoplasms appear on CT images as nonspecific opacification that may or may not be associated with destruction of bony tissue (Fig. 2–25A and B).

SPHENOID SINUS

The sphenoid sinus is the most posterior of the paranasal sinuses.

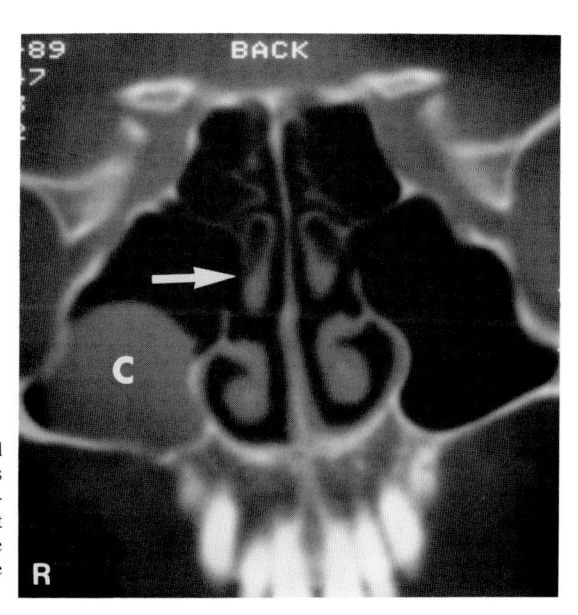

Figure 2–21. Coronal CT of a 53-year-old woman with a large right maxillary sinus mucous retention cyst (c). An accessory ostium in the posterior fontanelle is also present in the right maxillary antrum (arrow). The left maxillary antrum and ethmoid sinus are well pneumatized.

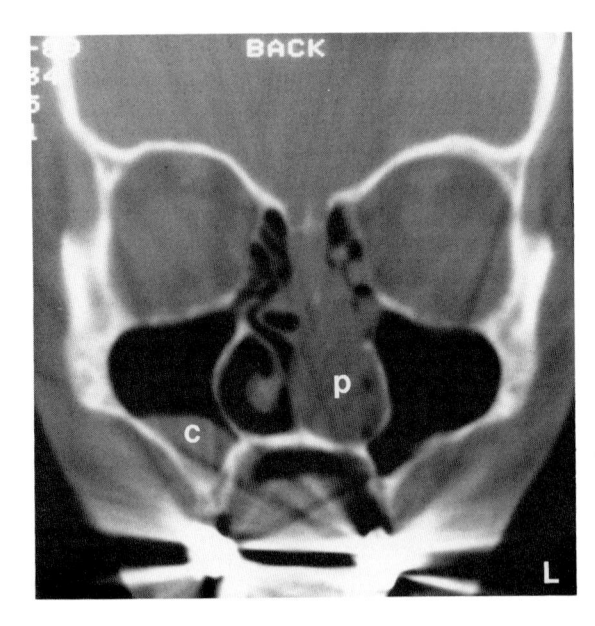

Figure 2–22. Coronal CT of a 75-year-old man with diffuse left nasal polyposis. The left nasal cavity is totally opacified (p). Soft tissue obstruction of the left ostiomeatal unit and mucoperiosteal thickening and a mucous retention cyst (c) in the right maxillary antrum are also present.

Anatomy

Pneumatization and septation of the sphenoid sinus is variable (Fig. 2–26). In some cases the air cells extend laterally from the body of the sphenoid into the greater wings, pterygoid plates, or the anterior clinoid processes. Pneumatization anteriorly can extend into the nasal septum and, rarely, posteriorly into the clivus.

Pathology

Opacification of the sphenoid sinus is most often due to retention of mucus or purulent secretions (Fig. 2–27). Benign or malignant *tumors* may also involve the sphenoid sinus. In general these masses cause nonspecific changes on CT, although when destruction of sphenoid sinus bone is noted, the cause is most often a malignant tumor (Fig. 2–28). Sphenoid sinus *mucoceles* and mycotic lesions generally cause bone expansion.

ADJACENT VITAL STRUCTURES

The anatomy and relationships to the paranasal sinuses of adjacent vital structures such as the internal carotid artery, frontal lobe, and orbital contents should be taken into consideration by the sinus surgeon.

Internal Carotid Artery

The cavernous segment of the internal carotid artery ascends in the more posterior portion of the cavernous sinus. Thus, this portion of the artery is immediately adjacent to the

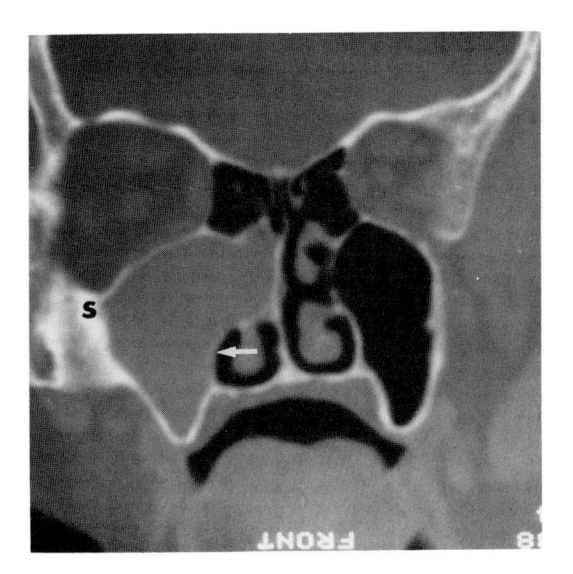

Figure 2–23. Coronal CT of an 80-year-old woman. The right maxillary antrum is completely opacified, bony expansion is present, the lateral wall is sclerotic (s), and the medial wall is eroded (arrow). The diagnosis of inverted papilloma was made at biopsy.

posterolateral aspect of the sphenoid sinus. Only a thin, bony plate may separate the artery from the lumen of the sphenoid sinus, and in some cases this bone may be completely dehiscent over the artery. Furthermore, the course of the internal carotid artery may be variable or anomalous. The relationship of the carotid artery to the sphenoid sinus is best demonstrated on an axial CT scan (Fig. 2–29).

Because of the high risk of injuring the internal carotid artery during surgery in the sphenoid sinus, axial CT images should be obtained whenever coronal CT images indicate that disease is present in the sphenoid sinus.

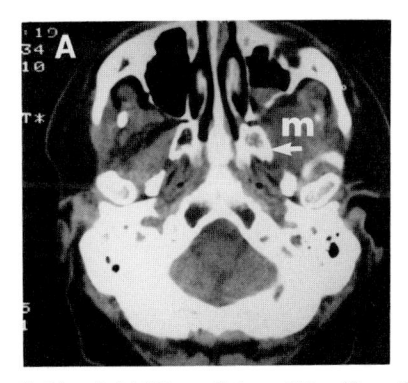

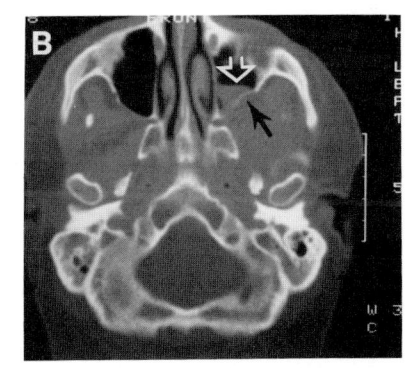

Figure 2–24. Axial CT on soft tissue (A) and bone (B) settings in a 26-year-old man with lymphoma. **A:** Tumor is present in the left infratemporal fossa (m), and the left lateral pterygoid plate is sclerotic (arrow). **B:** The posterolateral left maxillary sinus wall has been destroyed (black arrow), and an air-fluid level can be seen in the maxillary antrum (open arrow).

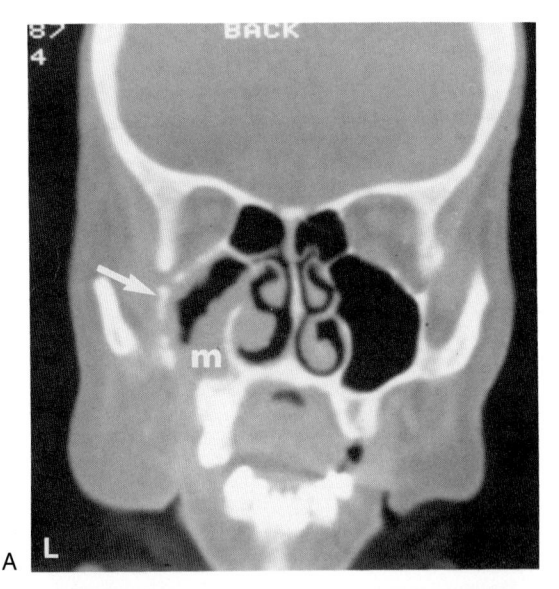

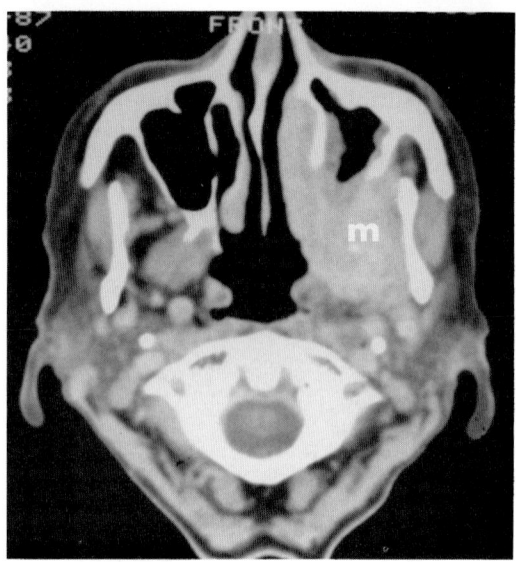

Figure 2–25. CT of the sinuses in a 76-year-old patient with carcinoma of the left maxillary sinus. **A**: In the coronal plane (patient's left is on left of photograph) a soft tissue mass can be seen to involve the left maxillary antrum (m) with destruction of the lateral wall of the left maxillary antrum (arrow). **B**: Axial CT shows part of tumor in the left infratemporal fossa (m) with bone erosion and soft tissue changes extending into the left maxillary antrum.

Frontal Lobe

The *roof of the ethmoid sinus* separates the ethmoid air cells from the overlying orbital gyri and the gyri recti of the frontal lobes. The anterior medial wall of the roof of the ethmoid sinus is very thin and is separated from the cribriform plate only by the anterior superior attachment of the middle turbinate (Figs. 2–3 and 2–10). These anatomic relationships put the frontal lobe at risk when surgery involves the roof of the ethmoid sinus.

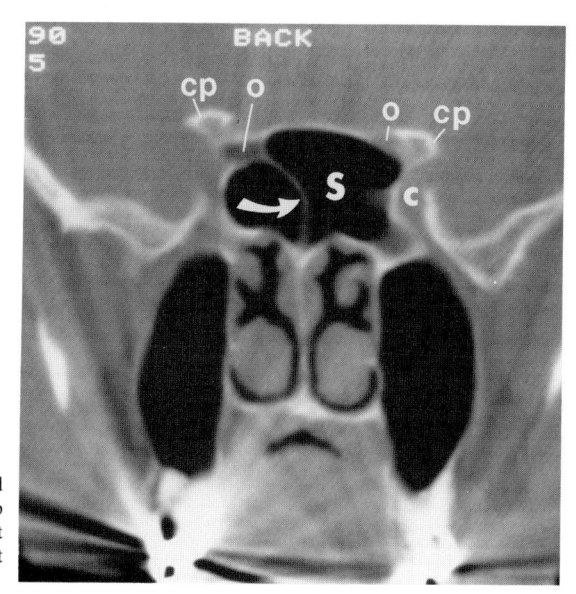

Figure 2–26. Coronal CT through septated (arrow) sphenoid sinus (S). Note relationship of left carotid canal (c) to lateral wall of left sphenoid sinus. The optic nerves (o) are just medial to the clinoid processes (cp).

Orbital Contents

The *lamina papyracea*, the medial wall of the orbit, forms the lateral margin of the ethmoid sinus. Penetration of this paper-thin wall may lead to intraorbital bleeding or injury of the medial rectus muscle, which lies close to the ethmoid air cells.

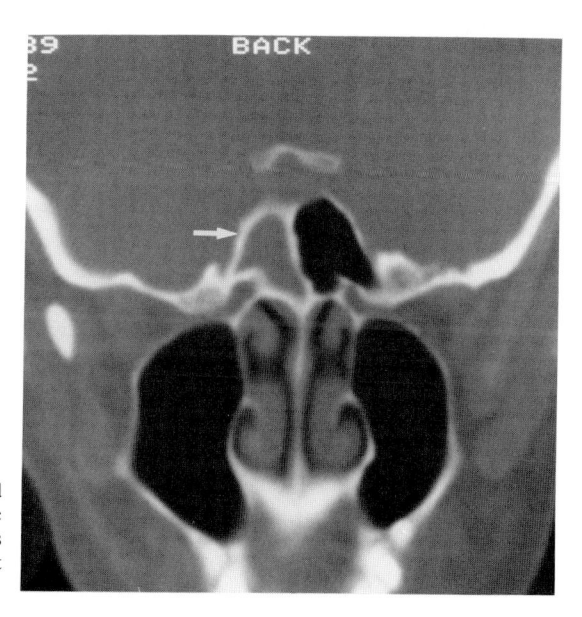

Figure 2–27. Coronal CT of a 41-year-old man with chronic headaches related to chronic sphenoid sinusitis. Lateral wall of the sinus is sclerotic on the right (arrow) and the right side of the septated sinus is opacified.

48 *Endoscopic Sinus Surgery*

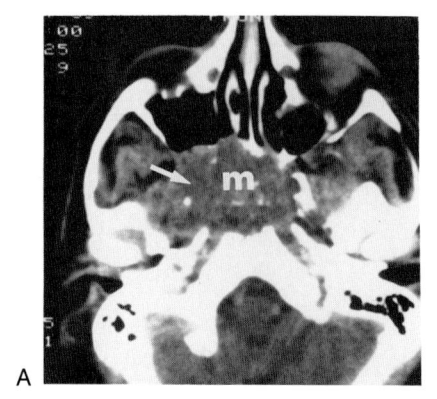

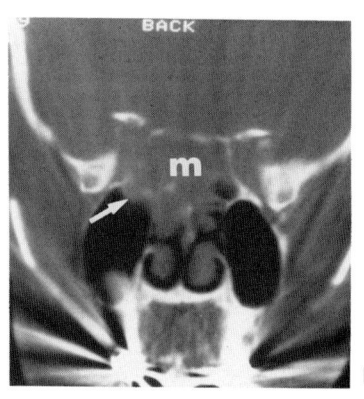

Figure 2–28. CT of a 66-year-old man with chordoma of the clivus invading the base of the skull and the sphenoid sinus. **A**: On axial CT the tumor (m) can be seen to have destroyed the medial and lateral pterygoid plates and the posterior wall of the right maxillary antrum (arrow). **B**: In the coronal plane the tumor mass (m) can be seen in the sphenoid sinus with erosion of the superior/posterior wall of the maxillary sinus (arrow).

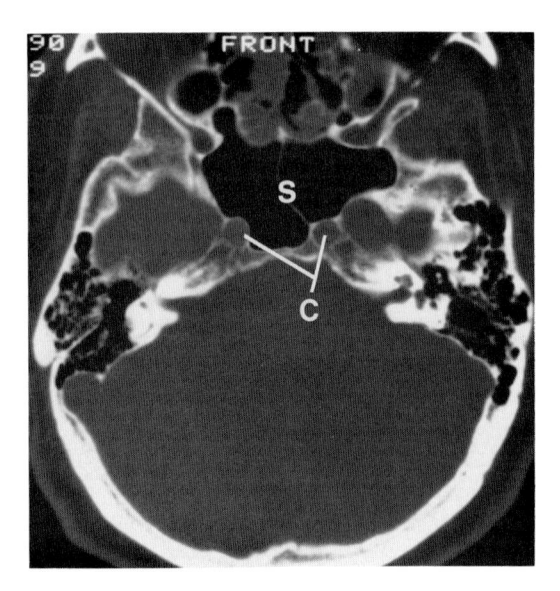

Figure 2–29. Axial CT of a 57-year-old man. Only a thin bony plate separates the carotid artery canal (c) and the posterolateral wall of the sphenoid sinus (S). This patient's sinus contains a septum that extends to the carotid artery canal; removal of this bony septum risks inadvertent injury to the carotid artery with massive hemorrhage and possibly death.

SECTION 2: ADVANCES IN PARANASAL SINUS IMAGING: SCREENING COMPUTED TOMOGRAPHY, 3-D RECONSTRUCTION, AND MAGNETIC RESONANCE IMAGING

Charles F. Lanzieri, M.D., and Mae Urso, M.D.

Rapid advances over the past decade in techniques for imaging the paranasal sinuses[17,18] led, by the mid 1980s, to direct coronal CT becoming the standard method for examining the paranasal sinuses. These advances were welcomed by the growing number of endoscopic sinus surgeons, who found that they now required much more detailed information about the anatomy and pathology of the lateral nasal wall and septum.

New imaging techniques found helpful in providing the surgeon with more accurate and specific information about detailed anatomy in each patient include screening CT, surface-rendered three-dimensional (3D) reconstruction, and magnetic resonance imaging (MRI). This part of the chapter focuses on the use of these new methods to obtain images of paranasal sinuses.

SCREENING COMPUTED TOMOGRAPHY OF PARANASAL SINUSES

Today many patients in whom problems of the paranasal sinuses are suspected undergo screening CT examinations (Fig. 2–30).

Technique for Screening Computed Tomography

To identify the locations at which screening axial CT images will be obtained, a lateral scan is obtained. On this scan, the radiologist measures the distance between the hard palate and the top of the frontal sinus and divides this distance by five (or by six if the frontal sinuses are quite large). Then, an axial image is obtained at each location. Because of the relatively high incidence of dental disease affecting the maxillary sinus, the most inferior image should be obtained in the plane that just grazes the hard palate.

50 *Endoscopic Sinus Surgery*

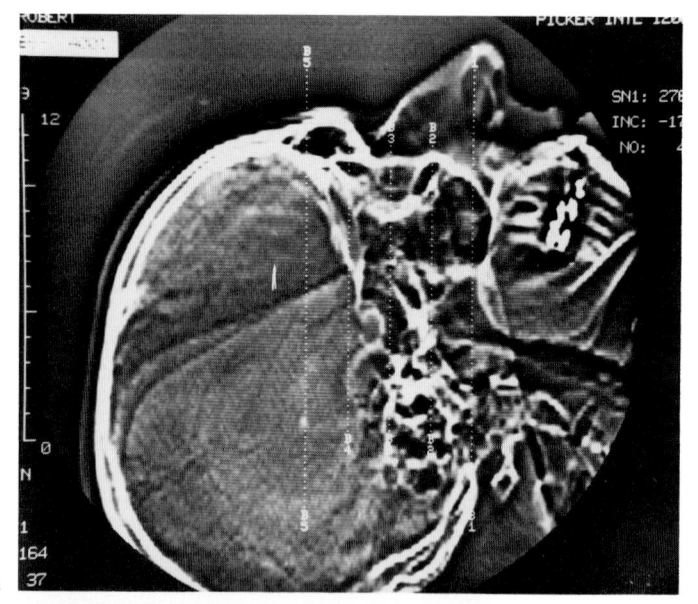

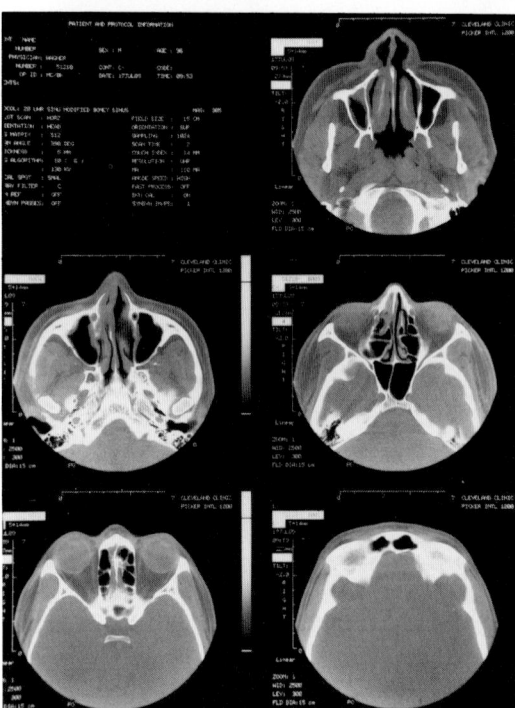

Figure 2–30. Screening CT of the paranasal sinuses. **A**: An axial, 5 mm thick section is obtained at each of five (or when the frontal sinus is large, six) locations from the roof of the palate to the top of the frontal sinus. **B**: The results of this screening CT study can be displayed on a single film for ease of interpretation and reproduction.

Advantages of Screening Computed Tomography

Screening CT has many advantages over traditional sinus film series for the evaluation of paranasal sinus anatomy and pathology. Most importantly, because five or six distinct images are obtained rather than a single view in which all sinuses are seen at once, screening CT provides a much clearer image of individual sinuses and their boundaries. In addition, concentrations of metal, soft tissue, air, and fat can be distinguished on CT by their various densities. CT images also lack the artifacts present on standard films. And the results of screening CT are easier to interpret and reproduce because they are presented on a single film.

Because screening CT requires only 15 minutes to perform, flexible scheduling is possible. The CT examination can usually be performed at the time of the patient's clinic visit and with minimal waiting time for the patient. This is cost effective for the clinic and the charge to the patient for screening CT is approximately the same as for a standard radiologic examination of the paranasal sinuses.

The dose of radiation the patient receives during screening CT is lower than the dose received during a typical paranasal sinus x-ray study consisting of four views (anteroposterior, Caldwell, Waters, and lateral)—20 mrad for a CT study versus 25 mrad for a four-view standard radiology study.

Screening CT of the paranasal sinuses is an appropriate first step in evaluating suspected paranasal disease. If the results of screening CT are abnormal, the radiologist orders a more detailed examination, including coronal views, with intravenous contrast when appropriate. The last advantage of screening CT over traditional roentgenographic studies is that these additional CT studies can be performed at the same visit as the screening CT, and, indeed, without even moving the patient on the scanner bed.

SURFACE-RENDERED THREE-DIMENSIONAL RECONSTRUCTION

The most recent advance in the clinical evaluation of intranasal and paranasal sinus anatomy and pathology involves using a series of small endoscopes to view structures in the nose directly. While encouraging otolaryngologists to perform more conservative procedures, this development has challenged radiologists to produce even more accurate and reliable images of intranasal and paranasal sinus structures.

Coincidentally, techniques for reformatting two-dimensional CT images as surface-rendered 3D reconstructions have become commercially available. Believing that the images obtained by this method would be more helpful to surgeons than series of planar images in conceptualizing complex anatomy, we recently evaluated surface-rendered 3D reconstructions of lateral nasal wall anatomy with regard to their usefulness in planning endoscopic endonasal surgery.[19]

We overlapped 4-mm coronal CT sections of the lateral nasal wall from patients with inflammatory disease to generate surface-rendered sagittal 3D images (Fig. 2–31A and B). We excluded the middle turbinate from the reconstructions so that structures in the middle meatus could be seen: the uncinate process, hiatus semilunaris, bulla ethmoidalis, and sinus ostia. These structures, and the nasolacrimal duct, are important landmarks for the endoscopic sinus surgeon.

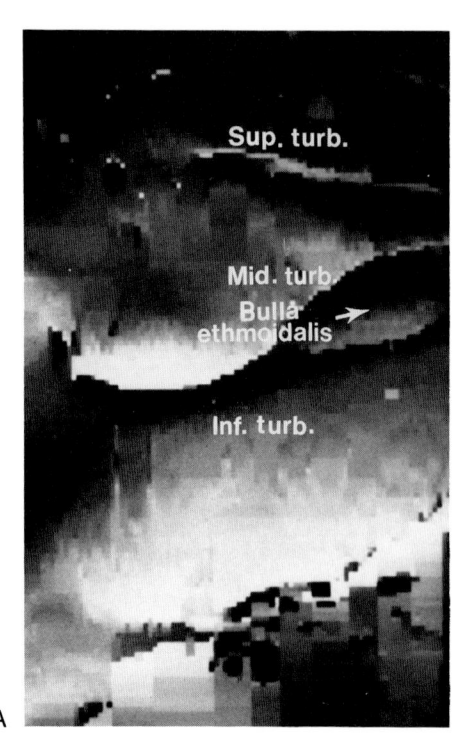

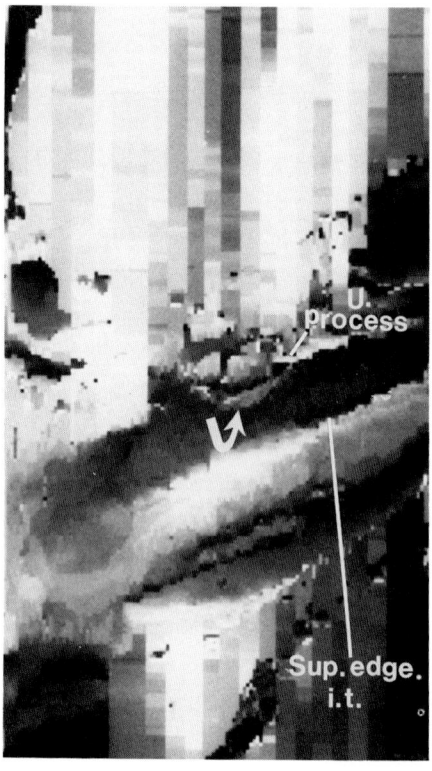

Figure 2–31. Surface-rendered 3D reconstructions of right lateral nasal wall. The nasal vestibule is to the left on these images. **A:** The turbinates and bulla ethmoidalis are visible. Inf. turb.: inferior turbinate; Mid.: middle; Sup.: superior. **B:** The middle turbinate has been removed electronically to show the uncinate (U.) process (curved arrow). i.t.: inferior turbinate; Sup.: superior.

Subtle medial protrusions from the lateral nasal wall, including the agger nasi cells, can also be demonstrated by 3D reconstruction, which permits them to be distinguished from the uncinate process (Fig. 2–32).

Nasal endoscopy is the method best suited for detailed evaluation of local sinus disease and the important anatomic variations that may influence sinus drainage. CT, however, provides the most useful information about the paranasal sinuses themselves. The en face view of the lateral nasal wall provided by 3D reconstruction may become a vital adjunct to CT and nasal endoscopy because it helps the surgeon visualize how the anatomy of the uncinate process, concha bullosa, paradoxical turbinates, and bulla ethmoidalis relates to obstruction of nasosinus drainage.

MAGNETIC RESONANCE IMAGING

When MRI first became clinically available in the mid 1980s, some radiologists expected that histologic diagnoses would soon be made solely on the basis of tissue characteristics identified on MRI. This is not yet possible, but MRI results can provide valuable information about paranasal sinus pathologic conditions.[20] In particular, MRI may help the radiologist distinguish neoplastic from inflammatory disease in this region.[21]

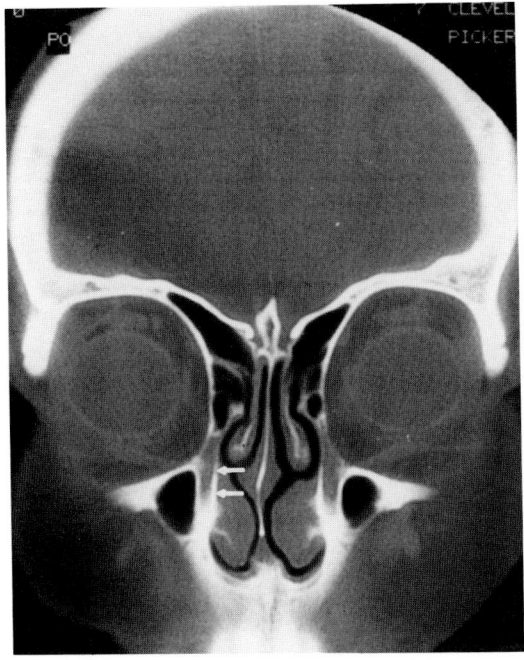

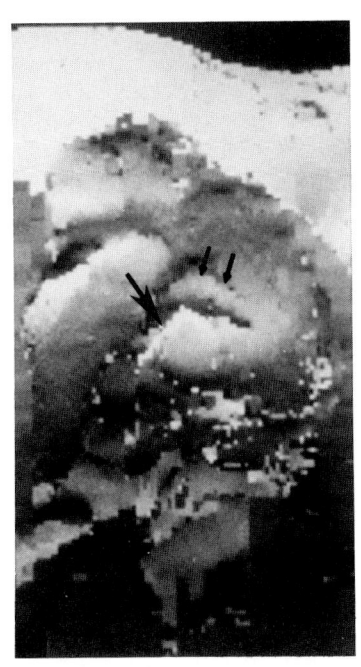

Figure 2–32. Nasolacrimal duct. **A**: Coronal CT. Occasionally, the nasolacrimal duct (double arrows) may protrude into the middle meatus and obscure or be mistaken for the uncinate process. **B**: Surface-rendered 3D reconstruction of **A** representing a parasagittal section through the patient's right lateral nasal wall. The nasolacrimal duct (double arrows) and middle turbinate (larger arrow) can be seen.

The intensity of the T_2-weighted MRI signal is directly proportional to the amount of water in the tissues. Thus, highly vascular tissues and interstitial tissues with high water content appear white on MR images, whereas air-filled areas appear black. The high water content of nasal mucosa and the mucoperiosteum lining the paranasal sinuses would thus be expected to give off high-intensity signals in these areas on T_2-weighted MR images. Normal mucoperiosteum is so thin, however, that no signal is seen (Fig. 2–33) unless mucosa covering the turbinates is highly edematous.

Inflammatory Disease

Edematous nasal mucosa will give a signal on MRI that is bright and varies with the nasal cycle. Polyps also produce strong signals on T_2-weighted images. Inflammatory disease affecting the paranasal sinuses is manifested on MR images as smooth or polypoid mucosal thickening that gives an intense signal on T_2-weighted images. Retained secretions also are high in water content, however, so it is not usually possible to differentiate between retained secretions and nasal polyps on MRI (Fig. 2–34).

A *mucocele*, because it is an airless expanded cyst that contains secretions produced by the mucosal lining of the sinus, usually gives a bright signal on T_2-weighted MR images. In addition, paranasal sinus mucoceles often give strong signals on T_1-weighted images because they have a high protein content. These two discrete signal patterns on MRI[22,23] are

54 *Endoscopic Sinus Surgery*

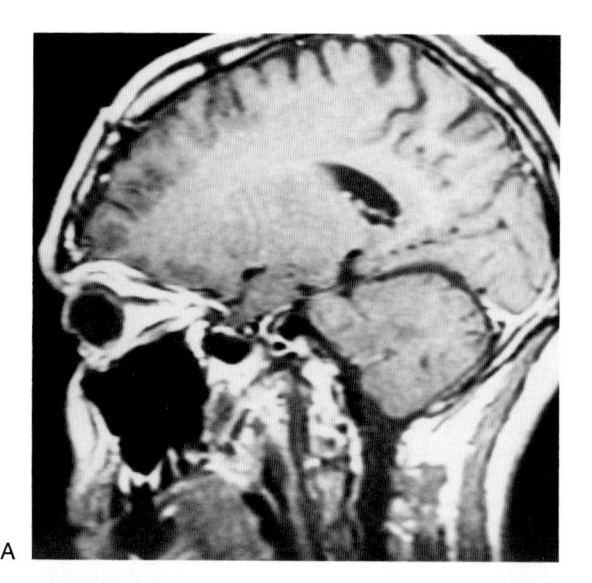

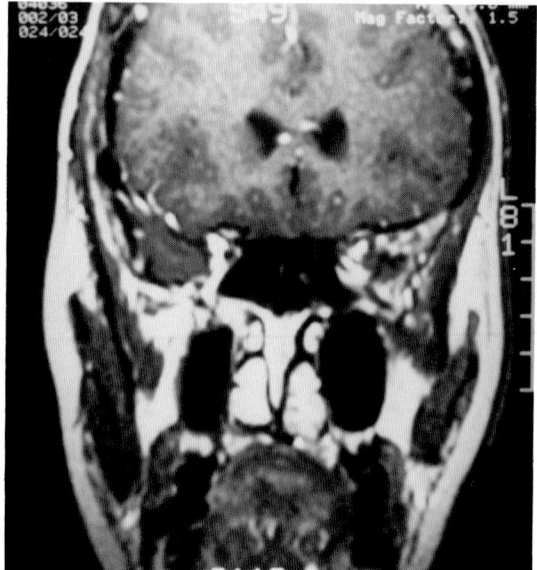

Figure 2–33. Sagittal (**A**) and coronal (**B**) magnetic resonance images of normal sinuses. Even after administration of gadolinium for contrast, the mucoperiosteum of this patient's paranasal sinuses is too thin to be visible as a bright band on these T_1-weighted images.

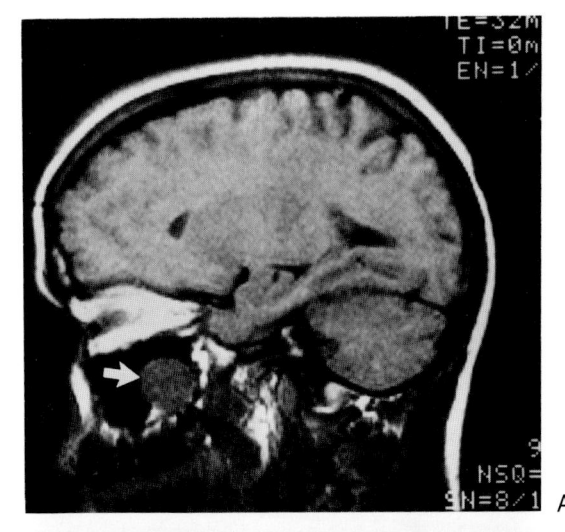

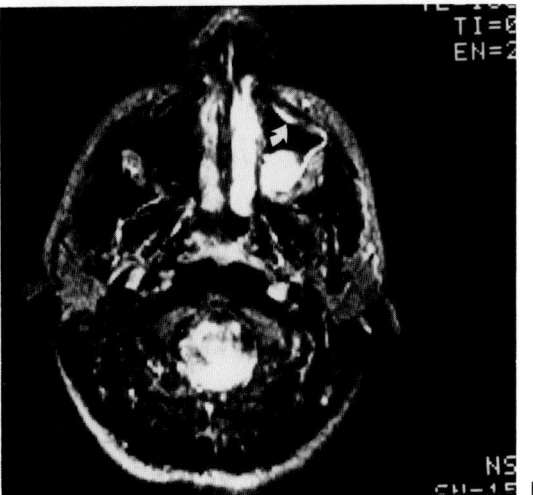

Figure 2–34. Magnetic resonance images of inflammatory paranasal sinus disease. **A**: A T_1-weighted sagittal section shows the typical appearance of an antral polyp (arrow). **B**: A T_2-weighted image shows polyp as a high-intensity (because of its high water content) signal in the right maxillary antrum; inflammation of antral mucoperiosteum is also visible (curved arrow).

not always seen with mucoceles, however. In fact, as greater numbers of MR images of patients with mucoceles are studied, an ever-widening range of variation is being identified in T_2-weighted signal intensity, and by implication in the hydration, of mucocele contents.

Mucoceles that give a less intense than expected or no T_2-weighted signal on MRI have been found at surgery to contain inspissated or dehydrated secretions. Corresponding CT findings have included a slightly dense central space or a pattern of fine calcifications in the mucocele.

A decreased MRI signal has also been noted from sinuses found to be infected by fungi such as *Aspergillus*. Some loss of T_2-weighted signal intensity in these cases could be due to the presence of Charcot-Leyden crystals, ferromagnetic particles concentrated by the fungus, and fungal hyphae in the mucocele; however, the hypointensity on T_2-weighted images is more likely due to inspissated mucus.

Neoplastic Disease

About 95% of all sinonasal tumors, including the most common ones (squamous cell carcinomas, lymphomas, and sarcomas), tend to be histologically uniform. Thus, they tend to produce uniform MRI signals, usually of intermediate intensity (both T_1- and T_2-weighted) (Fig. 2–35). The tendencies of tumors to produce signals of intermediate to low intensity and of inflammatory tissue to produce high-intensity signals make MRI of particular help to radiologists in differentiating tumor from inflammatory changes in the paranasal sinuses.

Not all tumors are alike, however. Tumors of minor salivary gland origin are more diverse in composition, some of them containing solid, serous, and mucous gland elements. Thus, some parotid tumors appear on T_2-weighted images as areas of homogeneous intermediate-intensity signals, but others give off nonuniform high-intensity signals.

One of the challenges for the radiologist interpreting MRI of the head and neck is differentiating recurrent tumor from postradiation inflammatory changes when both give off intermediate-intensity signals on T_2-weighted images. In such cases the patient may be given the contrast agent gadolinium-DTPA intravenously and then the MRI is repeated. Although both the tumor and the obstructed sinus will be enhanced on this second series of images, the patterns of enhancement are different: the tumor will enhance uniformly so that it appears as a solid mass, while the mucocele will show more peripheral enhancement (Fig. 2–36).

Limitations of Magnetic Resonance Imaging

Magnetic resonance imaging is not sensitive to calcifications and it does not demonstrate fine details of bony structures. Although it may distinguish between tumor and inflammatory processes, it does not provide enough information for the radiologist to distinguish among the many types of inflammatory changes that can occur in the paranasal sinuses. For these reasons, MRI is unlikely to become a primary imaging technique for evaluating benign paranasal sinus pathology.

Radiology of the Paranasal Sinuses 57

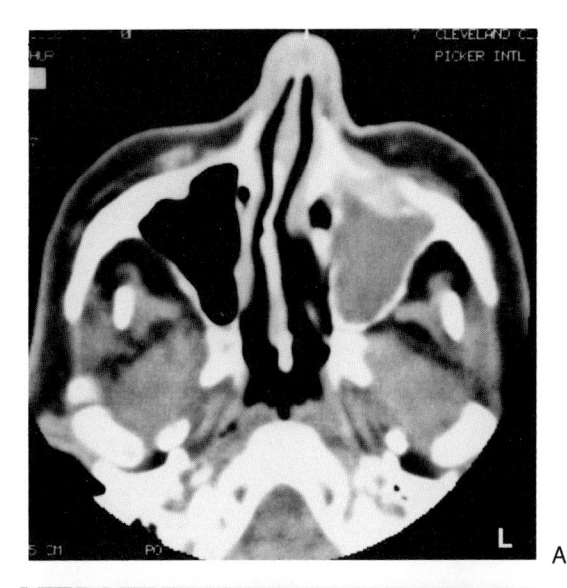

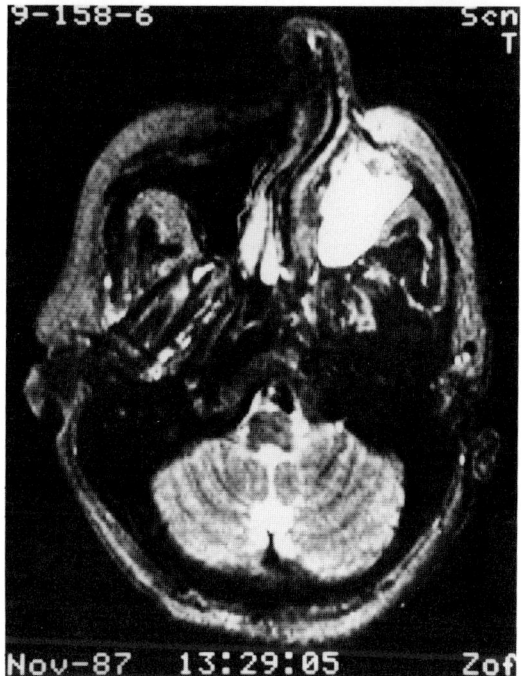

Figure 2–35. Squamous cell carcinoma and obstructed sinus. **A**: Nonenhanced CT through the maxillary sinuses shows complete opacification and slight expansion of the left maxillary sinus by a mucoid density suggestive of a mucocele. A soft tissue mass that had destroyed bone in the anterior wall proved on biopsy to be a squamous cell carcinoma. **B**: Corresponding T_2-weighted magnetic resonance image shows abnormalities corresponding to those seen on CT: high-water-content mucoid secretions gave off a high-intensity signal that appears as a white area on the image, and highly cellular tumor gave off a signal of intermediate intensity.

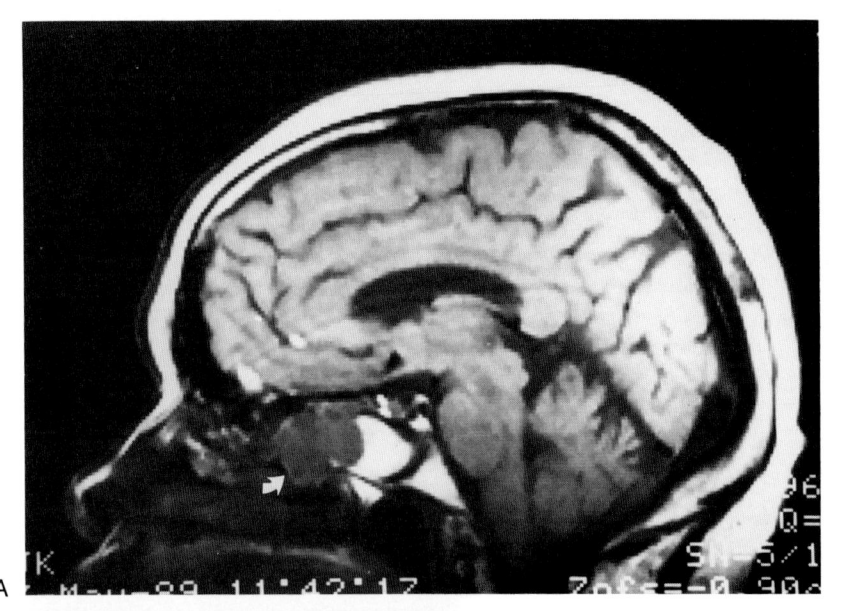

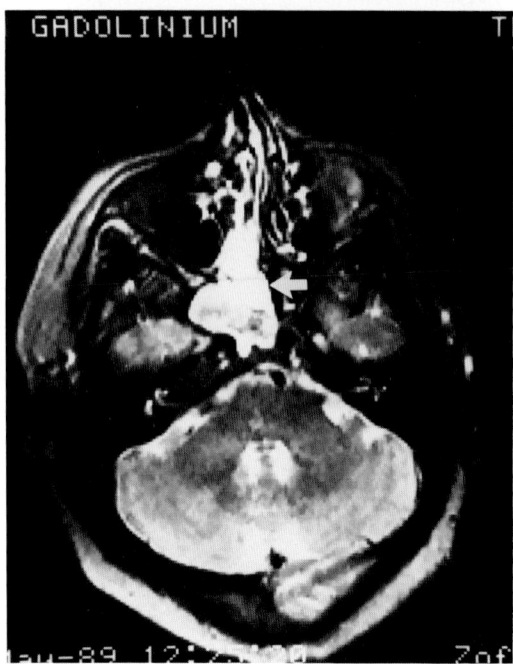

Figure 2–36. Gadolinium-enhanced magnetic resonance images of intranasal schwannoma. **A**: A sagittal T_1-weighted image shows a soft tissue mass of intermediate signal in the nasal cavity (arrow) and retained secretions in the sphenoid sinus posteriorly (white area of high signal intensity). **B**: After injection of contrast material, the mass in the nasal cavity shows homogeneous enhancement (arrow) and peripheral enhancement of the mucosa in the obstructed sphenoid sinus.

SUMMARY

CT images provide the surgeon with far more detailed information about the paranasal sinuses and adjacent vital structures than is available from standard roentgenograms. By studying serial CT images of the paranasal sinuses, the sinus surgeon can identify the subtle anatomic variations and pathologic alterations so essential to planning and performing endonasal endoscopic sinus surgery.

Newer techniques for paranasal sinus imaging can have a positive impact on the care of patients with suspected disease in this region. Screening CT provides many advantages over standard x-ray screening techniques, and surface-rendered 3D reconstruction may provide additional information to the endoscopic sinus surgeon. MRI has also proven useful in distinguishing inflammatory from neoplastic disease in the paranasal sinuses.

REFERENCES

1. Zinreich SJ, Kennedy DW, Rosenbaum AE, et al: Paranasal sinuses: CT imaging requirements for endoscopic surgery. Radiology 163:769–775, 1987.
2. Bolger W, Butzin C, Parson D: Paranasal sinus bony anatomic variations and mucosal abnormalities: CT analysis for endoscopic sinus surgery. Laryngoscope 101:55–64, 1991.
3. Price HI, Danzinger A: Computerized tomographic findings in mucoceles of the frontal and ethmoid sinuses. Clin Radiol 31:169–174, 1980.
4. Russell EJ, Czervionke L, Huckman M, et al: CT of the inferomedial orbit and the lacrimal drainage apparatus: Normal and pathologic anatomy. AJR 145:1147–1154, 1985.
5. Som PM, Lawson W, Biller HF, Lanzieri CF: Ethmoid sinus disease: CT evaluation in 400 cases. I. Nonsurgical patients. Radiology 159:591–597, 1986.
6. Terrier F, Weber W, Ruefenacht D, Porcellini B: Anatomy of the ethmoid: CT, endoscopic and macroscopic. Am J Rhinol 1:493–500, 1985.
7. Teatini G, Simonetti G, Salvolini U, et al: Computed tomography of the ethmoid labyrinth and adjacent structures. I. Normal anatomy and most common variants. Ann Otolaryngol 96:239–250, 1987.
8. Zinreich SJ, Mattox DE, Kennedy DW: Concha bullosa: CT evaluation. J Comput Assist Tomogr 12:778–784, 1988.
9. Som PM, Lawson W, Biller HF, Lanzieri CF: Ethmoid sinus disease: CT evaluation in 400 cases. II. Postoperative findings. Radiology 159:599–604, 1986.
10. Modic M, Weinstein MA, Berlin AJ, Duchesneau PM: Maxillary sinus hypoplasia visualized with computed tomography. Radiology 135:383–385, 1980.
11. Bolger WF, Woodruff WW Jr, Morehead J, Parsons DS: Maxillary sinus hypoplasia: Classification and description of associated uncinate process hypoplasia. Otolaryngol Head Neck Surg 103:759–765, 1990.
12. Furin MJ, Zinreich SJ, Kennedy DW: The atelectatic maxillary sinus. Am J Rhinol 5.79–83, 1991.
13. Silver AJ, Baredes S, Bello JA, et al: The opacified maxillary sinus: CT findings in chronic sinusitis and malignant tumors. Radiology 163:205–210, 1987.
14. Stammberger H, Jakse R, Beaufort F: Aspergillosis of the paranasal sinuses: X-ray diagnosis, histopathology and clinical aspects. Ann Otol Rhinol Laryngol 93:251–256, 1984.
15. Zinreich S, Kennedy D, Malat J, et al: Fungal sinusitis, diagnosis with CT and MR imaging. Head Neck Radiol 169:439–444, 1988.
16. Som PM, Shugar JMA: Antral mucoceles: A new look. J Comput Assist Tomogr 4:484–488, 1980.
17. Som PM: CT of the paranasal sinuses. Neuroradiology 27:189–201, 1985.
18. Som PM: The paranasal sinuses. In: Bergeron RT, Osborn AG, Som PM (eds): Head and Neck Imaging Excluding the Brain. St. Louis: CV Mosby, 1984, pp 1–142.
19. Lanzieri CF, Levine HL, Rosenbloom SA, et al: Three dimensional surface rendering of nasal anatomy from CT data. Arch Otolaryngol Head Neck Surg 115:1444–1446, 1989.
20. Council on Scientific Affairs, Report of the Panel on Magnetic Resonance Imaging: Magnetic resonance imaging of the head and neck region. JAMA 260:3313–3326, 1988.
21. Som PM, Shapiro MD, Biller HF, et al: Sinonasal tumors and inflammatory tissues: Differentiation with MR imaging. Radiology 167:803–808, 1988.
22. Van Tassel P, Lee Ya-Yen, Jing Bao-Shan, DePena CA: Mucoceles of the paranasal sinuses. AJNR 10:607–612, 1989.
23. Dawson RC, Horton JA: MR imaging of mucoceles of the sphenoid sinus. AJNR 10:613–614, 1989.

3
Office Evaluation of Nasosinus Disorders: Patient Selection for Endoscopic Sinus Surgery

MARK MAY, M.D., F.A.C.S.
SARA J. MESTER R.T.(R)
HOWARD L. LEVINE, M.D., F.A.C.S.

The availability of rigid nasal endoscopes as well as the use of paranasal computed tomography (CT) has permitted diagnosis and treatment of nasosinus disorders that were unrecognized previously. This chapter describes our methods for evaluating and recommending management of complaints related to the sinuses. Patients are offered endoscopic sinus surgery (ESS) selectively based on the results of the history, endoscopic examination, and radiologic studies, with the history, particularly the sinus symptom history, being the most important.

We follow a detailed Endoscopic Sinus Surgery Protocol (Appendix) to evaluate sinus symptoms and to plan and evaluate the results of surgery.

HISTORY

Because the goal of surgical therapy for nasosinus disease is to relieve the symptoms by eliminating disease, aerating the sinuses, and restoring mucociliary flow, patients are questioned closely about each symptom that may be present. The lack of any objective means to measure the severity of disease for degree to which symptoms interfere with the patient's lifestyle means that both the decision for surgery and the success of surgery are subjective. These evaluations are made by the patient.

Chief Complaint

The patient's chief complaint usually includes one or more of the symptoms listed on "page 3" (Fig. 3–1) of the Endoscopic Sinus Surgery Protocol (Appendix, page 259). Other complaints may include inability to sleep at night, the need to sleep in the sitting position, dry mouth or burning tongue, loss of appetite, weight loss, or irritability. Patients may also present with vague complaints involving almost every structure in the head and neck.

Symptom History

Mark + next to each symptom if present preoperatively on a chronic or recurrent basis. Rate the most bothersome three symptoms in red. Rate symptoms for each postoperative visit: W = Worse   I = Improved   S = Same   O = Gone

	Date	Date	Date	Date	Date	Date	Date	Date	Date
Nasal Stuffiness									
Nasal Airway Obstruction									
Postnasal Drainage									
Runny Nose									
Bloody Nose									
Puffy Eyes									
Eye Pressure/Pain									
Ear Pressure/Popping									
Headaches									
Facial Pressure									
Hoarseness									
Sore Throat									
Bad Breath									
Aching Teeth									
Taste/Smell Changes									
General Fatigue									
Dizziness/Lightheadedness									
Chronic Cough									
Itchy Nose									
Watery Eyes									
Red Eyes									
Scratchy Throat									
Frequent Throat Clearing									
Sneezing									
Other									

Figure 3–1.   Endoscopic Sinus Surgery Protocol, page 259.

History of the Present Illness

Table 3–1 lists the symptoms most often reported by patients, with nasal stuffiness, postnasal discharge, and headache being the most frequent. Patients are asked whether they have each symptom on the list, and after all symptoms have been reviewed they are asked to indicate the three that are most severe.

Past Medical and Surgical History

A survey of our first 400 patients operated on for ostiomeatal complex (OMC) disease showed that almost half had a history of chronic or recurrent suppurative sinusitis, and a large proportion had nasal polyposis (Table 3–2). More than one third had previously undergone nasoseptoplasty, and nearly one fourth had undergone sinus surgery previously (Table 3–2). Reactive airway disease occurred in slightly less than one fifth of patients.

Medications

The patient's current medications may affect the severity of sinus disease or its surgical management, or both.

Many patients with asthma use steroid medications chronically. These medications may mask symptoms of allergy, or temporarily control the size and extent of nasal polyps, and thus create a transient sense of well-being. In addition, steroid medications may need to be administered perioperatively to patients who have been taking steroids.

Patients with asthma and polyposis may have Samter's syndrome (also called ASA

Table 3–1 Symptoms of Sinus Disease Most Often Reported by 400 Patients Treated Consecutively by Endonasal Sinus Surgery

SYMPTOM	PATIENTS REPORTING SYMPTOM (%) PREOPERATIVELY	POSTOPERATIVELY*
Stuffy nose	92	14
Postnasal discharge	79	12
Headache (frontal, periorbital, facial)	63	13
Facial pressure	57	7
Runny nose	51	8
Taste and smell altered	45	5
Eye pain	42	1
Fatigue	35	4
Sore throat	31	6
Bad breath	24	1
Ear popping or fullness	22	9
Hoarseness	21	2
Lightheadedness	21	0
Nosebleed	12	6

*Based on patients' reports of symptoms during follow-up of 8 to 40 months.

Table 3–2 Past Medical and Surgical History: Most Common Factors Noted on Survey of 400 Patients with Ostiomeatal Complex Disease

FACTOR	PATIENTS REPORTING (%)
Sinusitis (chronic or recurrent suppurative)	47
Polyps	39
Previous nasoseptoplasty	37
Previous sinus surgery	24
Reactive airway disease	18
Samter's syndrome (polyps, asthma, aspirin sensitivity)	9.5

triad: asthma, polyposis, and aspirin sensitivity), in which taking aspirin may aggravate sinus symptoms. These patients must be cautioned to avoid aspirin and aspirin-containing products.

Patients who have been taking aspirin, nonsteroidal anti-inflammatory drugs (NSAIDs), or other medications that increase coagulation time should discontinue these medications at an appropriate time before surgery to avoid perioperative or postoperative bleeding (Table 3–3).[1] Warfarin, which is not listed in Table 3–3, should be discontinued 7 to 10 days before surgery if medically possible; furthermore, bleeding time, as indicated by results of partial thromboplastin and prothrombin time testing, should be in the normal range.

Other associations between pharmaceutical agents and the appearance and function of nasal mucosa include chronic use of: (1) topical nasal decongestants, marijuana, or cocaine; (2) steroids, decongestants, or antihistamines; and (3) estrogen compounds or beta-adrenergic receptor-blocking medications. Agents in group 1 may be responsible for nasosinus complaints, agents in group 2 can cause shrinking or even atrophy of the mucous membranes in the nose, and agents in group 3 can cause engorgement of the mucosa. It is important for the surgeon to be aware of a patient's use of any of these medications and to

Table 3–3 Recommended Waiting Period Between Cessation of Drug Therapy and Surgery*

DRUG	PERIOD BEFORE SURGERY (DAYS)
Aspirin	7–10
Diclofenac (Voltaren)	1
Diflunisal (Dolobid)	1
Ibuprofen (Motrin, Advil)	1
Indomethacin (Indocin)	1
Sulindac (Clinoril)	1
Tolmetin (Tolectin)	2
Naproxen (Naprosyn)	4
Piroxicam (Feldene)	14

*Guidelines of American Academy of Otolaryngology—Head and Neck Surgery (Committee on Medical Devices and Drugs), 1989.[1]

have the patient discontinue them before surgery. To achieve optimal results of surgery, the effects of these agents must be treated before surgery in some cases.

Symptom History

Symptoms of chronic sinusitis are most often due to impairment of mucociliary flow, which may be caused by one or more of the following: (1) anatomic deformity, (2) chronic infection, and (3) allergy. The symptoms list (Fig. 3–1) in the Endoscopic Sinus Surgery Protocol (Appendix) is designed to provide the patient's disease profile at a glance. The first eight symptoms are most often associated with obstructive changes, and the last six named symptoms suggest allergy. The symptoms in the middle—headaches through chronic cough—are noted with chronic infection.

The grouping of symptoms in the protocol (Fig. 3–1) was based on the observation that certain symptoms are often seen in combination and can point to a diagnosis. Thus, an itchy nose, watery or red eyes, a scratchy throat, and sneezing suggest allergy. Many patients with allergy also have nasal polyposis, which may be suspected if the patient complains of nasal obstruction and discharge and alterations in taste and smell. Headache, bad breath, aching teeth, and general fatigue suggest chronic suppurative sinusitis. When dental pain involves the maxillary molars or premolars, it could indicate primary maxillary sinus disease. Such pain may also be of dental origin, however, so in such cases a dental consultation should be obtained.

Of all the symptoms noted, postnasal discharge, chronic cough, and headache, as isolated symptoms, were the least likely to be relieved by sinus surgery.

Postnasal Discharge

Thickened mucous discharge may be due to a mucous membrane alteration, such as chronic mucositis, uninfluenced by surgical management.

Cough

The cough in patients with reactive airway disease or Samter's syndrome (ASA triad) often persisted in spite of surgical therapy. Although chronic cough may be associated with OMC disease, a primary pulmonary problem must be considered. Patients with chronic cough should not undergo sinus surgery unless it is indicated to relieve complaints related to nasosinus disease because in our experience sinus surgery did not relieve symptoms, such as bronchospasm or cough, of lower airway dysfunction.

Headache

Likewise, patients with an isolated or major complaint of headache with few or no symptoms related to the sinuses were unlikely to have the symptom relieved by ESS. The type of headache usually reported by patients with frontal, maxillary, or ethmoid sinus disease is characterized as dull, aching, pressure around the midface, eyes, and forehead. The pain is characteristically influenced by the patient's position and changes in barometric pressure. When the pain localizes to the top or back of the head, disease in the sphenoid sinus must be suspected.

MEDICAL MANAGEMENT OF SINUSITIS

Chronic Symptoms

Chronic sinus symptoms associated with sinusitis may be constant, intermittent, fluctuating, or recurrent. Before surgery is considered to treat chronic symptoms of sinus disease, medical management of allergic and other conditions must have been tried.

No strict guidelines can be established as to what constitutes an adequate trial of medical therapy, because often patients who consult a surgeon for management of subjective complaints have already decided that the complaints interfere with their quality of life sufficiently to consider accepting the risks of surgery. In most cases, antibiotic, decongestant, or antihistamine agents and steroid sprays, alone or in combination, have been tried without satisfactory results. In some instances the side effects or cost of these medications is unacceptable to the patient and surgery is preferred rather than another trial of medication.

Allergy

The physician should first seek to identify a possible allergen or allergens when sinus symptoms are suspected to be due to allergy, as indicated by a history in the patient or the patient's family of allergies and the presence of nasomucosal changes suggestive of allergy. In such cases, even if no allergen is identified, symptoms should be treated medically before suggesting sinus surgery. Medical management may include a course of steroid or antihistamine medication and environmental control of suspected allergens. Many patients whose sinus symptoms are due to allergy have been referred for surgery after medical management has failed, and the combination of medical and surgical management has been more effective in relieving symptoms than either modality alone.

Acute Suppurative Sinusitis

A diagnosis of acute suppurative sinusitis can be suspected from the history. Pus noted at the endoscopic examination helps to confirm the diagnosis. The origin of such pus correlates with the sinus involved: if pus is found in the nasofrontal recess just inferior to the anterior attachment of the middle turbinate, frontal sinusitis is likely; pus in the middle meatal region, especially if from the hiatus semilunaris, indicates likely maxillary or anterior ethmoid sinusitis, or both; and a purulent discharge in the sphenoethmoid recess is diagnostic of posterior ethmoid or sphenoid sinus infection or both.

Another useful diagnostic aid is locating the site of mucopus and its relationship to the torus tubarius. The flow of mucopus below the torus tubarius is associated with anterior OMC infection, whereas flow of mucopus above the torus tubarius is noted with posterior OMC (posterior ethmoid or sphenoid sinus) disease (see Chapter 1, Fig. 1–4B). A specimen for culture can be obtained by using the endoscope to locate the area of pus precisely and then sampling the infected material with a middle-ear wire culture tip (Calgiswab Type I, Spectrum Diagnostics, Glenwood, IL; Mini-tip Culturette, Becton Dickinson Microbiology Systems, Cockeysville, MD).

A clinical impression of acute maxillary and frontal sinusitis may be confirmed and documented by the results of roentgenographic examination. Plain sinus roentgenographs usually clearly define involvement of the maxillary and frontal sinuses but are most often inadequate to demonstrate involvement of the sphenoid and ethmoid sinuses. If the sinuses appear normal on plain roentgenographs and there is still suspicion that the symptoms are due to sinus disease, CT is the diagnostic modality of choice, although it is usually not needed for most patients with acute sinusitis.

Treatment of Acute Suppurative Sinusitis

Treatment of acute suppurative sinusitis will vary with the age of the patient, the severity of symptoms, and whether there are complications.

Medical Treatment

Usually the patient is prescribed a decongestant (such as oxymetazoline hydrochloride) every 8 hours for 3 days and an antibiotic (amoxicillin, cefaclor, minocycline, or trimethoprim-sulfamethoxazole) for a minimum of 10 and a maximum of 21 days. If symptoms resolve and the results of endoscopic examination are normal, the patient no longer requires care.

If the symptoms persist, a second course of antibiotic medication is prescribed or an alternative antibiotic is prescribed (a second-generation cephalosporin such as cefaclor, an augmented penicillin such as amoxicillin and clavulanic acid, or, occasionally, a fluoroquinolone such as ciprofloxacin). These antibiotics have enhanced activity against *Staphylococcus* and *Haemophilus influenzae*. Should symptoms not resolve after this second course of medication, surgery should be considered.

Considerations for Surgical Treatment

Acute sinusitis usually resolves with adequate medical treatment. When it does not, surgery should be considered if one of the following is true: (1) the diagnosis is not acute sinusitis but rather an acute exacerbation of a chronic sinus condition, (2) anatomic abnormalities of the septum or lateral nasal wall are causing obstruction of the OMC (Fig. 3–2), or (3) fungal sinusitis is present, which may be suspected by noting, on a CT scan, radiodense material in an opaque maxillary sinus (Fig. 3–3).

If symptoms persist and abnormalities are present on the CT scan or noted on endoscopic examination, surgical management is discussed with the patient. Patients who are reluctant or who are not suitable candidates to undergo surgery are hospitalized for intravenous administration of cefuroxime axetil, or clindamycin for those allergic to penicillin. If this treatment fails, then surgery should be considered based on the risk/benefit ratio for continued medical versus surgical treatment.

Endoscopic Management

Classically, acute suppurative sinusitis was evaluated and treated by puncturing the sinus with a needle inserted through a transnasal inferior meatal or transcanine fossa antrotomy to obtain aspirate for culture and to permit irrigation of the sinus with saline solution. Endoscopes are now used to evaluate the sinuses and manage sinus disease.

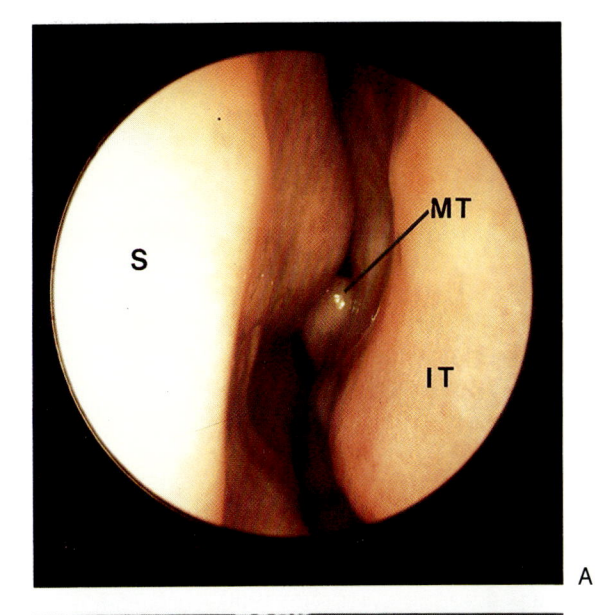

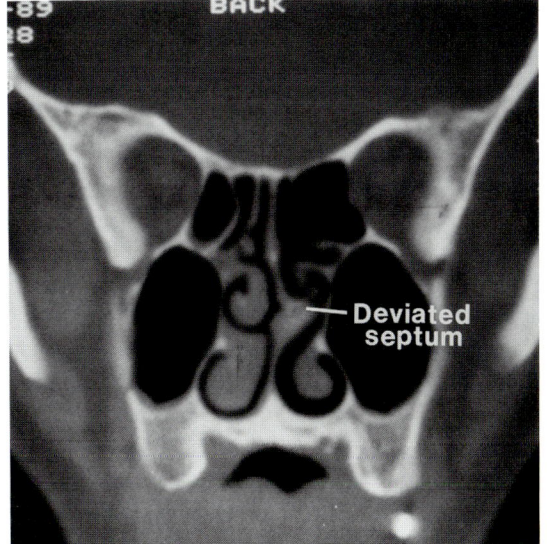

Figure 3–2. **A**: Endoscopic view, left nasal cavity. Note septal deformity with lateral displacement of a paradoxical turbinate compressing the ostiomeatal complex. IT: inferior turbinate; MT: middle turbinate; S: septum. **B**: Coronal CT. Septum deviated to the left of midline is compressing the middle turbinate into the ostiomeatal complex.

Endoscopic endonasal surgery performed over the past 4 years on seven patients with acute frontal sinusitis unresponsive to medical therapy has been proven an effective means to remove obstructing inflamed tissue from and promote excellent drainage of the nasofrontal recess and agger nasi area. A direct endoscopic approach to open the anterior OMC in 12 patients with acute maxillary sinus involvement or to treat an obstructed sphenoid sinus in 10 patients has also been effective.

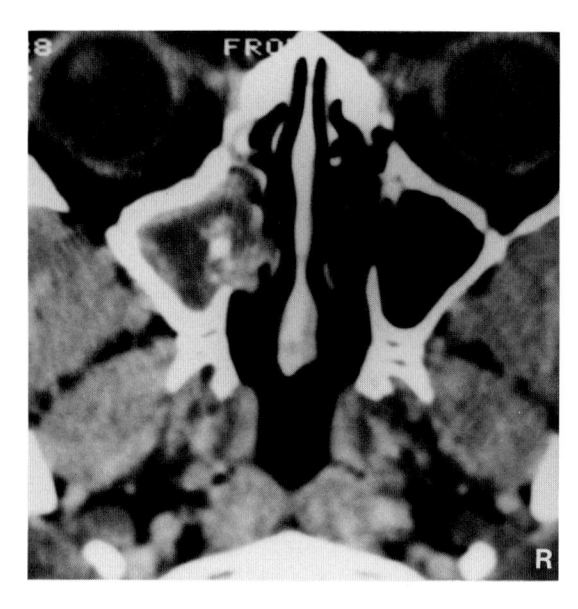

Figure 3–3. Axial CT through maxillary sinuses. Fungal sinusitis was suspected from review of CT image and confirmed at time of surgery. Note hypercalcification within opacified right maxillary sinus.

NASAL EXAMINATION

External Inspection

Examination of the nose begins with observation of any external deformities and their relationship to other facial landmarks. A crooked or twisted nose is usually associated with disturbance of function, and if the external nose is badly deformed the nasal septum is usually markedly deviated and the turbinates are abnormal.

A deviated nasal septum may often cause lateral compression of the middle turbinate and in turn obstruction of the OMC (Fig. 3–2A and B). If the bony and cartilaginous pyramid and the nasal tip are badly twisted, the internal nasal valve (between the septum and the caudal edge of the upper lateral cartilage) may be narrowed, causing obstruction that may occasionally be associated with OMC narrowing.

Internal Examination

Anterior rhinoscopy is performed with a head mirror or headlight and a nasal speculum. The turbinates are examined in a general manner to determine whether there is any enlargement that may be causing nasal symptoms and whether this enlargement is due to a vasoactive turbinate or bony enlargement. The relationship between the middle turbinate and the nasal septum may not be appreciated by inspection with a headlight and nasal speculum, however. This relationship may only become evident after nasal endoscopy.

As the internal nose is examined with the headlight and speculum, the presence and character of secretions and the color and turgor of the mucosa are noted, as well as septal deflections. An effort is made to inspect the space between the middle turbinate and lateral nasal wall, although often this cannot be accomplished until decongestants are applied. Examination of the compartment between the middle turbinate and lateral wall will provide the information most crucial to diagnosis in the majority of patients with nasosinus disorders.

Posterior Rhinoscopy

Posterior rhinoscopy is performed with a tongue depressor and nasopharyngeal mirror. The goals of this examination are to determine the character of the mucosa of the nasopharynx, whether adenoid tissue is present, and if the posterior tips of the inferior turbinates are polypoid or obstruct the nasal cavity.

Endoscopy

After anterior and posterior rhinoscopy are performed, the same areas are examined using the endoscope. More than one third of patients with nasosinus symptoms with no evidence of disease on anterior and posterior rhinoscopy will have abnormal findings on nasal endoscopy.[2] Endoscopic findings can be documented with videotape and photographs or 35 mm slides.

Equipment

Instruments used to examine the sinuses endoscopically and to document findings are listed in Tables 3–4 and 3–5; Figures 3–4 through 3–6 show how the equipment is set up. The

Table 3–4 Office Endonasal Endoscopy Equipment

MANUFACTURER*	DESCRIPTION	MODEL/CATALOG NO.
Storz	4 mm, 0° short endoscope	1215A
Storz	4 mm, 0° long endoscope	7200A
Storz	2.7 mm, 30° long endoscope	27018B
Storz	2.7 mm, 70° long endoscope	27018C
Storz	Miniature light source	481-C
Luxtec	Cables	495NL

*Karl Storz, 10111 W. Jefferson Blvd., Culver City, CA 99232. Luxtec Corporation, PO Box 225, Technology Park Road, Sturbridge, MA 01566-0225

Table 3–5 Equipment for Documentation of Endonasal Endoscopy

ITEM	MANUFACTURER AND MODEL NO.*
Camera	Olympus OM-2N
Lens	Karl Storz 593-T2
Film	Speed ASA 100, 35mm
Settings	Exposure ¹⁄₆₀ sec, 120 power
Video camera	Karl Storz model no. 9050B
Monitor	Karl Storz model no. TM22-V, color
Light source	Karl Storz xenon light source, 610
Cables	Luxtec 495 NL
Video cassette recorder	Panasonic AG 7350, ½-inch super VHS

*See Table 3–4 for manufacturers' addresses.

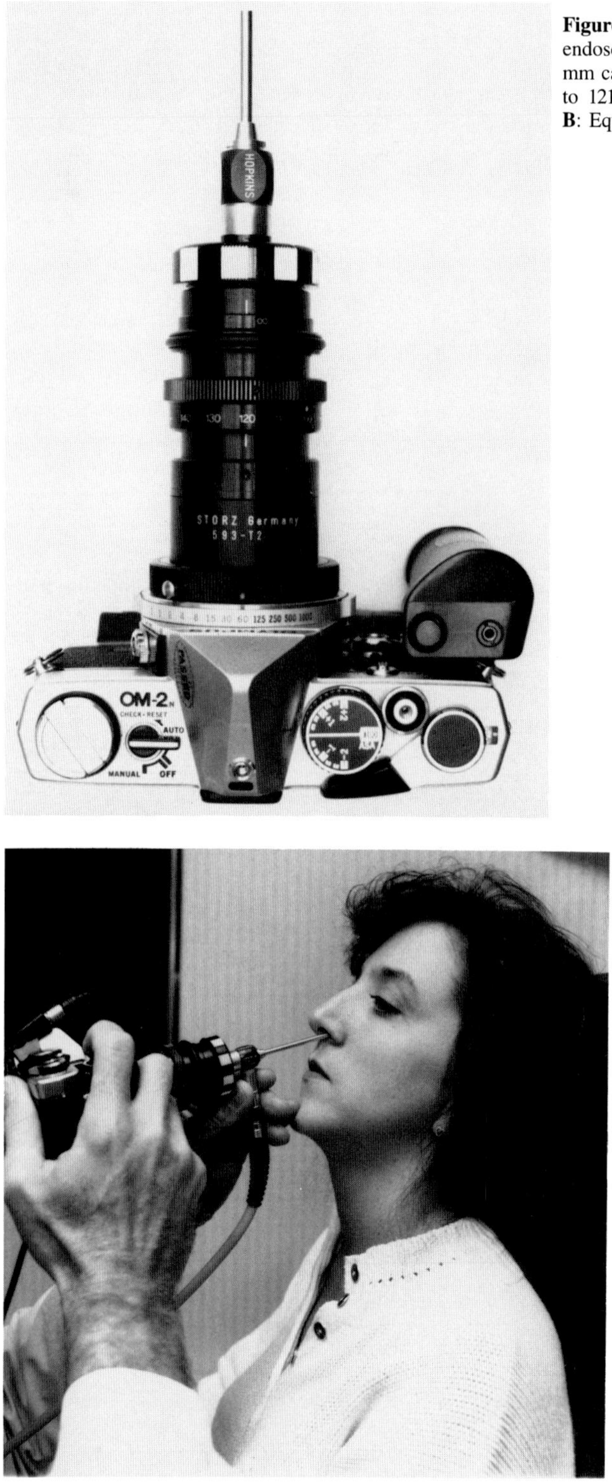

Figure 3–4. Equipment used to document endoscopy results. **A**: Olympus OM-2N 35 mm camera with Storz lens 593-T2 attached to 1217A 4 mm 0° short endoscopic lens. **B**: Equipment in use.

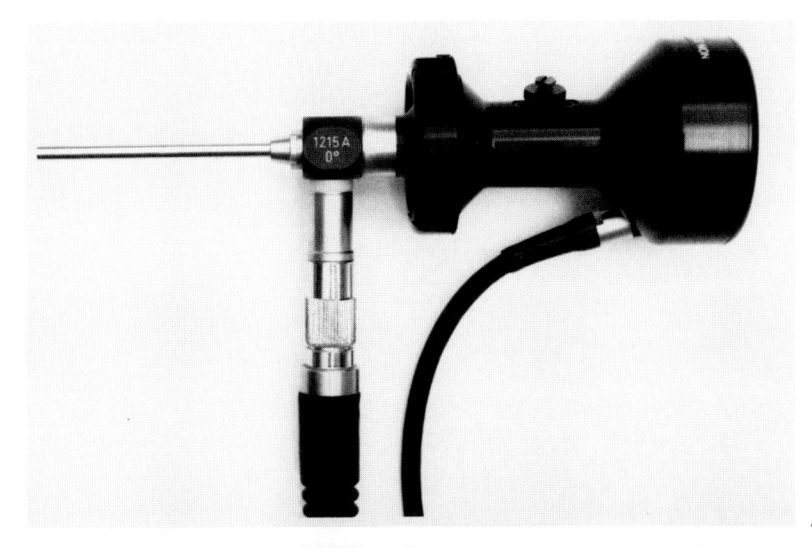

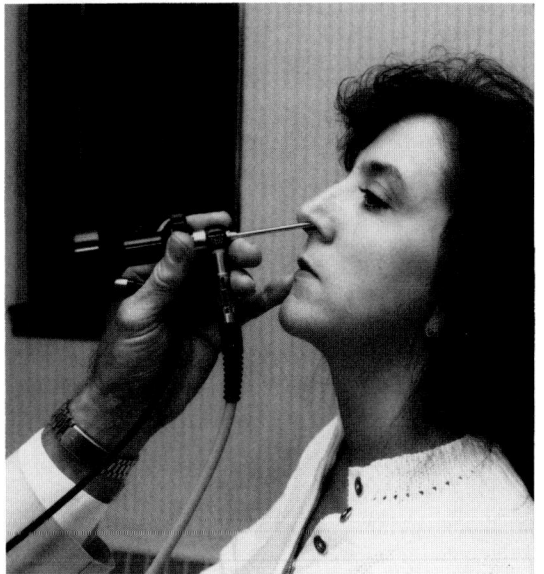

Figure 3–5. **A**: Video camera attached to endoscope. **B**: Equipment used to document endoscopy results.

1215A Storz 4 mm, 0° short endoscope is recommended to obtain a general overview of the nasal cavity. This endoscope is long enough to examine as far posteriorly as the nasopharynx, and the wide field of view, good illumination, and ease of handling that this instrument provides make it superior to longer endoscopes. The shorter endoscope is also ideal for intranasal photography and is less threatening to patients than a longer instrument.

Technique

The endoscope is inserted as far posteriorly as possible without causing the patient discomfort. Usually, it cannot be passed beyond the anterior attachment of the middle

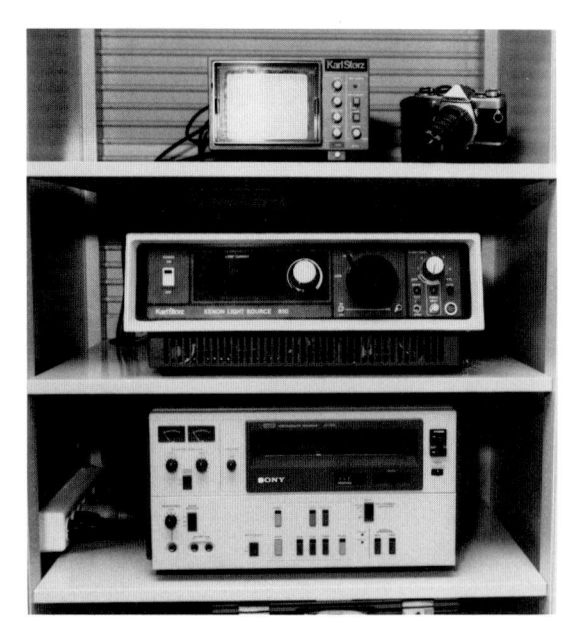

Figure 3-6. Equipment and set-up for video and photography.

turbinate, and therefore a local anesthetic and decongestant need to be applied. This is accomplished by placing a cotton pledget dampened with 2% tetracaine and 1% phenylephrine hydrochloride (Neo-Synephrine Nasal Spray) in the nose for approximately 5 minutes. For many patients, spraying the nose with 4% lidocaine and 1% phenylephrine hydrochloride will provide sufficient anesthesia to allow thorough nasal endoscopic examination.

Evaluating the Middle Turbinates and Septum

After application of the decongestant and anesthetic, the endoscope is used to reevaluate the same fields examined previously. The extent of turbinate decongestion is noted. Unless precluded by anatomic abnormalities, inspection of the uncinate process, hiatus semilunaris, bulla ethmoidalis, accessory ostia, superior turbinate, sphenoethmoid recess, torus tubarius, and nasopharynx is also carried out.

If it is difficult to pass the 4-mm, 0° endoscope between the middle turbinate and the lateral nasal wall, the 2.7 mm, 30° endoscope is used.

The relationship between the middle turbinate and the nasal septum is classified as TS 1, 2, or 3. This classification depends on whether, after the decongestant has been applied, the medial and lateral wall of the middle turbinate can be visualized (TS 1), part of the middle turbinate is obscured by septal deviation (TS 2), or septal deflection completely blocks the view of any portion of the middle turbinate (TS 3) (Fig. 3-7A, B, and C).

The results of the endoscopic examination help in planning surgery. For example, if the inferior turbinate is "boggy" and obstructs passage of the endoscope, even after application of decongestant, surgical reduction or laser photocoagulation[3] of this turbinate might be indicated. If an inferior nasoantral window was created previously, the maxillary sinus may often be inspected with a 30° or 70° endoscope. Often, purulent secretions are seen draining by gravity through this opening. The presence of purulent secretions within the maxillary

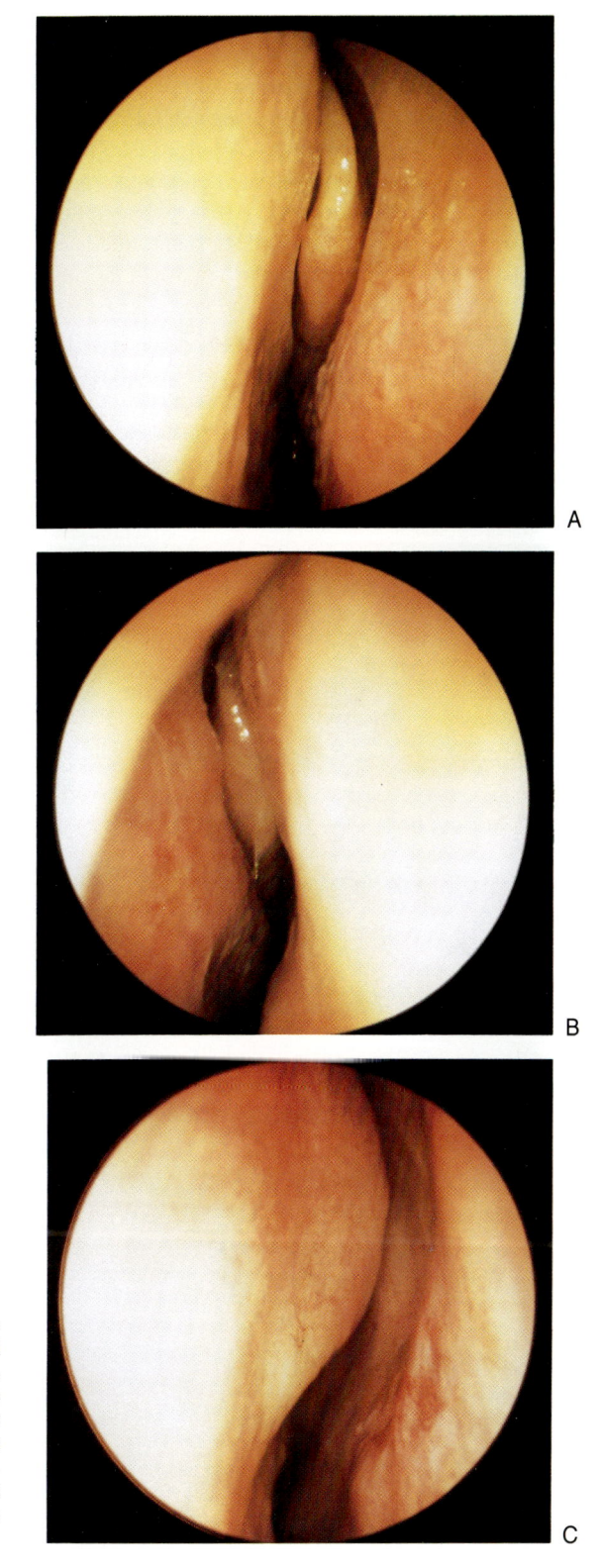

Figure 3–7. Endoscopic views, after decongestion of nasal mucosa, of turbinoseptal (TS) deformities. **A**: Left nasal cavity (TS-1). The medial and lateral borders of the middle turbinate can be seen. **B**: Right nasal cavity (TS-2). The view of the middle turbinate is partially obstructed by the septal deviation. **C**: Left nasal cavity (TS-3). The view of the middle turbinate is blocked completely by the septal deviation.

sinus in spite of a patent inferior meatal nasoantral window suggests obstruction of the natural ostium of the maxillary sinus.

The middle turbinate is evaluated for its shape and size as well as its relationship to the lateral nasal wall and septum. A bulge just above and anterior to the anterior attachment of the middle turbinate suggests enlarged agger nasi cells (Fig. 3–8A and B). Sometimes the anterior tip of the turbinate is triangular, which is of no clinical significance unless it obstructs the space between the turbinate and lateral wall (Fig. 3–9). Contact of the mucosa of the middle turbinate with the mucosa of the nasal septum, or of the mucosa of the middle turbinate with the mucosa of the lateral nasal wall, is often associated with OMC disease and sinus symptoms (Fig. 3–10A, B).

A middle turbinate that is concave medially rather than laterally is considered *paradoxical* (Fig. 3–11A, B). Presence of a paradoxical turbinate alone is not of clinical significance, but a paradoxical turbinate associated with symptoms or abnormal CT findings may need to be corrected. A paradoxical middle turbinate may be associated with ipsilateral deviation of the septum and bulbous enlargement of the contralateral turbinate

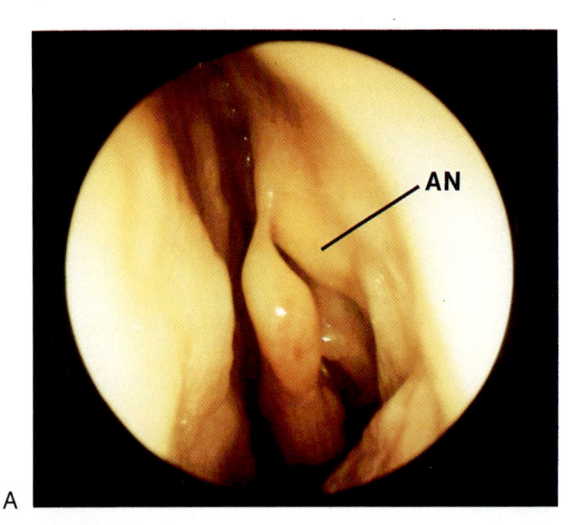

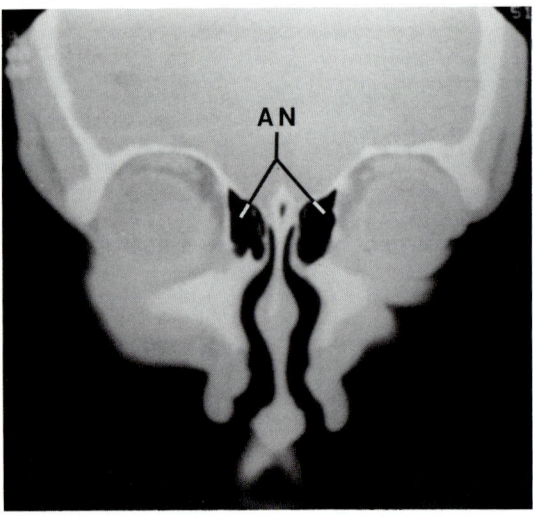

Figure 3–8. Agger nasi (AN) cell. **A**: Endoscopic view. Agger nasi cell appears as fullness in front of anterior attachment of middle turbinate. **B**: Coronal CT. Agger nasi cell is located just below the level of the frontal sinus.

Office Evaluation of Nasosinus Disorders 75

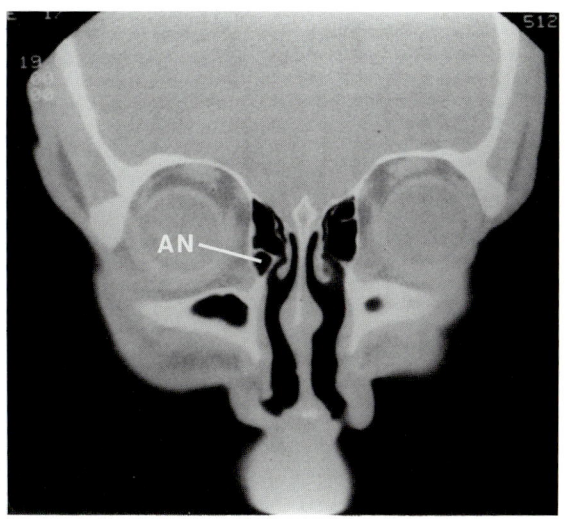

Figure 3–8. (*Continued*). **C**: Coronal CT. Agger nasi cell is in front of anterior attachment of middle turbinate.

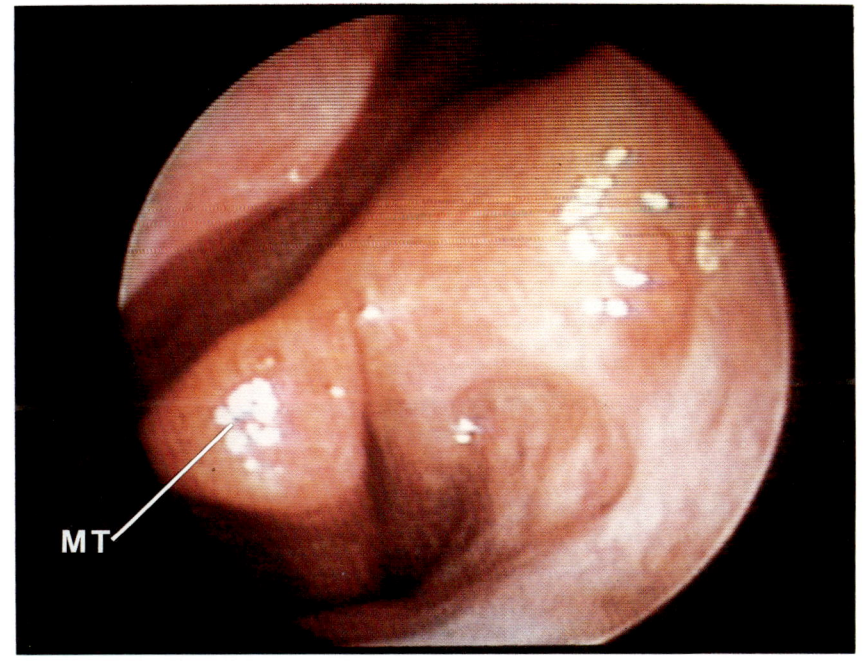

Figure 3–9. View through endoscope of triangular anterior edge of middle turbinate (MT).

76 Endoscopic Sinus Surgery

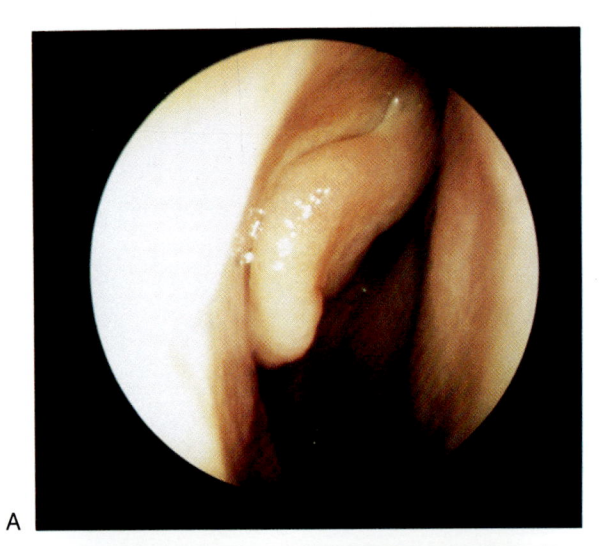

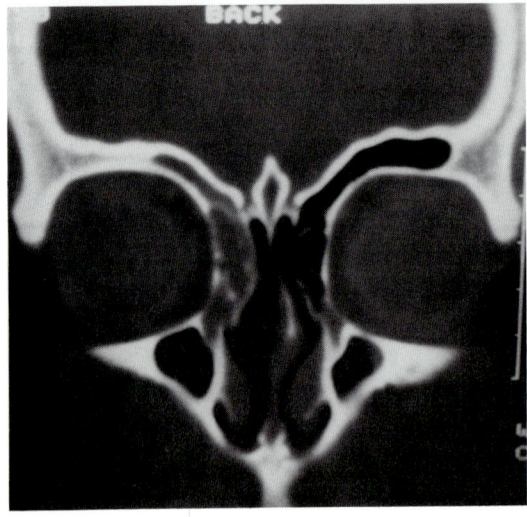

Figure 3–10. **A**: Endoscopic view of right nasal cavity. The middle turbinate is lateralized and its mucosa is in contact with the lateral nasal wall. **B**: Coronal CT of same area. Note opacity of anterior ethmoid sinus, nasofrontal recess, and frontal sinus on the right side due to obstruction of sinus drainage, the result of lateralization of middle turbinate.

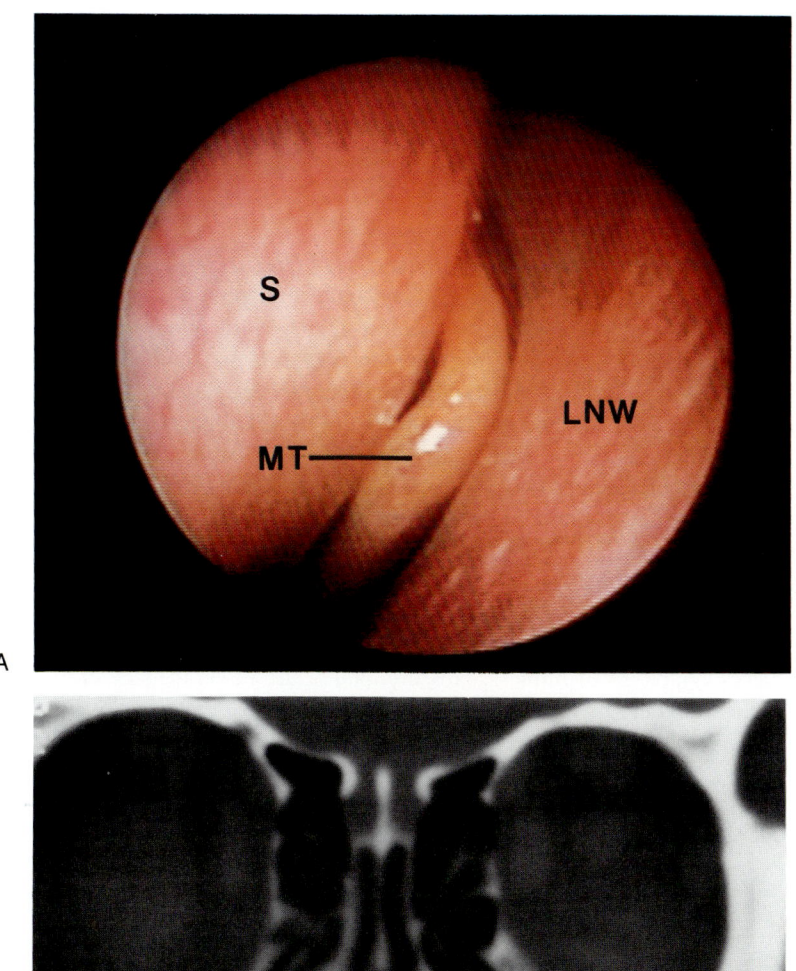

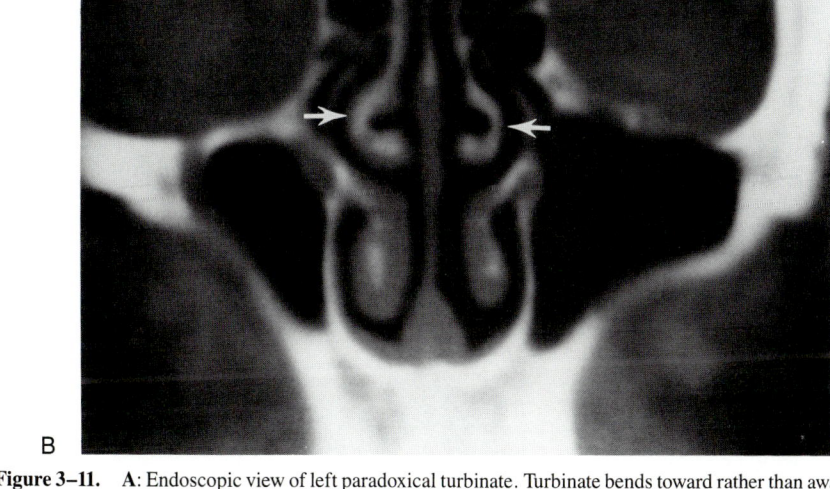

Figure 3–11. **A**: Endoscopic view of left paradoxical turbinate. Turbinate bends toward rather than away from the lateral nasal wall (LNW). MT: middle turbinate; S: septum. **B**: CT scan of same patient shows bilateral paradoxical middle turbinates (arrows).

(Fig. 3–12A, B). The paradoxical turbinate may be very thin and a partial turbinectomy may be indicated. Partial turbinectomy will be necessary if the patient requires OMC surgery because, if the turbinate should remain displaced laterally and adhere to the lateral nasal wall, the maxillary sinus ostium and nasofrontal recess would be obstructed after surgery (Fig. 3–13).

Concha Bullosa

A concha bullosa is an air-filled, cellular turbinate, most often the middle turbinate (Fig. 3–12A, B). The presence of a large concha bullosa should be suspected if the middle turbinate is bulbous and fills the space between the lateral wall of the nose and a septum deviated to the opposite side (Fig. 3–12A, B). This situation is often associated with a thin middle turbinate compressed against the lateral nasal wall on the contralateral side (Fig. 3–12B).

The presence of a concha bullosa can be confirmed by CT (Fig. 3–12B). About 30% of patients who undergo CT of this area are found to have an enlarged concha bullosa that is nevertheless normal and aerated and causes no symptoms. The concha bullosa can become problematic, however, if its drainage system becomes obstructed (Fig. 3–14A). In patients with isolated obstruction of the concha bullosa on one side, bivalving the concha and removing the lateral portion (Fig. 3–14B) provide complete relief of the complaint of pain in the medial canthal and lacrimal fossa region. In patients with ossification of the concha bullosa (Fig. 3–14A), probably due to chronic obstruction and inflammation, removal of the concha relieves symptoms of fullness, pressure, and headache on the side of the disease.

In patients who have had endonasal surgery previously, the middle turbinate and parts of the lamina papyracea or roof of the ethmoid sinus may have been removed. The patient

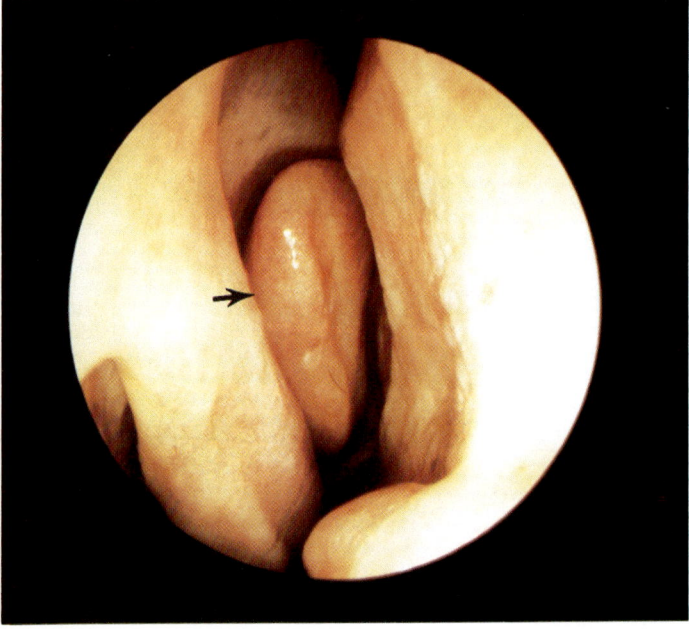

Figure 3–12. **A**: Endoscopic view of bulbous middle turbinate (concha bullosa) in right nasal cavity (arrow).

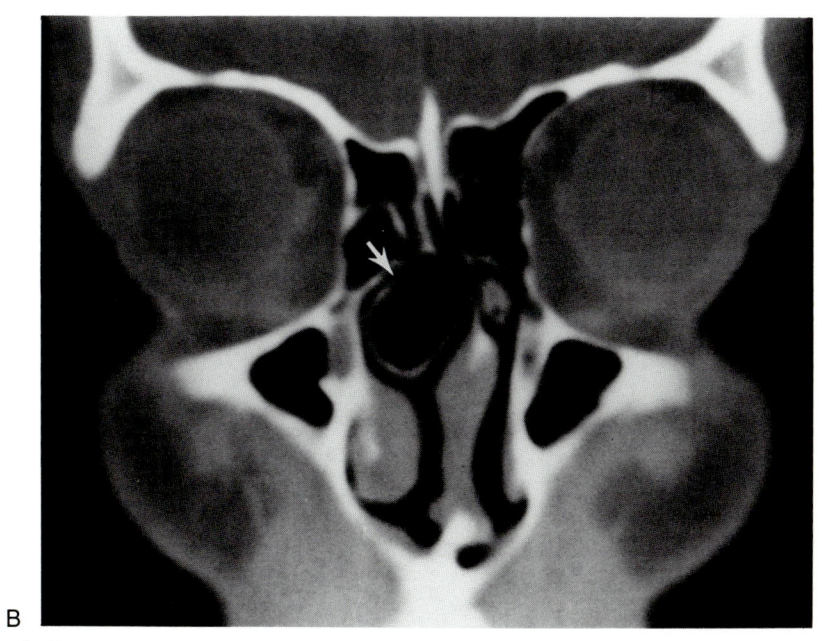

Figure 3–12. (*Continued*). **B**: CT of septum deviated to left side and paradoxical turbinate with concha bullosa on the right side (arrow).

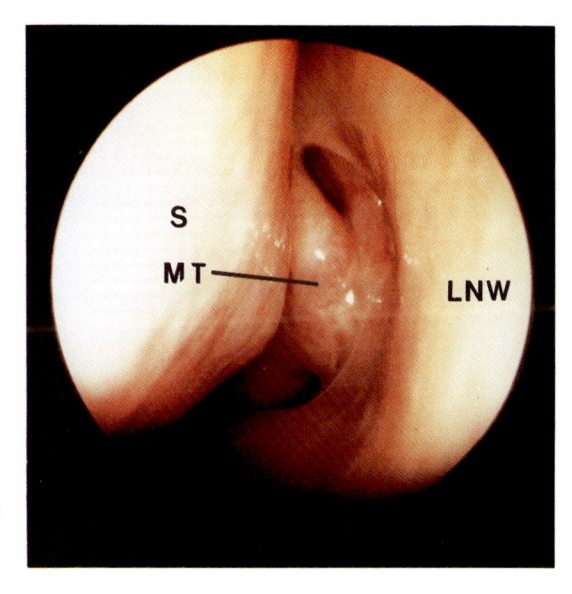

Figure 3–13. Endoscopic view of left middle turbinate (MT) adherent to lateral nasal wall (LNW) after ostiomeatal complex surgery. S: septum.

80   *Endoscopic Sinus Surgery*

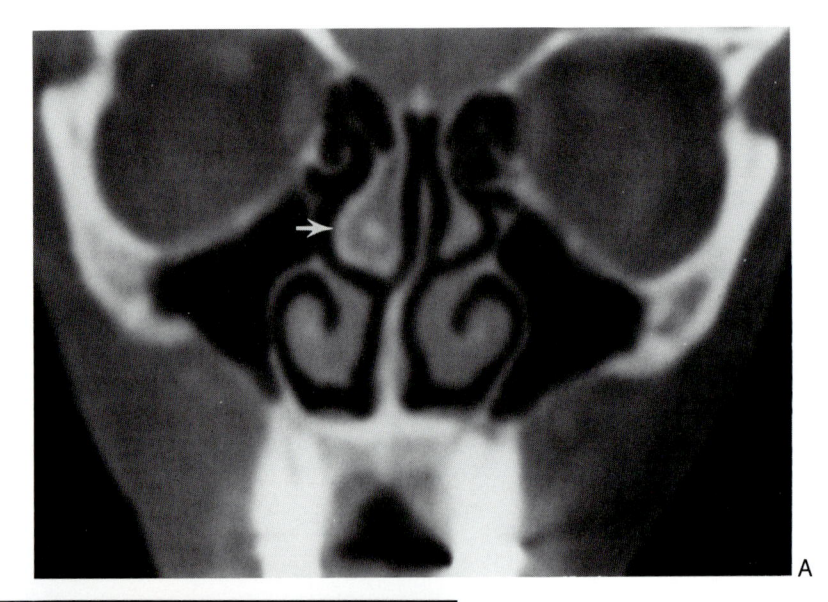

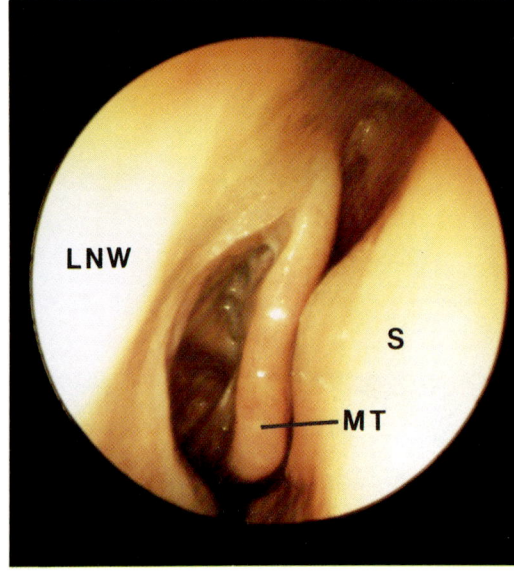

Figure 3–14. **A**: CT of obstructed, ossified, right-sided concha bullosa (arrow). **B**: Right middle turbinate (MT) healed after operative removal of lateral aspect. LNW: lateral nasal wall; S: septum.

may not know the details of the surgical procedure performed and details are often not given in operative reports, and so the removal of these structures may not be learned from a review of the patient's history. Because the absence of the middle turbinate may increase the risk of injury to the orbit or dura, it is important to assess for the presence of this landmark preoperatively.

Superior Turbinate

The surgeon should note whether a superior turbinate is present and should be careful to palpate it endoscopically to help distinguish it from a polyp or mass (Fig. 3–15). Because this turbinate attaches superiorly to the cribriform plate (Fig. 3–16A, B, and C), manipulation of the turbinate may cause the cribriform plate to crack, resulting in loss of smell and a possible cerebrospinal fluid (CSF) leak. The 4 mm 70° or the 2.7 mm 30° endoscope should be used to examine the superior turbinate and superior meatus to evaluate for posterior ethmoid and sphenoethmoid recess disease.

Lateral Nasal Wall

If the endoscope can be passed between the middle turbinate and the lateral nasal wall without discomfort to the patient, the uncinate process, hiatus semilunaris, and bulla ethmoidalis can usually be inspected. The uncinate process may be hypertrophied (Fig. 3–17), polypoid, or rotated laterally, a sign of OMC disease. Purulent material or polyps (Figs. 3–18 and 3–19) may extrude through the hiatus semilunaris, between the uncinate process

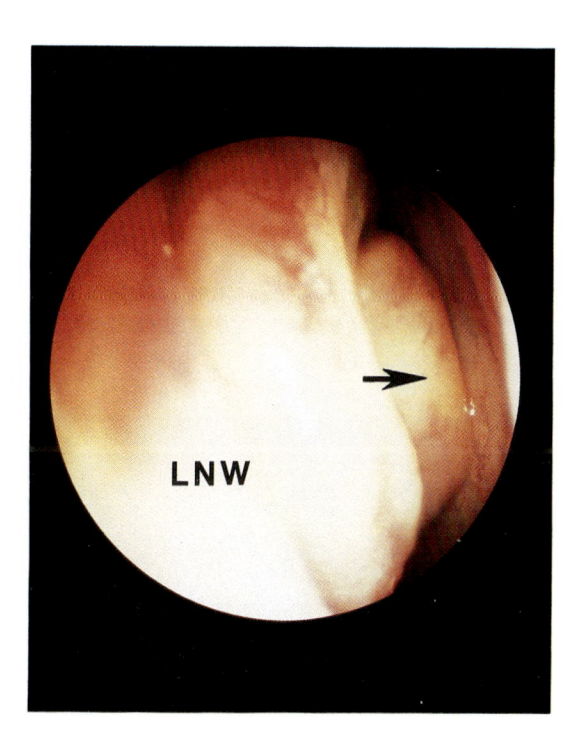

Figure 3–15. Endoscopic view of right superior turbinate (arrow). Note that turbinate may resemble a polyp or mass. LNW: lateral nasal wall.

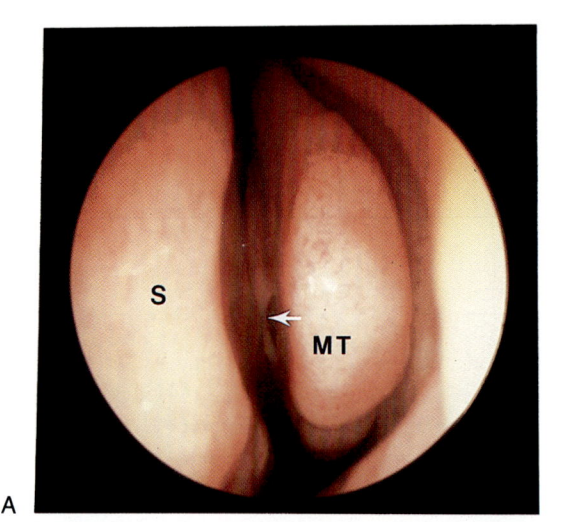

Figure 3–16. Left nasal cavity. **A**: Endoscopic view. The superior turbinate (arrow) may be seen above and behind the middle turbinate (MT). **B**: Closer endoscopic view. **C**: CT scan. Superior turbinates (arrows) are seen to attach to the cribriform plate. S: septum.

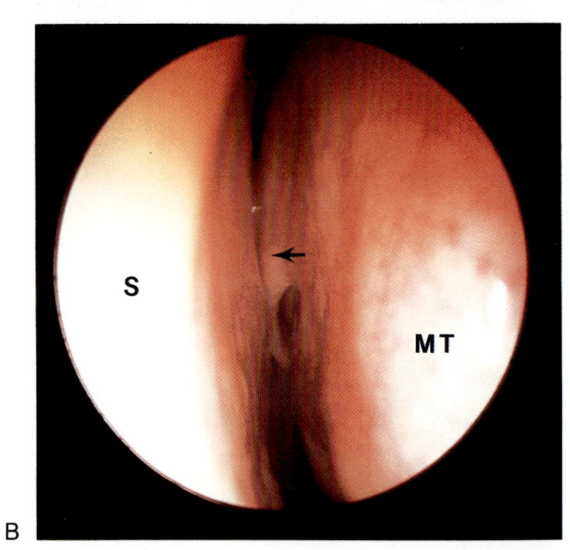

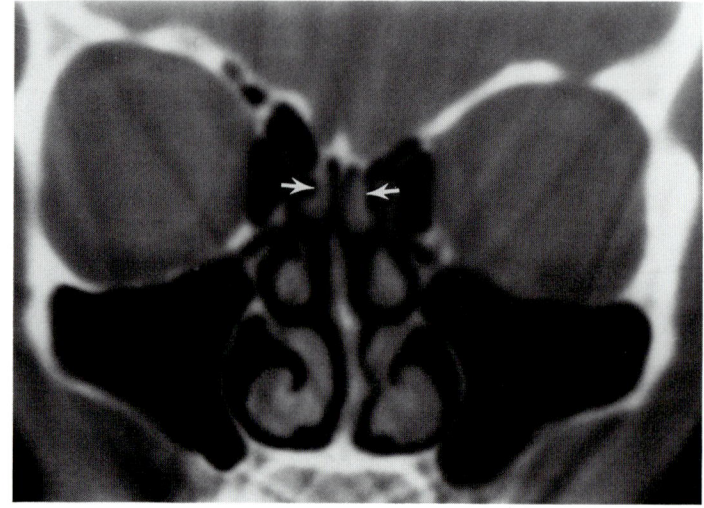

Office Evaluation of Nasosinus Disorders   83

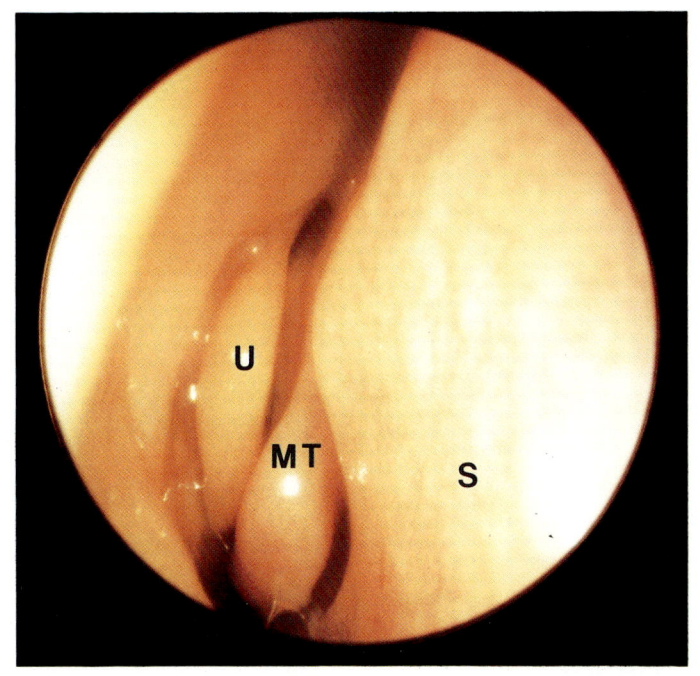

Figure 3–17.   Endoscopic view of right uncinate process (U) hypertrophy. MT: middle turbinate; S: septum.

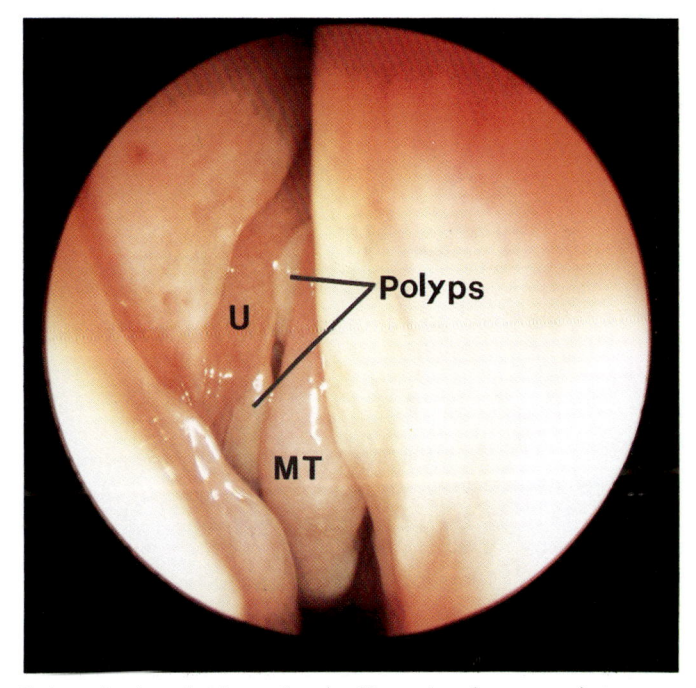

Figure 3–18.   Endoscopic view of right nasal cavity. Note polyps between uncinate process (U) and bulla ethmoidalis. MT: middle turbinate.

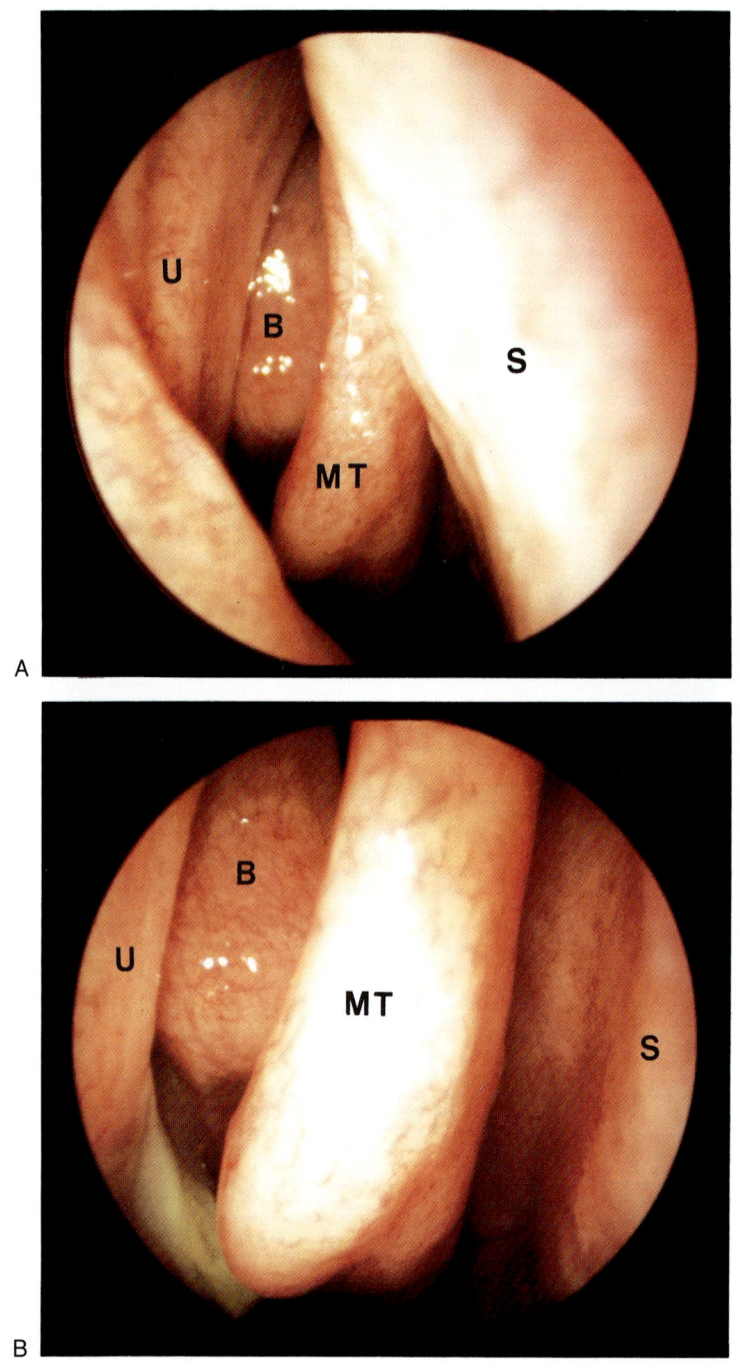

Figure 3–19. Endoscopic view of right nasal cavity. **A**: Note enlarged bulla ethmoidalis (B). **B**: Note purulent secretions between uncinate process (U) and bulla ethmoidalis. MT: middle turbinate; S: septum.

and bulla ethmoidalis. A bulla ethmoidalis that is anatomically enlarged or pathologically expanded (Fig. 3–19) is another finding associated with OMC disease.

As the endoscope is moved more posteriorly, the sphenoethmoid recess, torus tubarius, and nasopharynx can be inspected for purulent secretions (Fig. 3–20). When disease is present in the posterior ethmoid or sphenoid sinus, secretions are swept over the top of the torus tubarius. However, secretions will be found inferior to the torus tubarius if disease is present in the frontal, maxillary, and/or anterior ethmoid sinuses. Inflammation and engorgement of the torus tubarius is associated with the ear "popping," sensations of pressure in the ear, and even middle ear effusion often found in patients with acute or chronic sinusitis.

IMAGING OF THE SINUSES

Plain Sinus Roentgenography

A plain sinus roentgenographic survey is very helpful as a screening procedure for patients with acute or chronic sinusitis. When a single open-mouth (Waters) view is taken before and after surgery of the frontal and maxillary sinuses, a postoperative CT scan may not be needed to document the results of surgery.

Preoperative plain roentgenographs are also useful for making preoperative measurements. A lateral sinus view taken with the patient next to the film and the radiation source at least 36 inches away will give an undistorted, almost one-to-one, reproduction of the key structures that will be involved in endonasal sinus surgery.[4] The distance and angles from the nasal spine to the middle of the roof of the ethmoid sinus, ethmoid-sphenoid sinus junction, and anterior face of the sphenoid sinus can be measured with great accuracy (Figs. 3–21 through 3–23). These angles or measurements become critical during endonasal sinus surgery, and they will be described in greater detail in Chapter 5.

Although useful to make preoperative measurements, plain roentgenographs do not replace CT scans of the paranasal sinuses, because only a CT scan can provide the physician with an adequate view of the fine details of the paranasal sinuses required for diagnosis and planning surgery in this area.

Computed Tomography

Any patient with a nasosinus complaint whose symptoms are not responding to medical therapy, in whom the diagnosis is in question, or who is being considered for surgery should undergo CT in the coronal plane. When these CT scans show sphenoid sinus disease, the patient should undergo CT in the axial plane as well.

Details of CT scanning of the sinuses are given in Chapter 2. The system used to classify the CT findings is shown in the Endoscopic Sinus Surgery Protocol (page 261). This classification system is helpful in planning surgery.

The routine use of CT scans to plan surgery has changed some traditional procedures. For example, in the classic (nonendoscopic) endonasal approach to surgery on the sinuses, the ethmoid-sphenoid complex traditionally is marsupialized.[5] However, the results of CT

86 Endoscopic Sinus Surgery

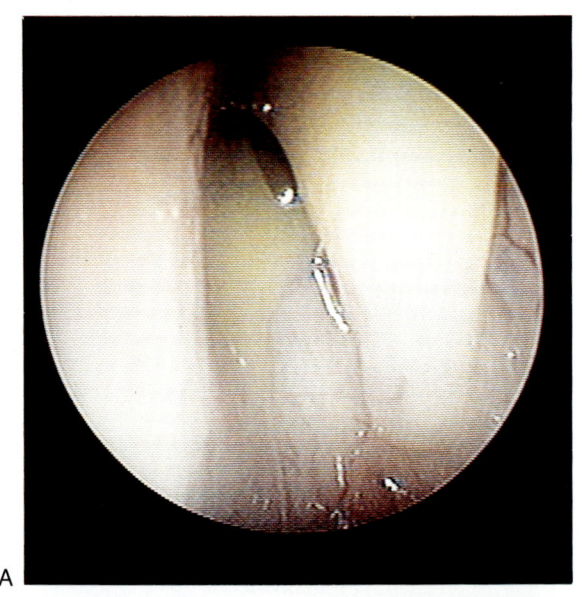

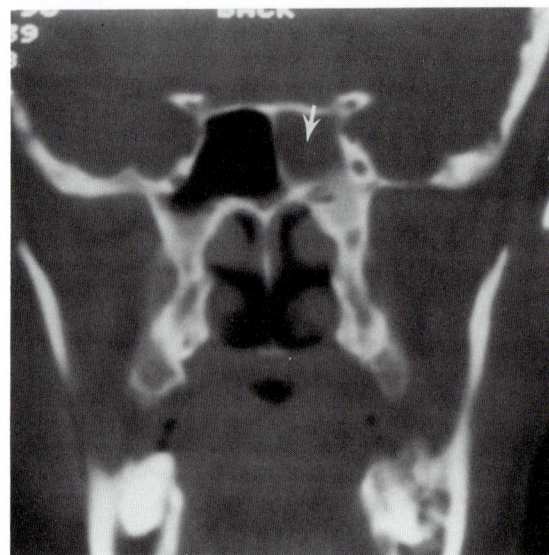

Figure 3-20. View of left sphenoethmoid recess through 70° endoscope. **A**: Purulent secretions in recess are associated with left-sided sphenoiditis. **B**: Diagnosis was confirmed by CT scan (arrow).

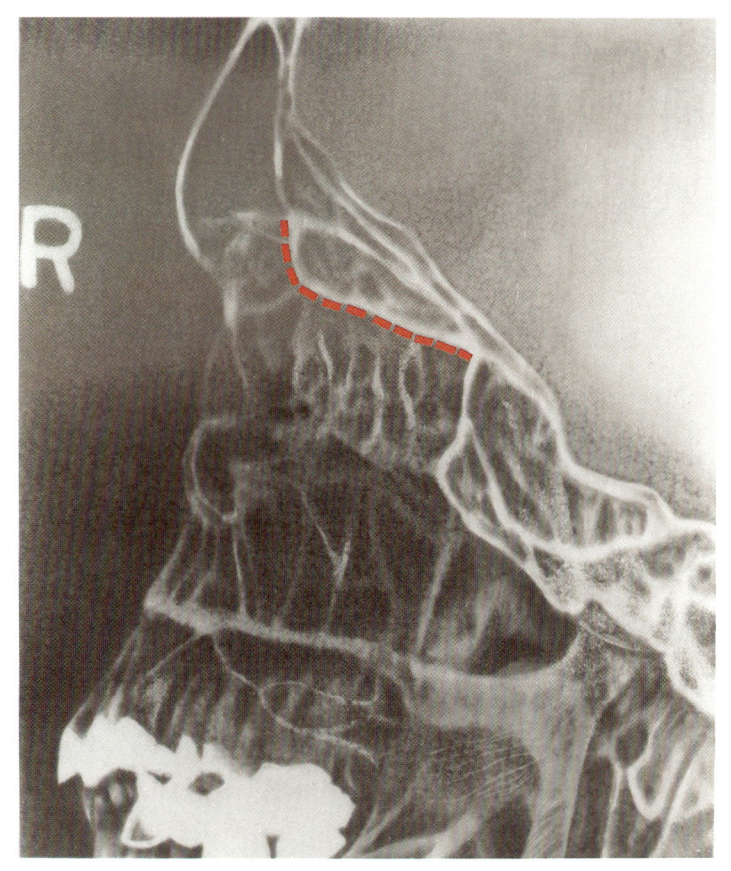

Figure 3–21. Lateral radiograph of the paranasal sinuses. The most inferior line connecting the posterior wall of the frontal sinus and the roof of the sphenoid sinus is selected to represent the roof of the ethmoid sinus (red).

show that the sphenoid and frontal sinuses are normal in two thirds of patients (Table 3–6). Thus, surgery in the region of the sphenoid and frontal sinuses is not always required.

CT is helpful in diagnosing anatomic abnormalities, not shown on plain sinus roentgenographs, that have obstructed the OMC. The decision to treat such a condition surgically is never based on the results of CT alone, but must be correlated with the patient's symptoms and endoscopic findings.

Finally, the results of CT scanning often aid the physician in diagnosing unusual causes of sinus symptoms. Such an example is the radiodense area within an opacity of the maxillary sinus in Figure 3–3, which is suggestive of fungal sinusitis.

CASE SELECTION FOR SURGERY

Informing the Patient

On completion of the evaluation, the findings from the history, endoscopic examination, and radiologic examinations are reviewed with the patient. When the patient's nasosinus

88 *Endoscopic Sinus Surgery*

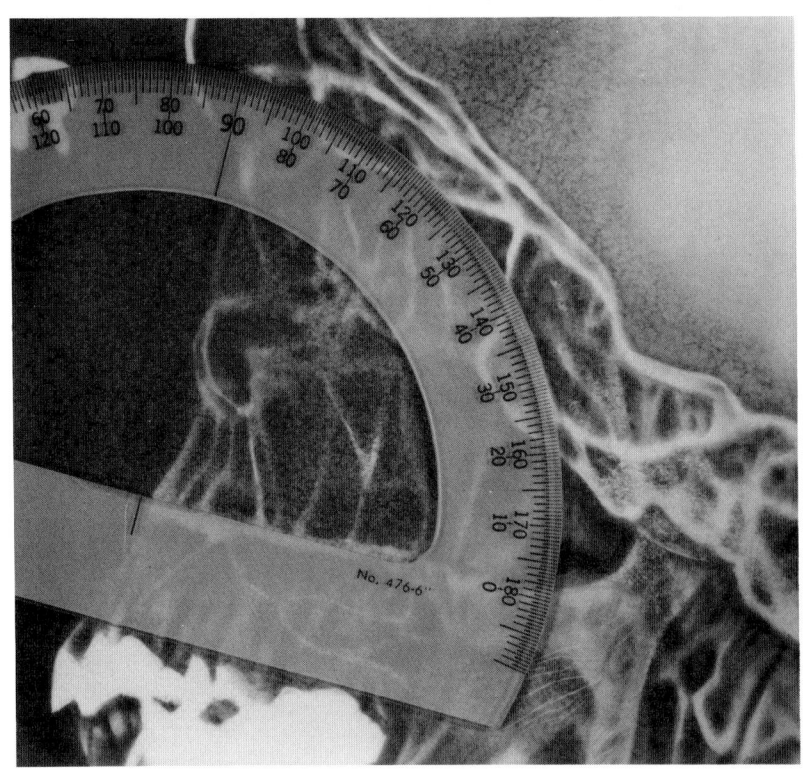

Figure 3–22.   A protractor is used to measure angles and distances from the nasal spine to key surgical areas.

Office Evaluation of Nasosinus Disorders   89

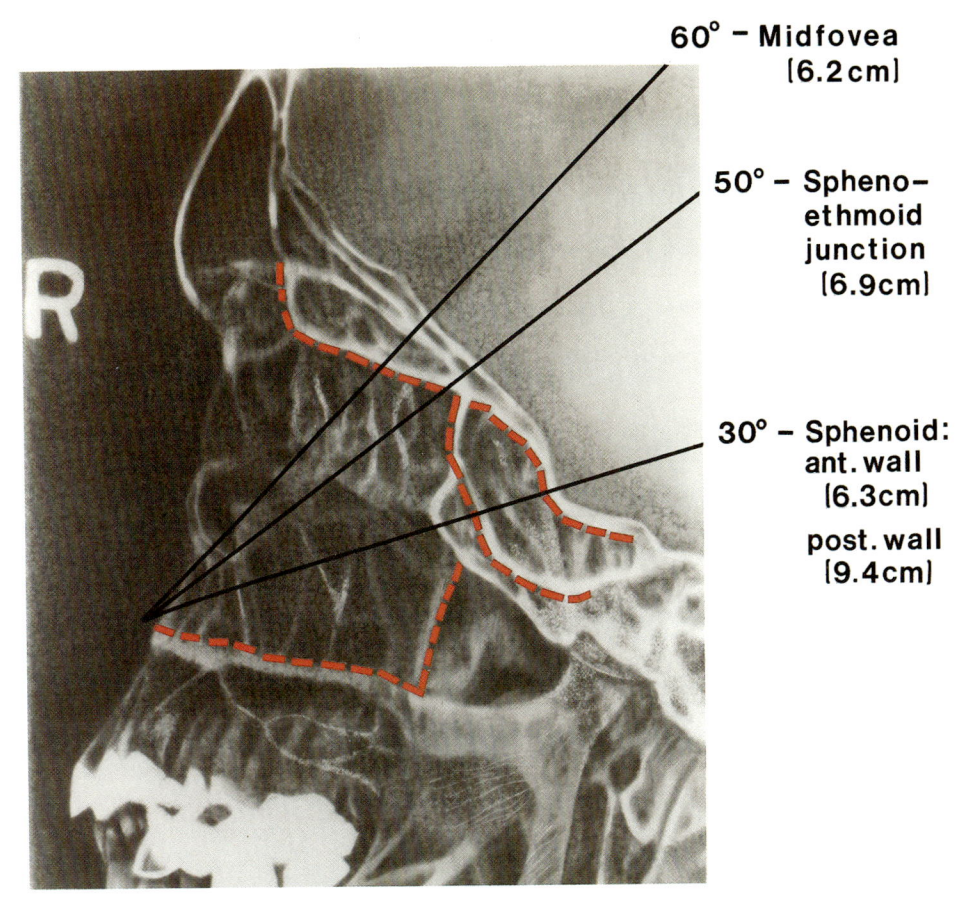

60° – Midfovea
(6.2 cm)

50° – Spheno-ethmoid junction
(6.9 cm)

30° – Sphenoid:
ant. wall
(6.3 cm)
post. wall
(9.4 cm)

Figure 3–23. The averages of values for three important surgical angles and four distances on the skull.

Table 3–6 Abnormal CT Findings in 184 Patients Evaluated Consecutively for Nasosinus Symptoms

SINUS CAVITY EXAMINED	PATIENTS WITH ABNORMAL FINDINGS (%)
Anterior ethmoid	88
Maxillary	82
Posterior ethmoid	73
Sphenoid	33
Frontal	31

condition has not responded well to appropriately administered medical therapy and the patient's symptoms are severe enough that he or she would consider surgery, a detailed explanation is provided of the surgical procedure and risks. It is emphasized that the surgery treats a condition that is generally not life-threatening, although it interferes with the patient's quality of life, and the potential complications of surgery can be life-threatening. These complications include bleeding; infection; sensory changes in the teeth, lip, or cheek; visual loss; CSF leak; and the possibility that additional surgery may be required (see Chapter 7).

Surgical Experience and Informed Consent

The weight given to each of the potential complications of surgery that are discussed with each patient depends on the type of surgery recommended for that patient.

SUMMARY

Arriving at an accurate diagnosis and making appropriate recommendations for treating nasosinus disorders require thorough history taking, endoscopic examination, and review of CT scans of the paranasal sinuses.

The history is the single most important factor in selecting which patients might be candidates for endoscopic sinus surgery. Surgery is reserved for patients whose symptoms of nasosinus disease persist despite appropriate medical management. Surgery is not considered, however, unless there are also abnormalities on endoscopic examination or on CT scans of the paranasal sinuses. In addition, patients' symptoms must interfere with their quality of life sufficiently to justify their informed consent to procedures that have the potential of life-threatening complications.

REFERENCES

1. Wasuesapack RW: Miscellania Medica, Committee on Medical Devices and Drugs. Bull Am Academy Otolaryngol Head Neck Surg 8:11, 1989.
2. Levine HL: The office diagnosis of nasal and sinus disorders using rigid nasal endoscopy. Otolaryngol Head Neck Surg 102:370–373, 1990.
3. Levine HL: The potassium-titanyl phosphate laser for treatment of turbinate dysfunction. Otolaryngol Head Neck Surg 104:247–251, 1991.
4. May M, Mester SJ, O'Daniel TG, Curtin HD: Decreasing the risks of endonasal endoscopic nasal surgery by imaging techniques. Op Tech Otolaryngol Head Neck Surg 1:89–91, 1990.
5. Friedman WH, Katsantonis GP, Rosenblum BN, et al: Sphenoethmoidectomy: A case for ethmoid marsupialization. Laryngoscope 90:473–479, 1983.

4
Anesthesia for Endoscopic Sinus Surgery

SAWSAN ALHADDAD, M.D.

Managing anesthesia for endoscopic sinus surgery (ESS) is a particular challenge for the anesthesiologist because the airway is "shared" with the surgeon and because patients undergoing this type of surgery may have a wide spectrum of medical problems. This chapter discusses preoperative anesthesia evaluation for ESS, and reviews patient monitoring, medications, techniques, and complications of local anesthesia and general anesthesia. Management strategies for patients with reactive airway disease are presented, as are criteria for hospital discharge.

EVALUATION AND PREPARATION FOR ANESTHESIA

Although most patients who undergo ESS are young to middle-aged adults, our patients ranged in age between 3 and 80 years. The most frequently seen medical problems in patients undergoing sinus surgery are asthma (present in 40 to 50%)[1] and multiple allergies (present in 30%)[2]; approximately 80% of patients with multiple polyps and asthma also have aspirin sensitivity.[3,4]

Anesthesia Evaluation

The preoperative anesthesia evaluation helps determine whether the patient will be scheduled to have ESS performed on an outpatient basis (patient is discharged the day of surgery) or will stay in the hospital the night after surgery.

A thorough preanesthesia history includes a history of the patient's past medical problems and surgical procedures and a history of anesthesia-related problems in the patient or family. Any medications the patient is taking and any drug allergies are noted.

Laboratory Tests

Few laboratory tests are needed to evaluate the anesthesia status of healthy, asymptomatic patients.[5] Preanesthesia laboratory tests ordered routinely at the Cleveland Clinic include complete blood count and levels of serum electrolytes, blood urea nitrogen, creatinine, glucose, bilirubin, transaminase, and lactate dehydrogenase. An electrocardiogram (ECG) tracing is obtained if the patient is older than 40 years or has a history of cardiac disease. A chest x-ray is obtained if the patient has a history of pulmonary disease.

Patients with asthma may need to undergo additional testing to ensure optimal outcome of anesthesia and surgery. Baseline spirometry with and without bronchodilators and an evaluation by an internist or pulmonologist are preferred for these patients. If a patient is actively wheezing before surgery, surgery is postponed until this is controlled.[6] Similarly, patients with hypertension are treated until their blood pressure is stabilized in a normal range before surgery.

Preoperative Medications

Bronchodilating medications (such as beta-adrenergic stimulants and theophylline) are continued for all asthmatic patients until the day of surgery. Other medications, such as antiarrhythmics and antihypertensives, are given with a sip of water on the morning of surgery.

Patients are usually given medications preoperatively to decrease anxiety (thus decreasing the doses of anesthetic and analgesic medications necessary during the procedure). They may also be given medications to reduce oral and respiratory secretions or to alter gastric secretory function to decrease the risk of aspiration pneumonitis.

Anxiolytic Medications

Because many patients who undergo endoscopic sinus surgery are sent home the same day, it is important to use the minimal amount of medication possible and to choose drugs that have short half-lives. The need for medication is minimized by allaying patients' fears regarding the procedure. Discussing thoroughly with the patient the anesthesia that will be administered and the expected course of events during administration and recovery from anesthesia is very helpful in this regard.

Because barbiturates and diazepam have long half-lives, these medications are avoided for sinus surgery patients. Midazolam and fentanyl have been shown not to delay recovery,[7–9] and at the Cleveland Clinic small doses of these medications (midazolam 2 to 3 mg intramuscularly [IM] or 1 to 2 mg intravenously [IV]; fentanyl 50 to 100 µg IV) have been used with success. Patients given larger doses of midazolam (0.07 mg/kg) may take longer to awaken after short surgical procedures than those given morphine (0.08 mg/kg).

Anticholinergic Medications

If an anticholinergic medication is required to reduce secretions, glycopyrrolate (0.2 mg IV) is used.

Prophylaxis for Aspiration Pneumonitis

The problem of pneumonitis resulting from aspiration during anesthesia of highly acidic (pH less than 2.5) gastric contents has been studied.[10,11] Patients who undergo surgery on an outpatient basis may be at increased risk of aspiration,[11] and prophylaxis has been recommended.[12,13]

Anxiety promotes increased secretion (more than 25 ml) of gastric juices, which contributes to the risk of aspiration. In addition to preoperative teaching and pharmacologic anxiolysis to reduce anxiety, prophylaxis is often given specifically to reduce gastric volume and to increase the pH of gastric secretions. To inhibit gastric secretions and reduce gastric volume, patients may be given metoclopramide (10 mg IV)[13] or an H_2-receptor-blocking agent such as ranitidine (150 mg orally [PO] the night before surgery and 50 mg IV the morning of surgery). To increase the pH of gastric secretions, patients may be given a nonparticulate antacid such as sodium citrate with citric acid (Bicitra, 30 ml PO).[13]

Preparations in the Operating Room

Contrary to arrangements for other types of head and neck surgery, for ESS the surgeon sits or stands at the side of the patient's head. To accommodate this arrangement, the patient is positioned with his or her feet at the head of the operating room table, and this means that during induction of anesthesia the anesthesiologist is not near the controls for tilting the table. To ensure that the position of the table can be changed rapidly during this time, for example if the patient vomits, the anesthesiologist may either instruct a nurse to stand at the controls and to be prepared to change the position of the operating room table on command from the anesthesiologist or use a remote control device, if this is available.

For ESS, the patient is positioned supine on the operating room table with a small roll under the shoulders and the head extended on a small circular pillow. Minimal monitoring apparatus to be placed on the patient includes ECG leads, a blood pressure cuff, a precordial stethoscope, a skin temperature probe, a pulse oximeter probe, and an analyzer to detect concentration of oxygen in inspired air.

After induction of anesthesia, the anesthesia machine is placed at the side of the operating room table next to the anesthesiologist.

LOCAL ANESTHESIA WITH SEDATION

At the Cleveland Clinic, we use local anesthesia with sedation, called monitored anesthesia care (MAC), for the majority of patients requiring ESS. MAC has two major advantages for the surgeon: (1) the possibility of earlier hospital discharge, and (2) a wider margin of safety in that patients receiving MAC will feel pain when the lamina papyracea, roof of the ethmoid sinus, or face of the sphenoid is palpated during surgery.[14]

MAC has disadvantages for the surgeon, however. These include: (1) increased risk, with increasing levels of sedation, that the patient will aspirate blood and secretions; (2) patient discomfort during surgery, even when the patient has been sedated and given adequate analgesia; and (3) the possibility that a patient with asthma will have severe bronchospasm, possibly due to anxiety or aspiration of blood or secretions.

Patient Oxygenation During Monitored Anesthesia Care

For patients undergoing MAC, nasal prongs are taped to direct supplemental oxygen into the patient's mouth, and oxygen is begun at 3 to 5 L/min to help maintain oxygen saturation of hemoglobin at safe levels. Patients usually tolerate this supplemental oxygen well, even though it causes mouth dryness. Even with supplemental oxygen, however, hypoventilation may occur due to the respiratory depressant effect of anesthesia medications. If oxygen saturation drops to below 90%, the patient is asked to take an occasional deep breath to improve ventilation.

Medications for Monitored Anesthesia Care

Doses of sedatives, narcotics, and antiemetics are titrated throughout MAC.

Sedation with Midazolam

An advantage of using midazolam for sedation is that it has an amnesic effect. In addition, this drug is especially well-suited for short procedures and same-day surgery because it has a short plasma half-life.[8,15]

Midazolam should be administered in titrated doses of 0.5 to 1.0 mg to provide a level of sedation that permits the patient to respond to verbal commands. Side effects of this drug include respiratory depression and apnea. In addition, depression of cardiovascular function has been reported in severely compromised patients and patients with sepsis given midazolam.

Patients who are oversedated with midazolam may become agitated and uncooperative, perhaps secondary to hypoxia or as a paradoxical reaction to the medication. Titration of midazolam to avoid oversedation is particularly important for patients undergoing ESS because narcotic drugs are used to provide pain relief during these procedures and potentiation of respiratory-depressant effects could lead to respiratory difficulties.

Narcotics

Fentanyl and alfentanil have been found useful for MAC during ESS procedures. *Fentanyl* is administered in 25- to 50-µg doses IV as needed during the course of the procedure. A total of 2 to 6 cc (100 to 300 µg) may be needed for the average hour-long procedure. Fentanyl is rapidly redistributed and eliminated, and, when administered in small doses throughout the procedure, the drug should not cause delayed respiratory depression. The most commonly seen side effects of fentanyl are nausea and vomiting, respiratory depression, and bradycardia.

Alfentanil is a very short-acting synthetic opioid. To provide a smooth, constant level of analgesia for ESS with MAC, a loading dose of 7.5 to 10 µg/kg is given IV, followed by a continuous infusion of 0.5 to 1.5 µg/kg/min.

Antiemetics

Administering a narcotic medication increases the risk that the patient will experience nausea and vomiting, which are the most common reasons for unplanned admissions of same-day surgery patients.[16] To decrease the possibility of this side effect of narcotics without greatly potentiating the sedative effect of other medications used during ESS, small doses of an antiemetic, such as droperidol (10 to 15 μg/kg IV), may be given.[9] A combination of metoclopramide (10 mg IV) and droperidol (10 to 20 μg/kg IV) has also been found effective for general anesthesia as well as MAC.[17]

Paradoxical reactions to droperidol have been reported in which the patient seems outwardly calm but expresses feelings of anxiety and panic.

Local Medications

The endoscopic sinus surgeon administers local anesthetic and vasoconstrictor medications (see Chapter 5), usually a combination of 1 or 2% lidocaine, 1/100,000 to 1/200,000 epinephrine, and 4% cocaine or oxymetazoline spray. Administering a vasoconstrictor medication with the local anesthetics reduces blood loss, improves visualization of structures in the operative field, and slows absorption of the local anesthetic so that anesthesia effects are prolonged and drug toxicity is reduced. Vasoconstriction is also helpful during general anesthesia.

Lidocaine

Lidocaine belongs to the amide group of local anesthetics and is often used for patients undergoing procedures involving the upper airway. The maximal safe dose of lidocaine is 4 mg/kg when this drug is used alone or 7 mg/kg when lidocaine is used in combination with epinephrine.[18]

Lidocaine toxicity is unlikely to occur at the concentrations (0.5 to 1%) and in the amounts used to provide local anesthesia for nasal surgery, unless the medication is accidentally injected into the bloodstream. Signs of lidocaine toxicity relate to the central nervous system and include tinnitus, lightheadedness, changes in vision and hearing, confusion, restlessness, slurred speech, and tremors. Greater degrees of toxicity are signaled by convulsions and seizures, and by depression of central nervous system function.[18]

Epinephrine

Epinephrine, a catecholamine with alpha and beta adrenergic effects, causes local vasoconstriction in concentrations between 1/200,000 and 1/100,000 (5 to 10 μg/ml). In addition, adding epinephrine to the lidocaine solution increases the allowable dose of lidocaine.

The greatest risk associated with using epinephrine for local anesthesia during ESS is accidental intravascular injection. The onset of symptoms is very rapid (within seconds after the injection) and includes palpitations, tachycardia, and hypertension. This response to intravascular injection of epinephrine is usually short-lived, but it can be dangerous in a patient with preexisting hypertension or coronary artery disease and if it persists should be treated with vasodilating and beta-adrenergic receptor-blocking medications (nitroglycerin, hydralazine, labetalol, or propranolol).

Phenylephrine may be used instead of epinephrine; it may be administered by adding it to the local anesthetic to reach a final concentration of 0.005% phenylephrine.[19] This drug is, however, an alpha-adrenergic receptor stimulant and so can cause severe hypertension with reflex bradycardia.

Cocaine

Cocaine, an ester local anesthetic and sympathomimetic, has been used for otolaryngologic surgery[20] mostly for its vasoconstrictive effects rather than for local anesthesia. The drug inhibits reuptake of catecholamines (endogenous or exogenous) into nerve endings, thus prolonging and potentiating endogenous and exogenous catecholamine activity both locally and systemically. Because of this mode of action, epinephrine should not be admixed with cocaine to delay the absorption of cocaine[21]; rather, cocaine should be applied topically before a solution of epinephrine and lidocaine is injected.[20]

The maximal allowable dose of cocaine is 4 mg/kg. This may be applied by soaking cotton pledgets with a 4% solution of the drug and leaving the pledgets in the nasal cavity, in contact with the mucosa, for 5 minutes. Alternatively, cocaine spray may be applied; because all of the spray is available for absorption by the nasal mucosa, whereas cotton pledgets will retain some of the solution, more cocaine will be absorbed when applied by spray than when the same volume of solution is applied on cotton pledgets.

Toxic effects of cocaine include nervousness, headache, tachycardia, hypertension, and restlessness. Hyperpyrexia may also occur with toxic doses of cocaine.

Complications During Monitored Anesthesia Care

Problems that may occur during MAC include changes in level of consciousness, respiratory depression, aspiration, hypertension, and bronchial spasm.

Restlessness and Confusion

Changes in level of consciousness during local anesthesia with sedation may be caused by local anesthetic toxicity, hypoxia, or an idiosyncratic response to medications. The patient who experiences toxicity to the local anesthetic should be given supportive care and supplemental oxygen, be monitored for oxygen levels, and be provided sedative medication, such as diazepam, to decrease the possibility of seizures. More severe toxicity may require administration of a muscle-paralyzing agent and intubation.[18]

Patients who do not have asthma may be given vasodilators and beta-adrenergic receptor blockers to manage the cardiac effects of cocaine or epinephrine toxicity.

Oversedation

Respiratory depression due to oversedation is best avoided by careful titration of sedative and narcotic medications. If oversedation does occur, it can often be managed by giving the patient supplemental oxygen and encouraging him or her to take deep breaths. If necessary, naloxone may be given IV in 40-µg boluses titrated to reverse the effects of narcotic medications; the effects of medications such as diazepam and midazolam may be reversed by physostigmine, 1 to 2 mg IV.

Aspiration

Oversedation may lead the patient to aspirate blood or secretions.

Hypertension

Hypertension may occur in patients operated on under MAC as a result of systemic absorption of epinephrine or cocaine or the accidental injection into the bloodstream of epinephrine-containing solutions. Hypertension may also result from hypoxia and hypercapnia due to respiratory depression. This condition should be managed early because it can lead to increased bleeding in the operative field, which makes endoscopic surgery very difficult, if not impossible, to perform.

The first step in managing hypertension is to determine its cause. If hypoxia or hypercapnia is present, this should be treated. If hypertension persists or is present in the absence of hypoxia or hypercapnia, it may be managed by administration of: (1) a vasodilator such as nitroglycerin (80-μg boluses IV) or hydralazine (2.5- to 5.0-mg boluses IV); (2) a calcium-channel blocking medication such as nifedipine (10 mg sublingually); or (3) a beta-adrenergic receptor-blocking medication such as propranolol or labetalol.

Bronchial Spasm

A severe asthmatic attack can occur during MAC in a patient whose asthma was previously well controlled. In some cases bronchial spasm may be triggered by patient anxiety; in other cases the attack may be related to drug-mediated release of histamine, although none of the medications described for MAC has appreciable histaminic effects. It is also possible that bronchial spasm occurs in response to mechanical stimulation of the airways secondary to aspiration of small amounts of blood in the pharynx.

Should the patient have a bronchial spasm during ESS with MAC, the procedure must be terminated immediately.

GENERAL ANESTHESIA

An "ideal general anesthetic" for ESS would, (1) not constrict the airway, (2) provide analgesia, amnesia, and suppression of reflex movement to noxious stimuli, (3) not affect blood pressure, (4) not interact with catecholamines or cocaine, (5) clear from the body rapidly to allow rapid emergence from anesthesia and return of reflexes, and (6) prevent bronchial smooth muscle spasm in asthmatic patients. Because no single medication is known that has all of the characteristics of an ideal general anesthetic, a combination of drugs is used during induction, maintenance, and reversal of general anesthesia in patients undergoing ESS.

Regardless of the types of medications given, all patients who undergo general anesthesia have at a minimum the level of monitoring described for those operated on under MAC. In addition, end tidal carbon dioxide is monitored by a capnograph or mass spectrometer, and breath sounds and temperature are monitored with an esophageal stethoscope.

A neuromuscular stimulator is used to monitor neuromuscular function when muscle relaxants are used.

Induction of Anesthesia

Anesthesia may be induced with inhalation agents or intravenous medications.

Inhalation Induction

Inhalation agents are usually used to induce anesthesia in children. Halothane is the most commonly used drug because it is the least irritating and thus best tolerated of the volatile agents. Halothane is, however, associated with increased risk of ventricular arrhythmias when cocaine and epinephrine are used,[22] so halothane may be discontinued after intubation.

Intravenous Induction

Intravenous agents, most often thiopental sodium (Pentothal) (3 to 5 mg/kg), are usually used to induce anesthesia in adults. Thiopental sodium may be used even when the patient has asthma if deep anesthesia is assured before instruments are inserted into the airway.[23]

Ketamine may be given in doses of 1 to 2 mg/kg as an alternative to thiopental sodium for induction of anesthesia. This sympathomimetic agent may help protect patients with asthma from bronchospasm.[23] When given to patients also receiving aminophylline, however, ketamine has been reported to cause lowering of the seizure threshold.[24] In addition, ketamine may potentiate the effects of topically applied cocaine and epinephrine, a drawback to its use in ESS.

Maintenance of Anesthesia

After general anesthesia has been induced, patients are given a muscle relaxant for intubation and anesthesia is maintained by an inhalation agent, alone or in combination with a muscle relaxant.

Muscle Relaxants

A muscle relaxant is given IV to facilitate intubation. For patients without asthma, succinylcholine (1 to 1.5 mg/kg), atracurium (0.5 mg/kg), or vecuronium (0.1 mg/kg) may be used.[25]

Because patients with asthma are at particular risk of bronchospasm during intubation and atracurium is known to cause histamine release at doses above 0.6 mg/kg, patients with asthma should be given succinylcholine or vecuronium or a reduced or divided dose of atracurium for muscle relaxation. In addition, the following steps should be taken to reduce airway reflex responses during insertion of the endotracheal tube in a patient with asthma: (1) achieve a deep level of anesthesia with an inhalation agent, (2) administer lidocaine (1 to 1.5 mg/kg IV) 1 to 2 minutes before intubation, and (3) block the response to intubation by administering a narcotic medication (fentanyl or, if the procedure is very short, alfentanil).

Inhalation Agents

An inhalation agent is usually used to maintain anesthesia. Agents that have been used include halothane, isoflurane, enflurane, and nitrous oxide. Halothane may not be the agent of first choice for ESS procedures, however.

All inhalation agents sensitize the myocardium to the effects of endogenous or exogenous catecholamines,[19,22] but halothane is the worst offender. Because of these potentiating effects, when halothane is used the maximal allowable dose of epinephrine with lidocaine is 1.5 μg/kg. In contrast, when isoflurane is used the maximal dose is 5 μg/kg and when enflurane is used the maximal allowable dose is 6 to 7 μg/kg.

Halothane also may not be the inhalation agent of choice for patients with asthma. Inhalation agents have been found equally effective in dilating bronchial smooth muscle,[26] and so halothane offers no advantage in this regard. In addition, using halothane for maintenance anesthesia in patients with asthma may be disadvantageous because administering halothane with sympathomimetic bronchodilators such as theophylline and epinephrine increases the risk of arrhythmias.[6,27]

Narcotic Anesthesia

Maintaining anesthesia with an inhalation agent alone results in prolongation of the emergence phase of anesthesia because to prevent the patient from moving he or she must be kept deeply anesthetized until the end of the operation. Addition of a muscle relaxant to the anesthetic regimen allows for a lighter level of anesthesia, but also increases blood pressure, which may increase bleeding from the operative site. To meet the need for lighter levels of anesthesia without elevating blood pressure, a technique using inhalation anesthesia and a narcotic medication was developed. At the Cleveland Clinic alfentanil is used for this "balanced anesthesia technique" because alfentanil has a very short (1.5 hours) half-life and small volume of distribution.[28,29]

The most practical way to administer alfentanil is with a Harvard infuser pump (such as the Bard 900 Mini-infuser, Bard Medsystems Division, Murray Hill, NJ). The narcotic may be infused continuously, which provides a more even level of anesthesia with a smaller total amount of drug, or by intermittent boluses.

Initiating Narcotic Anesthesia

Alfentanil is begun before induction of anesthesia with a loading dose of 20 to 30 μg/kg ideal body weight. This dosage is administered in divided doses over 5 minutes to allow for observation of the patient's response to this medication.

When a loading dose of alfentanil has been given, a smaller dose of thiopental sodium is given for induction of anesthesia.

Maintaining Anesthesia with Narcotics

Nitrous oxide is given for maintenance anesthesia with alfentanil.

After the patient has been intubated, if alfentanil will be given by *continuous infusion* the maintenance phase is begun at 0.25 to 1.5 μg/kg/min. The rate of infusion of alfentanil can be varied, according to the patient's heart rate, blood pressure, and other measures, to maintain anesthesia at the desired level; boluses (5 to 7.5 μg/kg) of alfentanil, very low levels of other inhalation agents, and a small dose of midazolam may also be given as needed. The alfentanil infusion should be discontinued 15 minutes before the anticipated end of the procedure.

When alfentanil will be given by *intermittent bolus* during the maintenance phase of anesthesia, doses of 5 to 10 μg/kg each are administered as needed to maintain anesthesia. The last bolus should be given not later than 15 to 20 minutes before the end of the procedure.

Side Effects and Advantages of Narcotic Anesthesia

Use of narcotic medications for anesthesia is associated with a high (45%) incidence of nausea and vomiting. Administering droperidol (20 μg/kg IV) and metoclopramide (10 mg IV) at the beginning of the procedure has been found to reduce the incidence of this adverse effect without unduly prolonging the patient's recovery from anesthesia.[29,30]

The narcotic anesthesia technique provides many advantages for ESS: (1) Analgesic effects of narcotic medications administered intraoperatively extend into the postoperative period; (2) the narcotic medication blunts changes in blood pressure that may occur with intubation, may decrease the hypertensive response to administration of epinephrine and cocaine, and may reduce blood loss; (3) patients emerge rapidly from narcotic anesthesia and experience return of reflexes by the end of the procedure; and (4) narcotic medications do not increase, and may decrease, airway responsiveness to mechanical stimulation.

Complications of General Anesthesia

Complications that may occur in patients given general anesthesia for ESS include: (1) catecholamine/inhalation anesthetic interaction; (2) hypertension and possible bleeding secondary to systemic effects of cocaine and epinephrine; (3) bronchospasm, and (4) nausea and vomiting.

Emergence from Anesthesia

At the end of an ESS procedure with general anesthesia, a medication is given to reverse the effects of muscle relaxant agents and the patient's airway is suctioned thoroughly to remove blood and secretions that have drained posteriorly from the nose. Neuromuscular function is monitored by observing how the patient responds when asked to lift the head or by using a neuromuscular stimulator. When the patient can cough and swallow and respond appropriately to verbal commands, the airway is considered secure enough for the endotracheal tube to be removed.

It has been recommended that, to avoid bronchospasm, patients who have asthma be extubated under deep anesthesia after spontaneous ventilatory function has returned. However, the blood that is present in the upper airway immediately after ESS poses the risk of airway obstruction or laryngospasm. Most patients with asthma are therefore extubated after their airway reflexes have returned. Occasionally, a patient will be considered at high risk for bronchospasm with awake extubation, and deep anesthesia will be induced for extubation of these patients. Before this is performed, any secretions present in the pharynx should be suctioned cautiously.

Patients who have undergone ESS should keep the head elevated 12 hours after surgery to decrease postoperative bleeding.

THE ASTHMATIC PATIENT

Mention has been made in this chapter of ways in which anesthesia management during ESS may need to be modified for patients with asthma. Kingston and Hirshman[6] reviewed the perioperative management of such patients, and their recommendations may be summarized as follows.

1. Preoperative assessment for patients with asthma should include spirometry, chest x-ray, and measurement of plasma theophylline level. The patient should be in optimal physical condition for surgery, and no elective procedure should be performed if the patient is wheezing actively.
2. Whether or not they are already on a steroid regimen, patients with asthma may be given a steroid perioperatively, either prednisone or hydrocortisone phosphate. Prednisone (30 to 60 mg/day PO) can be given for 1 to 2 days before the procedure and doses tapered over the first few postoperative days. Alternatively, a dose of hydrocortisone phosphate (100 to 150 mg IV) may be given on the morning of surgery[5] and tapered doses given orally for several days postoperatively.
3. Patients with asthma should continue to take all prescribed bronchodilator medications until the day of surgery.
4. Medications known to release histamine, such as morphine, curare, and atracurium, should be avoided in patients with asthma.
5. To avoid bronchospasm due to mechanical stimulation of the airway in a patient with asthma, an inhalation or narcotic technique should be used to achieve deep anesthesia before intubation for general anesthesia.
6. Bronchospasm that occurs during ESS under general anesthesia can be treated by deepening inhalation anesthesia or administering a beta-adrenergic receptor stimulant subcutaneously (SC) or by inhalation. Patients undergoing a procedure with MAC may be given a beta-adrenergic receptor stimulant.

Injectable beta-adrenergic receptor stimulants include terbutaline and epinephrine. Terbutaline is a $beta_2$-selective medication that has little effect on the myocardium, and to treat bronchospasm, a 0.25 mg SC dose may be given and repeated once in 15 to 30 minutes (maximal dose, 0.5 mg in 4 hours). Epinephrine (1/1000, 0.25 to 0.5 ml SC) has also been used to treat bronchospasm occurring intraoperatively, but epinephrine has both $beta_1$-adrenergic and $beta_2$-adrenergic receptor activity and thus may cause cardiovascular effects such as hypertension and tachycardia.[31]

Aerosolized sympathomimetics that may be used to treat intraoperative bronchospasm include albuterol, terbutaline, and isoetharine. Any of these $beta_2$-adrenergic receptor-selective medications may be given in a metered aerosol preparation or administered with a jet nebulizer by T-piece into the inspiratory limb of the anesthesia circuit.[6]

POSTANESTHESIA CARE

Anesthesia care after ESS is carried out in two phases. Immediately after surgery the patient is taken to the postanesthesia care unit and monitored according to the institution's routine protocol for same-day surgery or short-stay surgery patients. At the Cleveland Clinic, a modified Aldrete scoring system is used to assess the patient's recovery from anesthesia and readiness for discharge from the postanesthesia care unit. According to this system, a score of 0, 1, or 2 is given for level of activity, respiration, circulation, consciousness, and skin color; patients are ready for discharge when a score of 9 or 10 has been achieved and vital signs are stable.

When patients undergo ESS as outpatients at the Cleveland Clinic, they are discharged from the postanesthesia care unit to an outpatient recovery area. In this area they are given fluids by mouth and assessment continues.

Discharge Criteria

Various tests of cognitive and psychomotor function have been described to assess a patient's recovery from anesthesia, but such tests are too complicated and time-consuming to use in a busy outpatient setting; in addition, their ability to measure "street readiness" has been questioned.[32] After outpatient surgery at the Cleveland Clinic, patients may be discharged home when:

1. Vital signs are stable
2. Nausea and vomiting are minimal and under control
3. Pain can be well controlled by an oral medication prescribed by the surgeon
4. The patient is fully oriented and able to ambulate and void
5. Bleeding is not excessive
6. A responsible adult is available to accompany and stay with the patient at home.

Unplanned admissions to the hospital do occur occasionally after ESS. At the Cleveland Clinic, the most common reasons for admitting a patient after this type of procedure are repeated episodes of nausea and vomiting, excessive intraoperative or postoperative bleeding, more extensive surgery than planned, and intraoperative bronchospasm or aspiration.

Discharge Instructions

Patients and their escorts are given verbal and written instructions for continuing postoperative care at home. Patients are told to: (1) resume taking usual preoperative medications, (2) avoid for the next 24 hours activities that require muscle strength, coordination, and judgment (e.g., driving, using a stove, handling tools), (3) avoid for the next 24 hours making decisions that have legal ramifications, and (4) avoid alcoholic beverages for the next 24 hours.

The written instructions include telephone numbers where patients or their escorts can obtain help and further information during the postoperative period.

SUMMARY

ESS may be performed with local anesthetic with sedation, or with the patient under general anesthesia. The type of anesthesia and planned length of stay (same day or overnight after surgery) are determined based on the results of the preoperative anesthesia assessment; special precautions must be taken at all stages of anesthesia for patients who have asthma.

Medications given before ESS include anxiolytics and possibly anticholinergics and agents to decrease gastric secretion volume and acidity. Medications used for anesthesia and analgesia may include: (1) sedatives, which must be titrated carefully to prevent respiratory depression or apnea, especially when narcotics are used; (2) short-acting narcotics; (3) antiemetics, used as prophylaxis for narcotic-induced nausea and vomiting; (4) lidocaine, which causes central nervous system depression with toxic levels; (5) epinephrine, which may cause hypertension and cardiac arrhythmias if injected intravascularly; (6) cocaine, applied topically for vasoconstriction, which causes nervousness, headache, tachycardia, hypertension, and restlessness at toxic levels; (7) muscle relaxants for intubation; and (8) inhalation agents.

Precautions must be taken with general anesthesia to keep the airway clear of blood and secretions, maintain oxygenation, control blood pressure, and promote rapid emergence from anesthesia. Patients with asthma are at particular risk during intubation and extubation for general anesthesia because mechanical irritation of the airway during these maneuvers can induce bronchospasm.

REFERENCES

1. Eichel BS: The intranasal ethmoidectomy: A 12 year perspective. Otolaryngol Head Neck Surg 90:540–543, 1982.
2. Fairbanks DNF: Dental and allergic aspects of sinusitis and nasal polyposis: A review. Otolaryngol Head Neck Surg 90:527–533, 1982.
3. Friedman WH: Sphenoethmoidectomy: Its role in the asthmatic patient. Otolaryngol Head Neck Surg 90:171–177, 1982.
4. English GMH: Nasal polypectomy and sinus surgery in patients with asthma and aspirin idiosyncracy. Laryngoscope 96:374–380, 1986.
5. Roizen MF: Routine preoperative evaluation. In: Miller RD (ed): Anesthesia, 2nd ed. New York, Churchill Livingstone, 1986.
6. Kingston HG, Hirshman CA: Perioperative management of the patient with asthma. Anesth Analg 63:844–855, 1984.
7. Jacobsen H, Hertz JB, Johansen JR, et al: Premedication before day surgery. Br J Anaesth 57:300–305, 1985.
8. Smith MT: The pharmacokinetics of midazolam in man. Eur J Clin Pharmacol 19:271–278, 1981.
9. Epstein BS: Outpatient anesthesia. In: American Society of Anesthesiologists: Refresher Courses in Anesthesiology. Philadelphia: JB Lippincott, 12:85–95, 1984.
10. Modell JH: Aspiration pneumonitis. In: American Society of Anesthesiologists: Refresher Courses in Anesthesiology. Philadelphia: JB Lippincott, 10:163–170, 1982.
11. Ong BY, Palahniuk RS, Cumming M: Gastric volume and pH in outpatients. Can Anaesth Soc J 25:36–39, 1978.
12. Joyce TH: Prophylaxis for pulmonary acid aspiration. JAMA 83(Suppl 6A):46–52, 1987.
13. Manchikanti L, Grow JB, Colliver JA, et al: Bicitra (sodium citrate) and metoclopramide in outpatient anesthesia for prophylaxis against aspiration pneumonitis. Anesthesiology 63:378–384, 1985.
14. Maniglia AJN: Fatal and major complications secondary to nasal and sinus surgery. Laryngoscope 99:276–283, 1989.
15. Reves JG, Frazer RJ, Vinik HR, Greenblatt DJ: Midazolam: Pharmacology and uses. Anesthesiology 62:310–324, 1985.
16. White PF, Shafer A: Nausea and vomiting: Causes and prophylaxis. Semin Anesth 6:300–308, 1987.
17. Doze VA, Shafer A, White PF: Nausea and vomiting after outpatient anesthesia: Effectiveness of droperidol alone and in combination with metoclopramide. Anesth Analg 66(Suppl):S41, 1987.
18. Savarese JJ, Covino BG: Basic and clinical pharmacology of local anesthetic drugs. In: Miller RD (ed): Anesthesia, 2nd ed. New York: Churchill Livingstone, 1986.
19. Gallo JA: Catecholamine anesthetic interaction in ENT surgery. In: Brown RB (ed): Anesthesia and ENT Surgery, Contemporary Anesthesia Practice. Philadelphia: FA Davis, 1987.

20. Hashiasaki GT, Johns ME: Cocaine applications in otorhinolaryngologic anesthesia. In: Brown RG (ed): Anesthesia and ENT Surgery, Contemporary Anesthesia Practice. Philadelphia: FA Davis, 1987.
21. Schenck NL: Cocaine: Its use and misuse in otolaryngology. Trans Am Acad Ophthalmol Otolaryngol 80:343, 1975.
22. Johnston RR, Eger EL, Wilson C: Comparative interaction of epinephrine with enflurane, isoflurane and halothane in man. Anesth Analg (Cleve) 55:709–712, 1976.
23. Way WL, Trevor AJ: Pharmacology of intravenous nonnarcotic anesthetics. In: Miller RD (ed): Anesthesia, 2nd ed. New York: Churchill Livingstone, 1986.
24. Hirshman CA, Krieger W, Littlejohn G, et al: Ketamine-aminophylline-induced decrease in seizure threshold. Anesthesiology 56:464–467, 1982.
25. Miller RD: Clinical pharmacology of vecuronium and atracurium. Anesthesiology 61:444–453, 1984.
26. Hirshman CA, Edelstein G, Peetzs, et al: Mechanisms of action of inhalation anesthesia on airways. Anesthesiology 56:107–111, 1982.
27. Thiagarjah S, Grynsztejn M: Ventricular arrhythmias after terbutaline administration to patients anesthetized with halothane. Anesth Analg 65:417–418, 1986.
28. Bovill JG, Sebel PS, Blackburn CLH: The pharmacokinetics of alfentanil (R39209): A new opioid analgesic. Anesthesiology 57:439–443, 1982.
29. White PF, Coe V, Shafer A: Comparison of alfentanil with fentanyl for outpatient anesthesia. Anesthesiology 64:99–106, 1986.
30. Jorgensen NH, Coyle JP: Effects of intravenous droperidol upon nausea and recovery using alfentanil anesthesia. Anesthesiology 65(A):S139, 1989.
31. Daniele RPH: Asthma. In: Wyngaarden JB, Smith LH (eds): Cecil Textbook of Medicine, 16th ed. Philadelphia: WB Saunders, 1982.
32. Korttila K: How to assess recovery from outpatient anesthesia. In: American Society of Anesthesiologists: Refresher Courses in Anesthesiology. Philadelphia: JB Lippincott, 16:133–144, 1988.

5
Endoscopic Sinus Surgery

MARK MAY, M.D., F.A.C.S.
HOWARD L. LEVINE, M.D., F.A.C.S.
SARA J. MESTER, R.T.(R)
MARILYN PORTA, R.N.

Surgery to treat sinus disease has changed dramatically in the United States since 1985, when Kennedy et al[1,2] and Stammberger[3] reported on the use, based on earlier theory,[4] of endoscopes to diagnose and treat sinus disease. Nasal endoscopy with rigid instruments and computed tomography (CT) of the paranasal sinuses have helped physicians diagnose previously unrecognized disorders, and nasal endoscopes have allowed surgeons to approach the ostiomeatal complex (OMC)—the narrow anatomic area between the middle turbinate and the lateral nasal wall.

This complex anatomic compartment contains the drainage sites of three of the four paranasal sinuses: the maxillary, the ethmoid, and the frontal. It had been thought that surgeons should avoid the maxillary sinus ostium because violation of this "sacred" opening might result in chronic maxillary sinus infection. Messerklinger,[4] however, showed that maxillary sinusitis is most often due to obstruction of the maxillary sinus ostium and that the ostium must be patent to maintain mucociliary flow from the sinus into the nasal cavity.

On the basis of this analysis, Kennedy et al[1,2] and Stammberger[3] proposed a conservative type of sinus surgery they termed "functional endoscopic sinus surgery" (FESS). The single goal of FESS is to restore normal mucociliary flow in the region of the OMC.

This chapter describes preparations for endoscopic sinus surgery (ESS), procedures in the operating room, three surgical approaches to the ethmoid sinus complex, anesthesia from the surgeon's point of view, step-by-step technique for ESS, special considerations during surgery, prevention and management of bleeding, and postoperative care of the patient who has undergone ESS.

PREPARATIONS FOR SURGERY

The preoperative evaluation for ESS, including imaging studies to be performed, was discussed in Chapter 3 (see in particular Table 3–6). A review of plain radiographs as well as CT scans is especially important for planning surgery on the paranasal sinuses. Figure 5–1[5] shows how distances and angles between anatomic structures of importance during ESS are measured on a preoperative lateral sinus radiograph. Figure 5–2 shows the system used to classify CT findings; the implications of disease classification for the type of surgery planned were discussed in Chapter 3.

Special Preoperative Considerations

Special consideration must be given before ESS to patients with reactive airway disease, massive polyposis, suppurative sinusitis, hypertension, or medical therapy that prolongs bleeding.

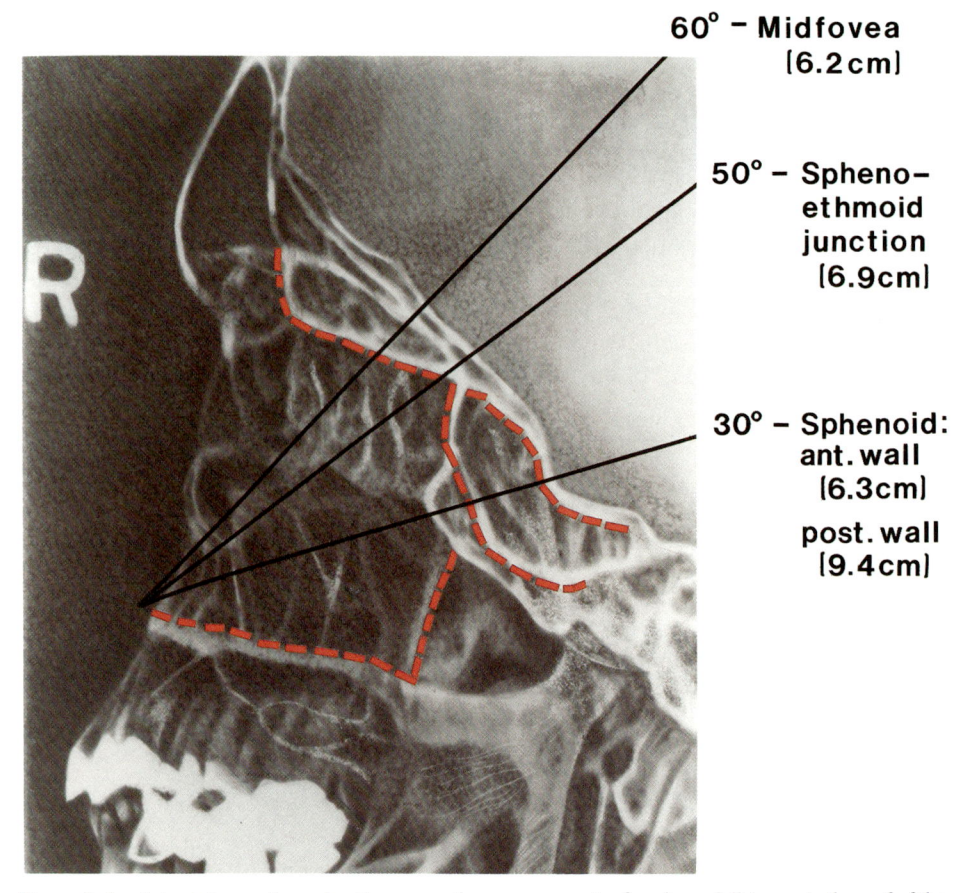

Figure 5–1. Lateral sinus radiograph with preoperative measurements of angles and distances to the roof of the ethmoid sinus. ant: anterior; post.: posterior. (Reprinted with permission from May et al.[5]).

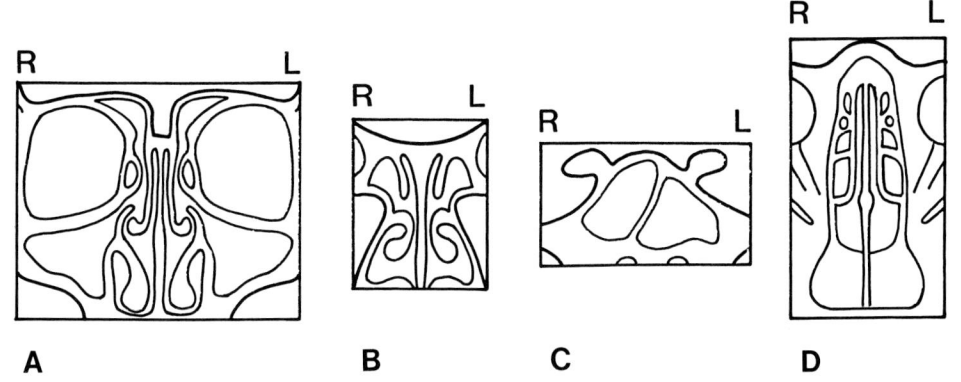

Figure 5–2. Representations of anatomy as seen on coronal CT scans for classification of findings. **A:** Frontal sinus and agger nasi, infundibulum with uncinate process, bulla ethmoidalis, maxillary sinus, and anterior ethmoid complex. **B:** Posterior ethmoid region. **C:** Sphenoid sinus. **D:** Axial CT scan to show relationship of ethmoid and sphenoid sinuses to optic nerve and carotid artery. Areas of involvement in each patient are noted on the office protocol (Appendix) and the extent of disease is classified on the right side, left side, or both sides as: 1+, limited to OMC; 2+, incomplete opacification of one or more sinuses (frontal, maxillary, sphenoid); 3+, total opacification of one or more sinuses but not all; or 4+, total opacification of all sinuses.

Some patients with reactive airway disease may need to be admitted the day before surgery to undergo aggressive pulmonary therapy. These patients, and those who are already taking steroid medications, should be given a bolus dose of a corticosteroid (100 mg hydrocortisone sodium succinate) intravenously (IV) preoperatively. Patients with massive polyposis should receive steroid therapy perioperatively on the following schedule: 80 mg/day for preoperative days 5 and 4; 60 mg/day for preoperative days 3 and 2; 40 mg/day for preoperative day 1 and postoperative day 1; and 30, 20, and 10 mg/day, respectively, on postoperative days 2, 3, and 4. Intraoperatively, patients with massive polyposis are given 40 mg methylprednisolone IV in preference to hydrocortisone because methylprednisolone has a longer half-life and fewer side effects.

Patients who have suppurative sinusitis should receive an appropriate antibiotic medication for 10 days before surgery.

Hypertension must be controlled before ESS. This disorder should be managed by a medical consultant, and surgery must be postponed until therapy has maintained blood pressure in an acceptable range for at least the day of surgery. Medications, such as aspirin or nonsteroidal anti-inflammatory drugs (NSAIDs), that prolong bleeding are discontinued before surgery (see Table 3–3, Chapter 3).

On-Call to the Operating Room

Approximately 20 minutes before being taken to the surgical suite, the patient is given a sedative and the decongestant oxymetazoline (Afrin 0.05%) is sprayed on the nasal mucosa. Decongestion of the nasal mucosa decreases bleeding and slows the systemic absorption of topical anesthetic agents that will be applied later.[6]

IN THE OPERATING ROOM

CT scans taken preoperatively are displayed on a view box in the operating room, so that the surgeon can refer to them as needed during the procedure.

When the patient arrives in the operating room, an intravenous infusion is begun. If the patient has an active infection, a dose of an antibiotic appropriate to the suspected cause of the infection may be administered IV at this time, and additional doses given IV during the perioperative period.

We do not cleanse the patient's face before the procedure, because the actual operative area inside the nose is not sterile.

The patient's eyes are left uncovered for ESS to allow for constant monitoring by palpating movement and observing for periorbital ecchymosis, subcutaneous emphysema, change in pupil size, limitation of extraocular movement, or increase in orbital tone. The patient's visual acuity should have been tested during the preoperative evaluation; pupil size, pupil reactivity, and extraocular muscle function are tested before anesthesia is administered and in the immediate postoperative period.

THREE APPROACHES TO SINUS SURGERY

Several approaches to sinus surgery have been developed. This section reports on three approaches that may be considered, depending on the type and severity of sinus disease present and the surgeon's preference.

Video Endoscopic Sinus Surgery, Two-Handed Technique

The "two-handed" technique developed by May et al.[7] for video ESS is a modification of the surgical approach described by others.[1-3]

Surgical Equipment and Materials

Figures 5–3 through 5–14 show a sample operating room arrangement for ESS and the instruments, endoscopic and video equipment, and materials used for performing ESS by the two-handed video technique. Table 5–1 lists the steps for proper care and handling of the video and endoscopic equipment.

Technique

With this two-handed video technique (Fig. 5–15),[7] the surgeon and the assistant watch the monitor as the assistant guides the endoscope to the surgical field. The surgeon continues to watch the monitor and directs the assistant to alter placement of the endoscope as needed during the procedure. By watching the monitor rather than being limited to the view through the endoscope, the surgeon has a better perspective than when looking through the endoscope of the position of the instruments relative to the patient's nose, orbit, and slope of the anterior skull base.

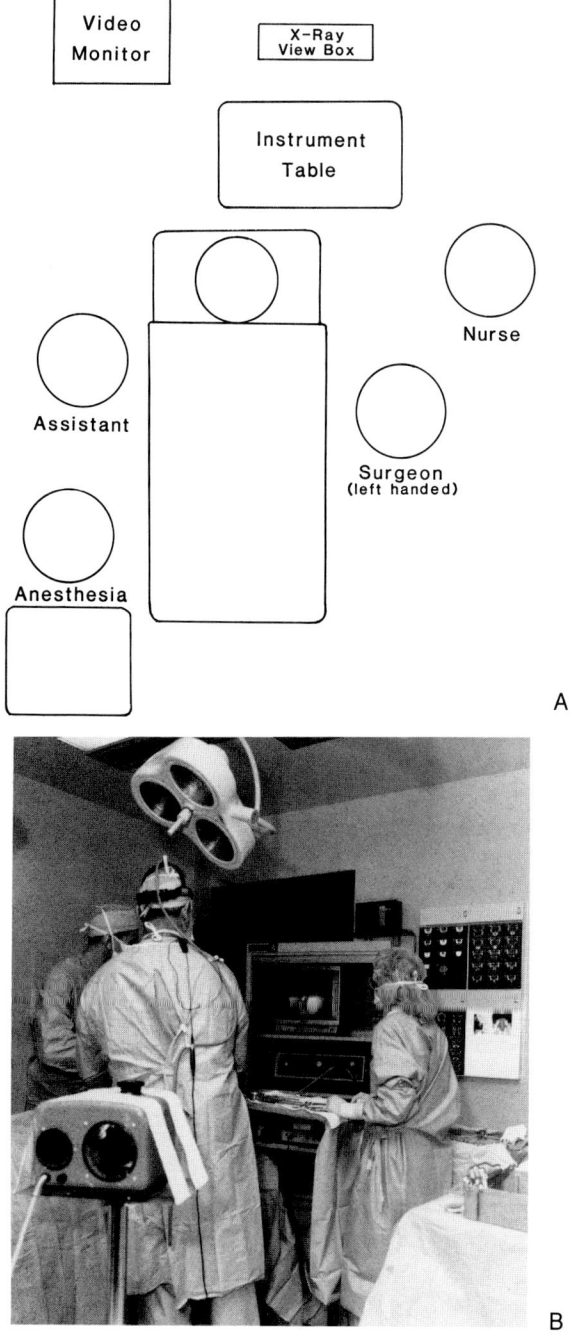

Figure 5–3. Sample operating room setup to permit surgeon's visualization of video monitor, x-ray view box, and anesthesia monitor. The surgeon should be positioned so that the patient is on the side of his or her dominant hand. **A**: Diagram of layout for left-handed surgeon. **B**: Left-handed surgeon performing video endonasal endoscopic sinus surgery.

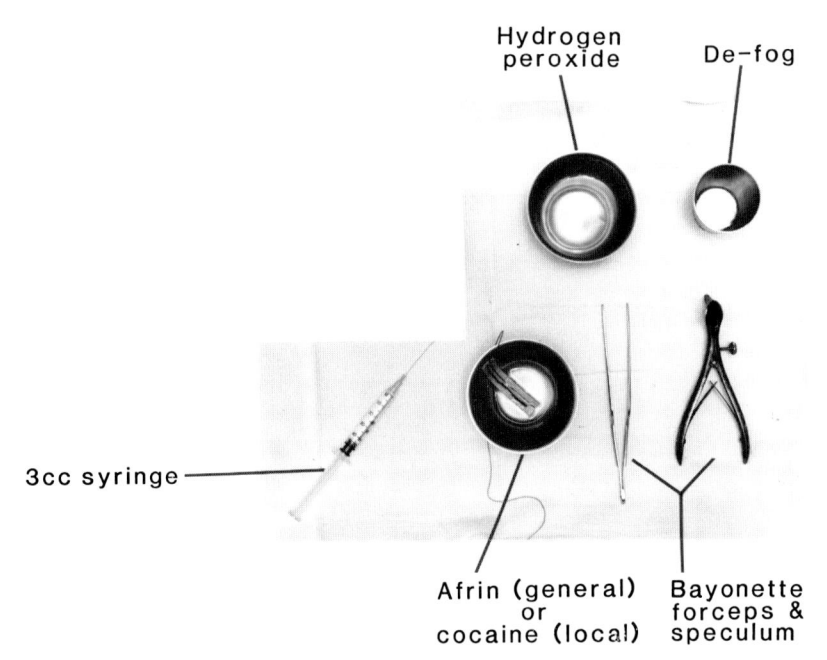

Figure 5–4. Medications used during surgery. Tip of 25 gauge, 1.5 inch needle on 3 cc syringe containing lidocaine and 1/100,000 epinephrine has been bent slightly to allow easier access to the lateral nasal wall. Cotton pledgets are used to apply oxymetazoline (Afrin) for hemostasis. Peroxide is used to clean the endoscope. Ultrastop (item 36212, Gynescope Corp., Willoughby, OH) is used to defog the endoscope.

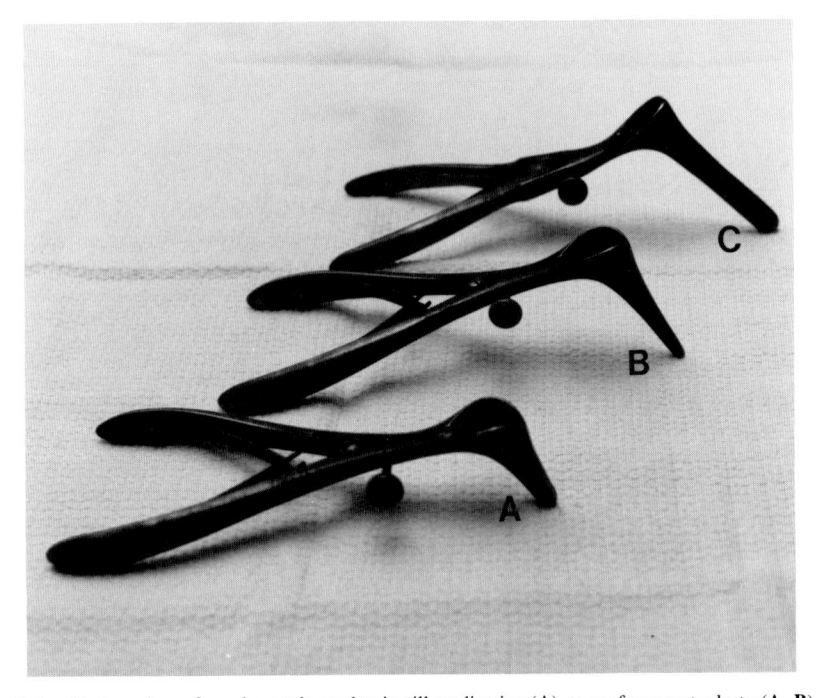

Figure 5–5. Various sizes of nasal specula used to instill medication (**A**), to perform septoplasty (**A**, **B**), and to displace septum or turbinate when greater exposure is needed (**C**).

110

Endoscopic Sinus Surgery   111

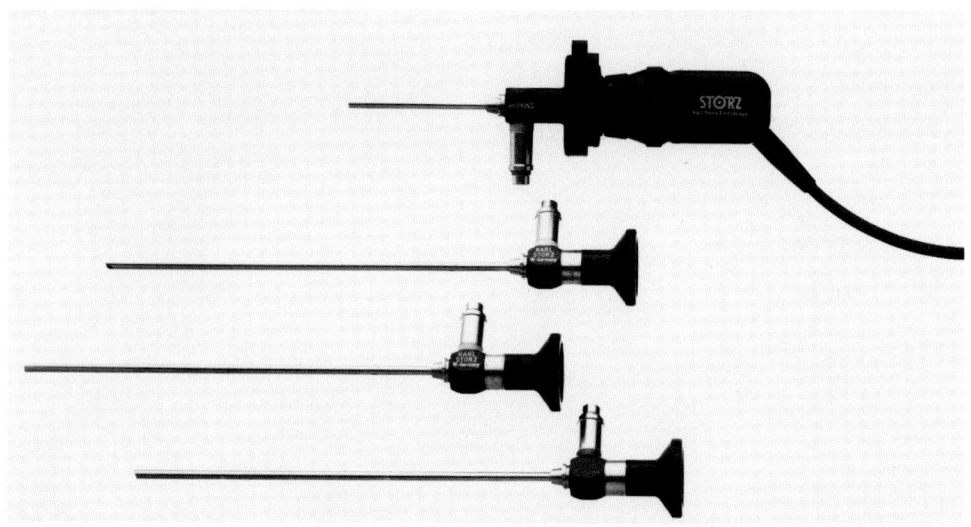

Figure 5–6. Equipment used for two-handed video-endoscopic technique. Top to bottom: video camera (item 9050B, Karl Storz Endoscopy-America, Culver City, CA), which the surgeon watches rather than viewing the operative field through the endoscope, attached to 0°, 4 mm straight endoscope (item 1215A, Karl Storz) used for photographic documentation. Next, 70°, 4 mm lateral endoscope (item 7200C, Karl Storz) is used to view the sphenoethmoid recess, nasofrontal recess, and maxillary sinus (through enlarged maxillary sinus ostium). Next, 0° 4 mm straight endoscope (item 7200A, Karl Storz) is the instrument most often used for ESS because it gives an undistorted image that does not become disoriented with rotation of the endoscope, as long as the camera is not rotated. Bottom, 30° 4 mm forward-oblique endoscope (item 7200B, Karl Storz) is used to view structures hidden by overhanging ledges, for example, in the nasofrontal recess and maxillary sinus. Not shown is the fiberoptic light cable (item 495NL, Karl Storz).

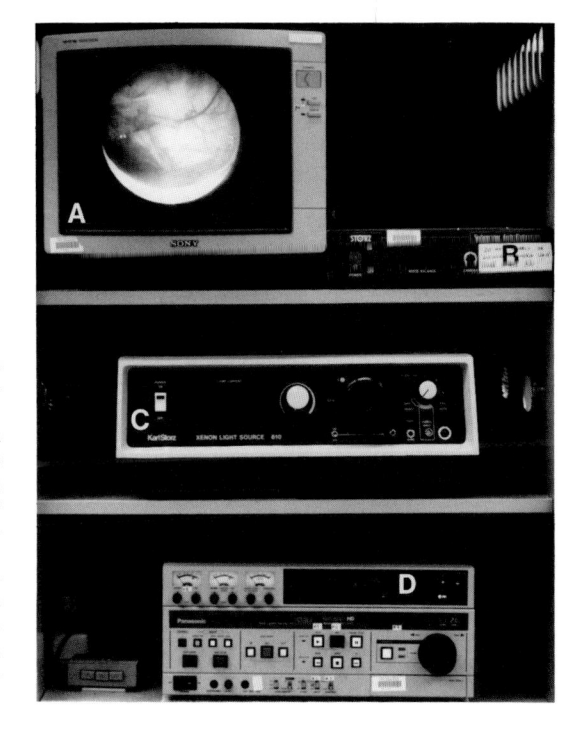

Figure 5–7. Equipment for viewing and recording endonasal endoscopic sinus surgery. **A**: Video monitor (Trinitron, Sony). **B**: Color-balance autoexposure video camera (Super Kam, Karl Storz). **C**: Light source (item 610C, Karl Storz). An automatic flash connection permits flash photography through the endoscope. **D**: Videocassette recorder, 1/2 inch super-VHS (item AG7500A, Panasonic). Not shown: A low-sensitivity microphone is clipped to surgeon's mask to record his or her comments without significant background noise, and a foot switch is positioned so the surgeon can turn video recording on and off.

112 *Endoscopic Sinus Surgery*

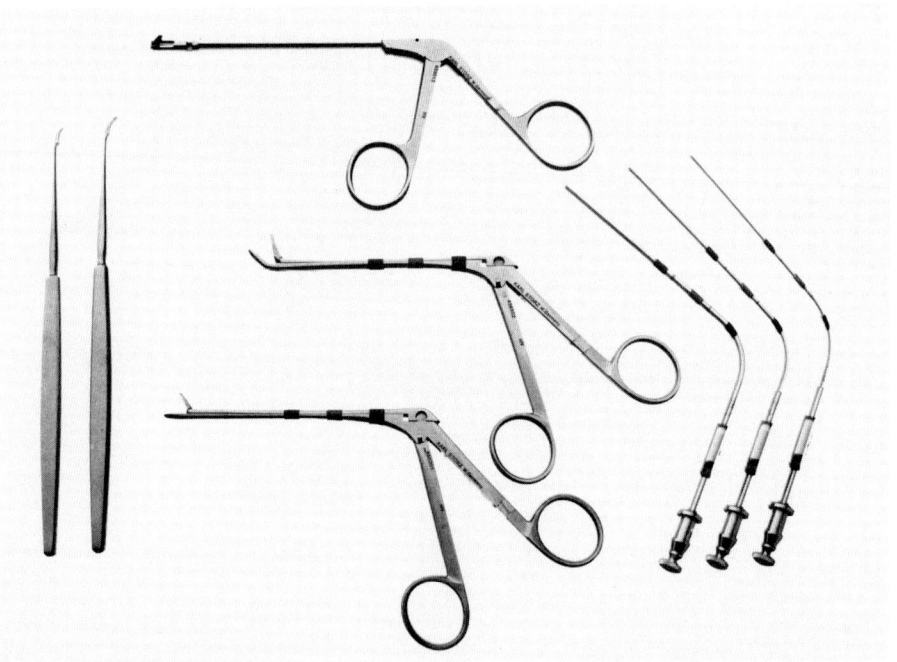

Figure 5–8. Instruments used most often for endoscopic sinus surgery. Left: Pointed sickle knife (item 668001, Storz Instrument Co., St. Louis MO) and blunt sickle knife or back knife (item 629002, Storz) used to incise the uncinate process. Center top: Stammberger antrum punch, small right-side cutting (item 459011, Storz; not shown: left-side cutting, item 459012), used to remove the remnant of uncinate process and inferior remnant of posterior fontanelle when enlarging the maxillary antrostomy. Center middle: Small Struempel-Boss upturned ethmoid forceps (item 457000S, Storz; not shown: large, item 4565025) used in the area of the maxillary sinus ostium, to take down the face of the bulla ethmoidalis, remove the basal lamella, and free the mucous membrane and polyps from ethmoid and sphenoid sinuses. Center bottom: Blakesley ethmoid forceps, size 1 (item 456001, Storz; not shown: size 4, item 456004) used to remove the uncinate process, enlarge the maxillary sinus ostium by removing part of the posterior fontanelle, take down the bulla ethmoidalis and basal lamella, and open the ethmoid and sphenoid cells. Right: Frazier suction cannulas no. 5, 7, and 9 F, 17.5 cm; the smallest (no. 5) is used when surgery begins in the anterior OMC and progressively larger suction cannulas are used as surgery moves toward the sphenoid sinus. Not shown here: double-ended maxillary sinus ostium seeker (item 629820, Storz), shown in Figure 5–21A, is used to displace lateralized uncinate process and to probe natural maxillary sinus ostium and nasofrontal channel and isthmus.

Endoscopic Sinus Surgery   113

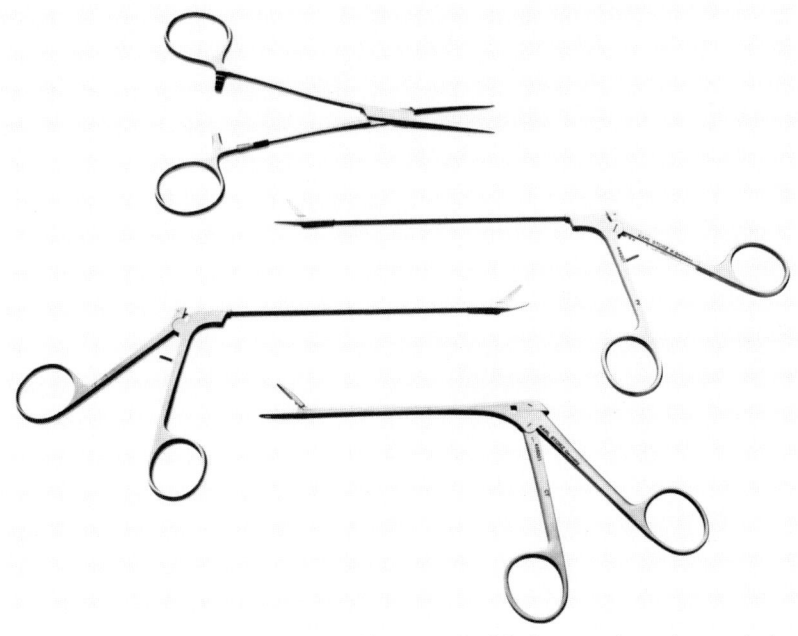

Figure 5–9. Instruments for partial middle turbinectomy. Straight hemostat is used to crush the superior attachment of the middle turbinate for hemostasis. Straight nasal scissors (item 449201, Storz) is used to cut across the crush line. Then a left (item 449203, Storz) or (not shown) right (item 440202, Storz) nasal scissors is used to connect the inferior edge of the middle turbinate to the superior cut to allow removal of the anterior third of the middle turbinate with the Ferris-Smith fragment forceps (item N545, Storz).

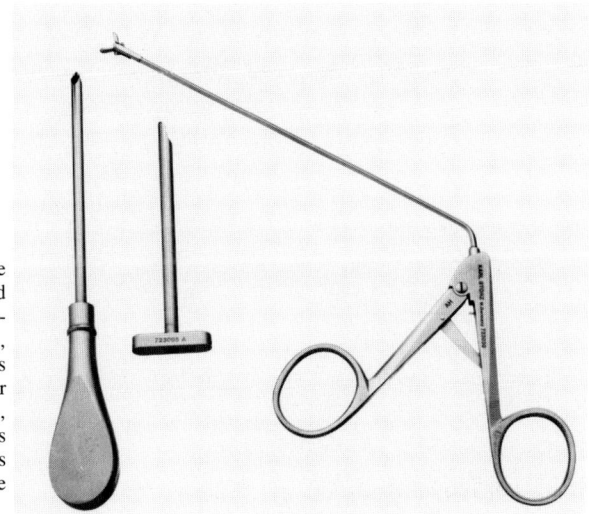

Figure 5–10. Instruments for transcanine fossa antrostomy, maxillary sinoscopy, and transcanine fossa surgery. Left to right: sinoscopy trocar and cannula (item 723005B, Storz) are used to access the maxillary sinus through a canine fossa puncture; the trocar cannula acts as a speculum for endoscopes, forceps, and suction tips. The cup forceps (item 723030, Storz) is designed to pass through the trocar cannula to remove tissue from the maxillary sinus.

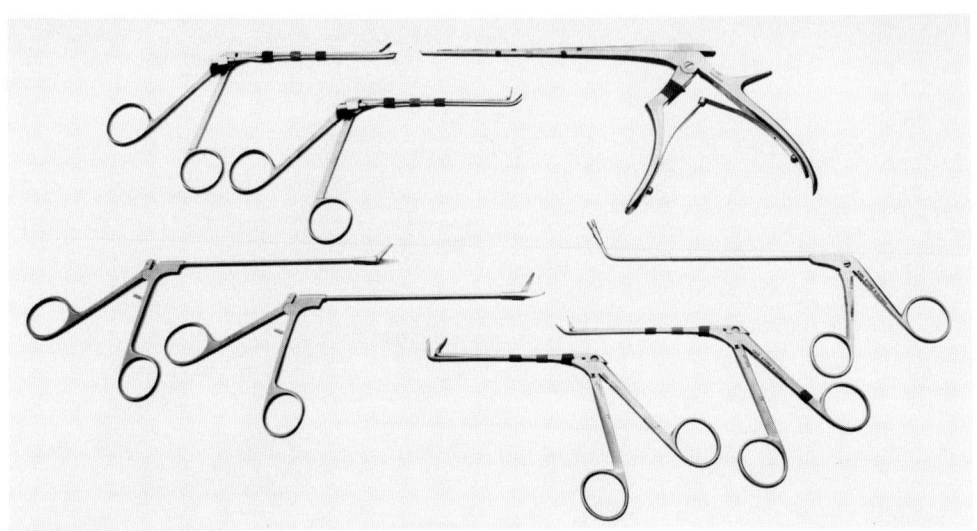

Figure 5–11. Instruments for special situations. Clockwise from top left: Kennedy suction forceps, upturned size 1 (item 650041, Storz) and straight size 1 (item 650031, Storz) are ideal to manage excessive bleeding. Micro-Kerrison forceps, 40° 2 mm upbiting (item R1647, Bruggels, North Quincy, MA; not shown: 2 mm downbiting, item R1646) are ideal for removing ethmoid cells along the roof of the ethmoid sinus, anterior wall of the sphenoid, nasofrontal recess, and agger nasi region. Giraffe sinus forceps (item 650212, Storz), used to remove tissue in the nasofrontal recess and maxillary sinus, can reach the anterior lateral walls of the maxillary sinus through an enlarged maxillary antrostomy with direct monitoring through a 30° or 70° endoscope. A 90° forceps (short, item 456803, Storz; not shown: long, item 131246) is used to work in the nasofrontal recess or maxillary sinus through an enlarged maxillary sinus antrostomy. Nasal scissors (see Fig. 5–9) are used to remove remnants of posterior aspect of the middle turbinate or to enlarge the maxillary sinus ostium by cutting the posterior fontanelle so that it flaps down into the nasal side. This flap ostioplasty ensures patency of the natural ostium. Not shown: Eicken antrum cannulas (3 mm short curved, item 586230, Storz; 4 mm short curved, item 588240; and 3 mm long curved, item 586030) are used for irrigation, suction, and probing in the nasofrontal recess and frontal sinus (long curved cannula) and the sphenoid and maxillary sinuses (short curved cannulae, although the long curved cannula may be used to reach the lateral recesses of these sinuses).

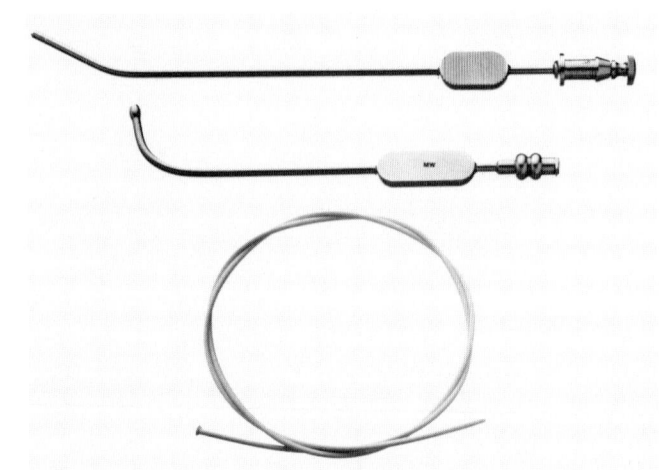

Figure 5–12. Instruments to cannulate the frontal sinus. Top: Siebenmann antrum cannula, 23 cm, size 0 (item 203903, Storz), can be bent to conform to the curvature of (middle) 3 mm, long, curved Eicken antrum cannula (item 586030, Storz). Bottom: blue 0.04 cm tip, 60 cm plastic catheter (item 15447, Becton-Dickinson, Rutherford, NC) is threaded through the Siebenmann cannula into the frontal sinus and the antrum cannula is withdrawn, leaving the catheter in place to keep the passage open with minimal likelihood of granulation tissue or crust forming.

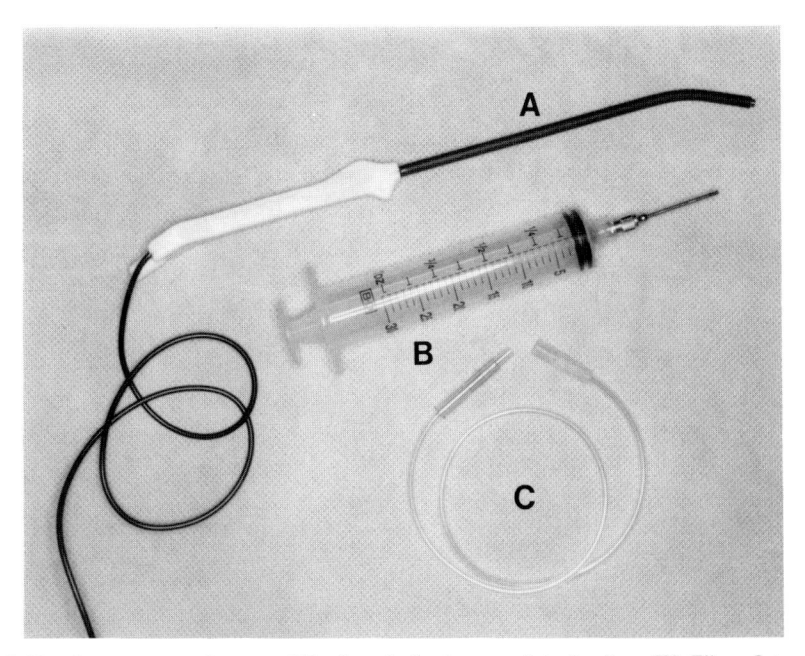

Figure 5–13. Instruments used to control bleeding. **A:** Suction coagulator (medium, H8, Ellman International, Hewlett, NY) can be bent slightly at the end for optimal control of bleeding from anterior and posterior ethmoid or sphenopalatine arteries. **B:** Syringe with 30 cc normal saline and 16 gauge blunt needle (item 7938, Popper and Sons, New Hyde Park, NY) is used for irrigation of the operative field and the endoscope lens to promote visibility. **C:** Hudson catheter (Hudson Oxygen Sales, Wadsworth, OH) is of small enough caliber to fit together with the blunt needle (**B**) placed through the trocar cannula that has been inserted into the maxillary sinus via a canine fossa approach. This sinus is irrigated by instilling saline with the syringe and aspirating fluid back through the catheter attached to suction.

116 *Endoscopic Sinus Surgery*

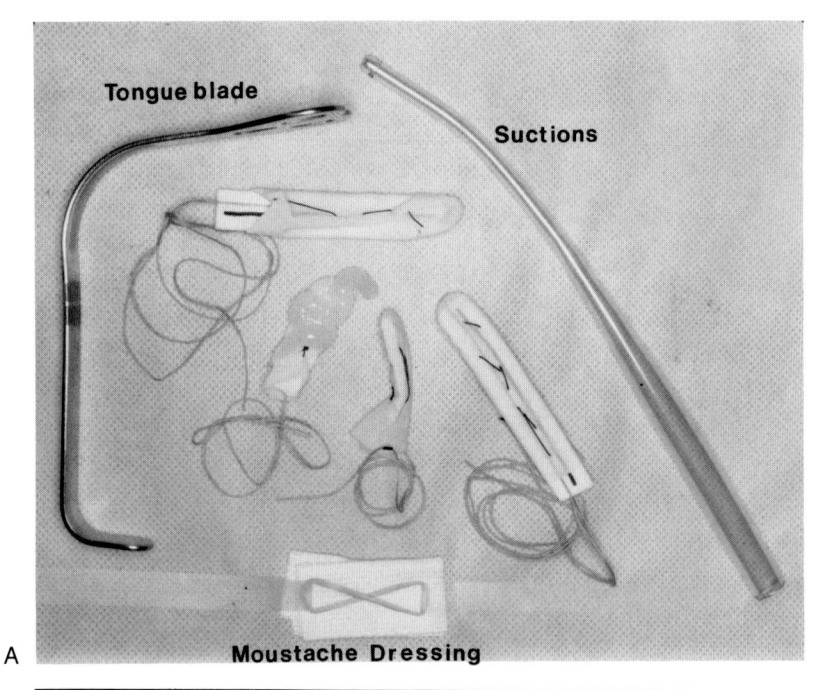

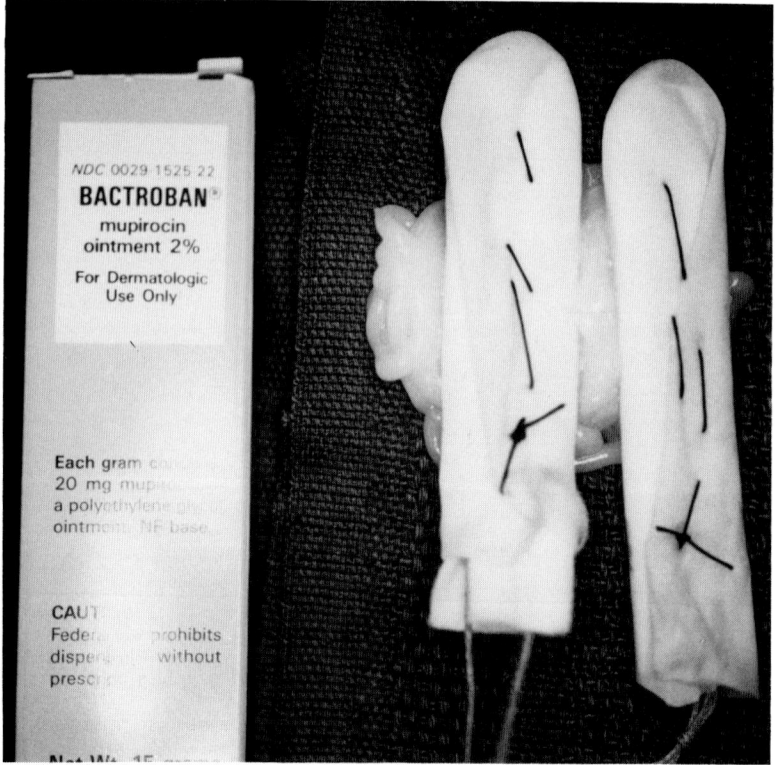

Figure 5–14. (Figure continued and legend on next page.)

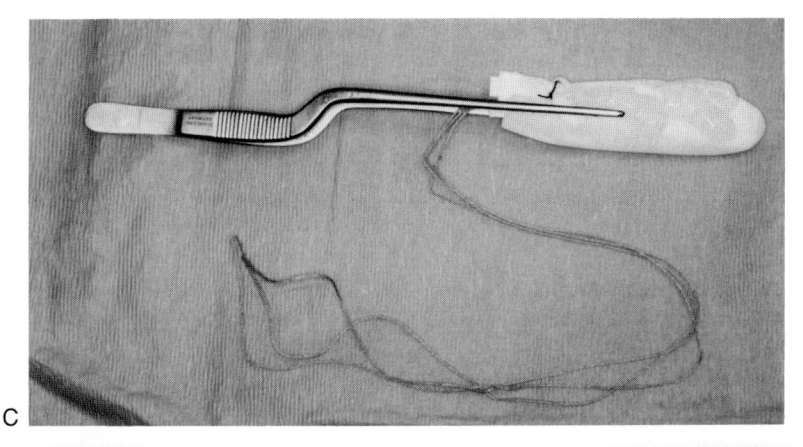

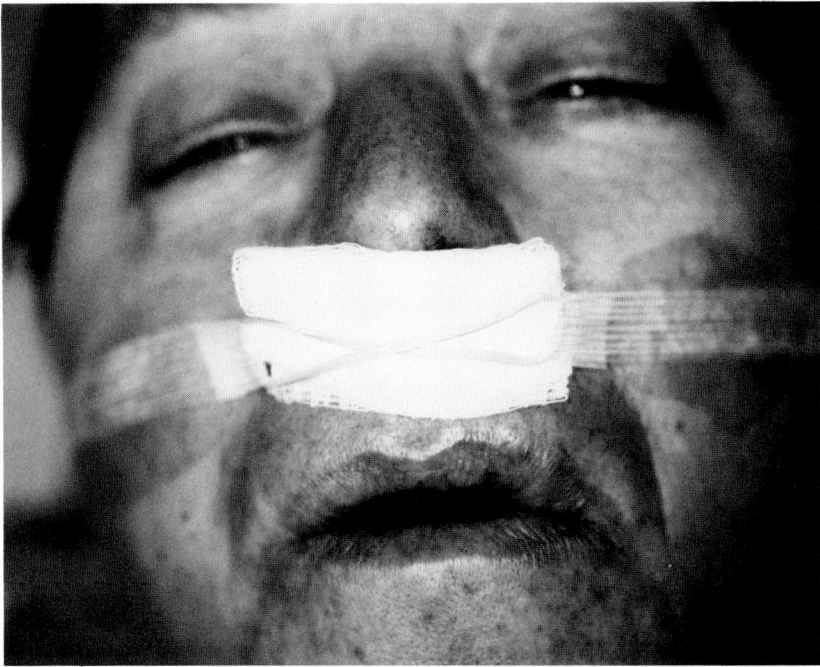

Figure 5–14. (*Continued*) **A**: Instruments and materials used at the completion of surgery. While the tongue is held out of the way with the tongue blade (item 46-1012, Pilling Co., Fort Washington, PA), the Yankower suction tip is used to remove secretions from the back of the oropharynx. **B, C**: An internal nasal dressing is placed between the middle turbinate and lateral nasal wall and left in place for 24 hours. If the middle turbinate is removed, the dressing is placed between the nasal septum and posterior aspect of the inferior turbinate. **D**: A moustache dressing placed under the nostrils and over the upper lip absorbs secretions. The dressing is a 2×2 inch gauze pad held in place by an elastic band attached to the patient's face in a figure 8 with paper tape. The elastic band holder permits the gauze pad to be replaced without removing the tape, which prevents irritation of the patient's skin.

Table 5-1 Sterilization and Handling of Video and Endoscopic Equipment

PROCEDURE	OPTIONS	ADVANTAGES/STEPS FOR BEST RESULTS
Sterilization	Steris System 1*	1. Rapid, low-temperature, liquid-chemical process that is safe for heat-sensitive, immersible instruments 2. Equal in efficacy to steam or ethylene oxide sterilization 3. Does not lead to fogging of the video camera or of the lens systems of endoscopes, as do traditional cleansing or antibiotic solutions, or to decomposition of the housing that holds the lens in place 4. Requires less time than soaking in a traditional cleansing solution for efficacy against hepatitis B virus; this permits use of a uniform sterilization technique for all patients and instruments
	Cidex solution/ gas sterilization	1. May be used if Steris System 1 is not available 2. Immediately after using video camera or endoscope AFFIX THE SOAKING CAP, wash with warm water (add a mild detergent if necessary), rinse thoroughly, and towel dry before placing in disinfectant; leave in disinfectant no longer than 10 minutes; rinse in sterile water as rapidly as possible; clean lenses with dry or alcohol-moistened cotton-tipped applicators 3. DO NOT steam any part of the camera or endoscopes
Handling	Endoscopes	1. Hold the endoscope by the eyepiece and support the distal end 2. Before and after use, inspect endoscopes for clouding, scratches, fingerprints, or residual debris 3. Avoid touching the lens 4. Avoid placing other instruments on top of the endoscope
	Light cables	1. Turn off the light source BEFORE disconnecting the endoscope from the light cable; heat from the cable can cause a burn or even start a fire 2. Bending fiberoptic cables sharply will damage the fibers; coil them loosely
	Camera	1. Store the camera with the soaking cap in place to protect the lens 2. Coil camera cable loosely to prevent damage
Troubleshooting	Loss of video image quality (fogging or out of focus)	1. Due to diminished light intensity; search for cause 2. Check settings on monitor and light source 3. Check for dirty or fogged eyepiece or distal lens; wipe moisture from eyepiece, dip end of endoscope in peroxide, wipe end, and dip end in defogging solution 4. Check for charring at end of instrument due to heat and carbon deposition; if charring is present, clean the instrument 5. Examine instrument for broken fiber bundles by reflecting a light over the end that plugs into the light source and looking for dark areas; if dark areas are present, replace the cable 6. Blood absorbs light; irrigate and suction the operative field and control oozing

*Karl Storz Endoscopy-America, 10111 W. Jefferson Blvd., Culver City, CA 90232-3578

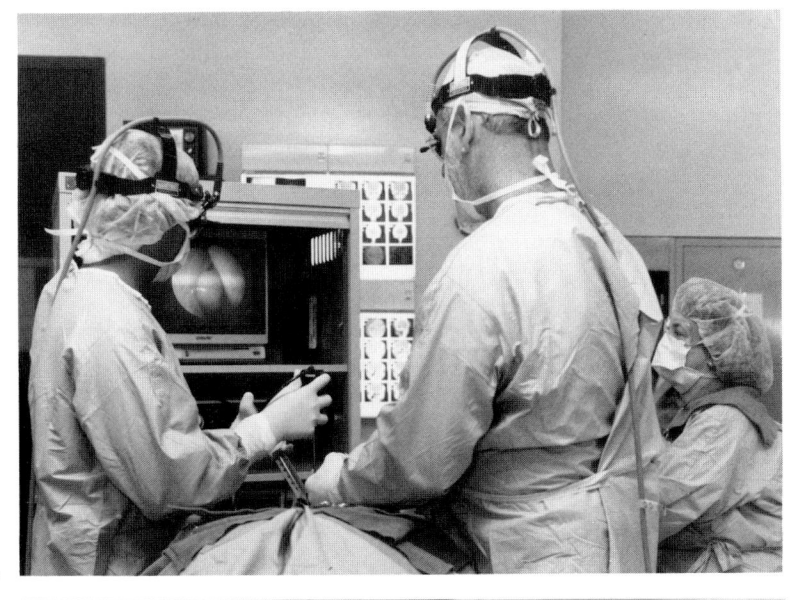

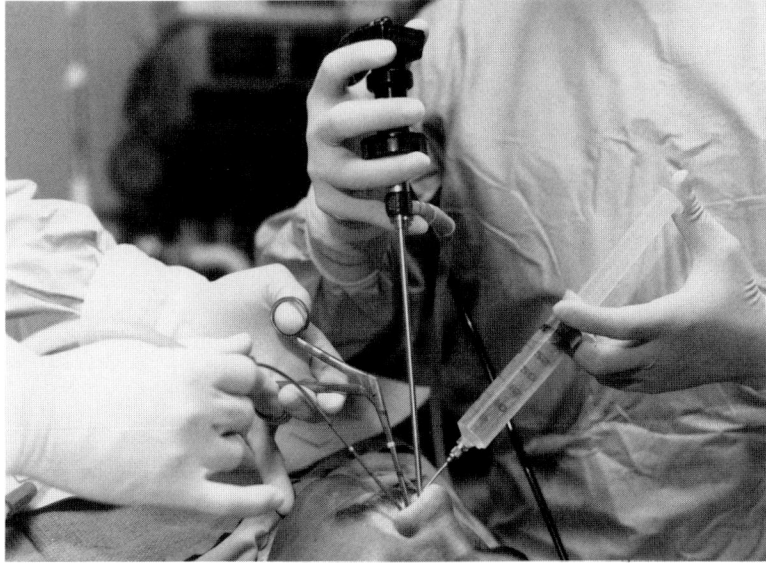

Figure 5–15. Two-handed technique for endoscopic sinus surgery. **A**: Surgeon and assistant working with aid of video camera and monitor. **B**: Close-up view of instruments and endoscope in use for technique. The surgeon directs the assistant to position the endoscope and irrigate with saline while the surgeon manipulates suction with one hand, forceps with the other (Reprinted with permission from May et al[7]).

In addition to manipulating the endoscope the assistant provides an additional hand (actually a four-handed technique) to irrigate the surgical field (Fig. 5–15B) with saline to keep the endoscope lens and surgical field clear. Another advantage of the two-handed technique is that because the assistant is holding the endoscope, the surgeon has a free hand to use the suction cannula to palpate, probe, retract, and suction blood away from the surgical site just as he or she would do during otologic surgery. The involvement of the assistant in the surgery and displaying the view through the endoscope on the video monitor make this technique an excellent vehicle for teaching ESS.

Furthermore, having an assistant hold the endoscope is helpful when the surgeon wishes to enlarge or connect an accessory ostium with the natural ostium of the maxillary sinus. For this procedure, the endoscope is placed in the maxillary sinus through a transcanine approach (Fig. 1–6). As Figure 5–16 shows, the pattern of maxillary sinus–nasal mucosa mucociliary flow is from the nasal mucosa into the maxillary sinus through the accessory ostium and back into the nose via the natural maxillary sinus ostium in a circular movement. By watching the view of the maxillary sinus cavity in the monitor, the surgeon, with an instrument placed in the nasal cavity, can enlarge the maxillary sinus ostium. In this way the surgeon can confirm that the opening being enlarged is the maxillary sinus ostium and not an accessory ostium in the fontanelle: if the surgeon notes a streak of blood or secretions flowing from the maxillary sinus through the ostium and into the nose, this is confirmation that it was the maxillary sinus ostium that was enlarged. The success of this procedure in diagnosing and managing sinus disease is shown in Figure 5–17, A–E.

Because the nasal side of the natural maxillary sinus ostium is just below the lamina papyracea,[8] direct visualization of the maxillary sinus ostium with the endoscope placed through the canine fossa helps orient the surgeon to the location of the orbit.

Two-Handed Endoscopic Versus Operating Microscope Technique

Draf[9] has described an endonasal sinus surgery technique using the binocular operating microscope. This technique provides the surgeon the advantages of magnification and a three-dimensional view of the operative field, as well as the use of two hands to perform surgical maneuvers.[10,11]

The binocular microscope does not, however, provide an angled view, as does the endoscope with a wide-angle lens. Furthermore, the view through the microscope is obscured by instruments in the field, whereas the view through the endoscope is unobstructed because the lens is actually close to the surgical field. Lastly, surgery usually cannot be performed with the patient under local anesthesia when the operating microscope is used, because pressure of the nasal speculum used to maintain exposure is too uncomfortable for the awake patient.

The endoscope cannot provide the three-dimensional view seen through the operating microscope, however. To compensate for this, the endoscopic surgeon can use the suction tip as a sort of "cat's whisker" to probe, sound, palpate, and measure the depths and widths of the anatomic-surgical box of the ethmoid complex.

When this endoscopic procedure is performed under local anesthesia, the assistant can irrigate the surgical area with saline solution that is prevented by a balloon catheter (Xomed Post Pac, Xomed, Jacksonville FL) (Fig. 5–18A)[12] from entering the pharynx. The balloon

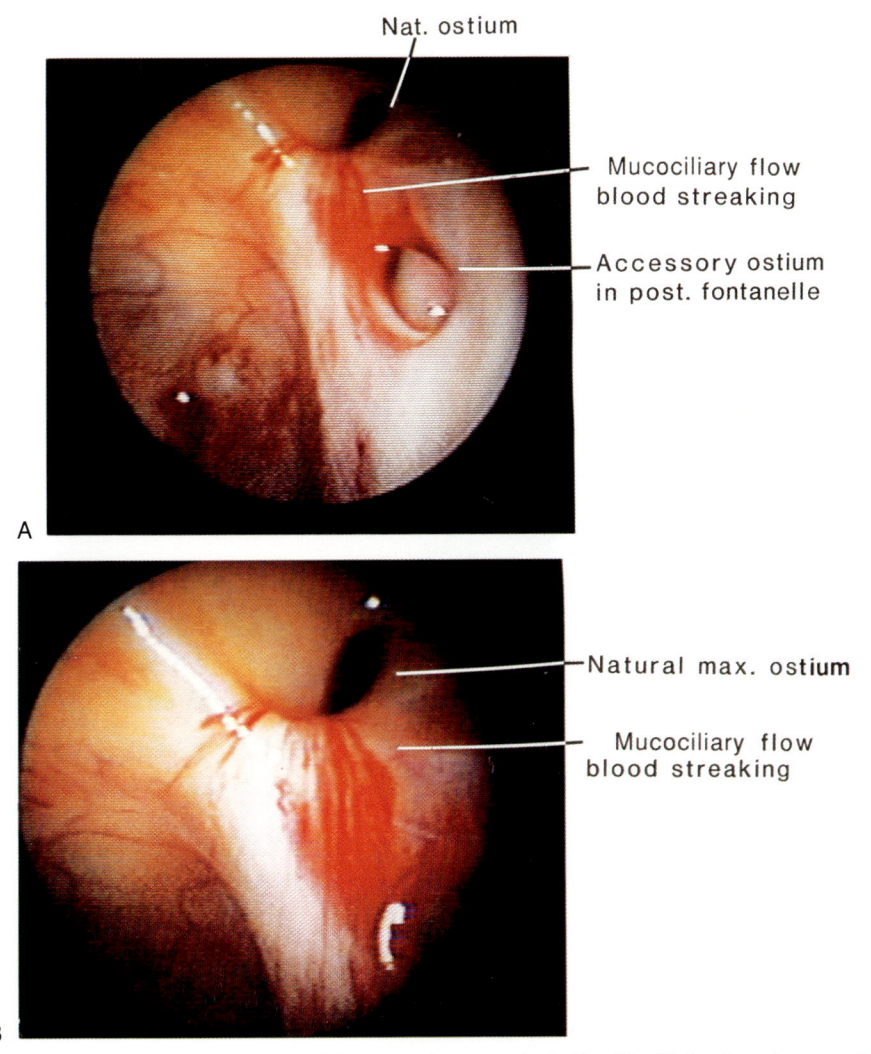

Figure 5–16. Endoscopic view through right transcanine approach. **A:** Note blood being drawn by mucociliary flow from the accessory ostium to the natural ostium. This circular movement of material from the nose through an accessory ostium into the maxillary sinus and back to the nose through the natural ostium is thought to be responsible for the symptoms of sinus disorder after a separate opening has been made in the posterior fontanelle. **B:** Close-up view of blood being drawn into the natural ostium.

122 *Endoscopic Sinus Surgery*

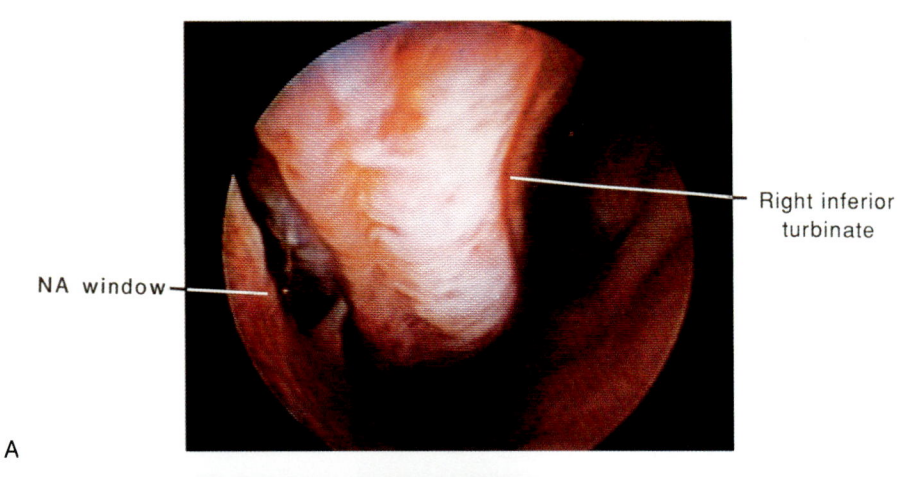

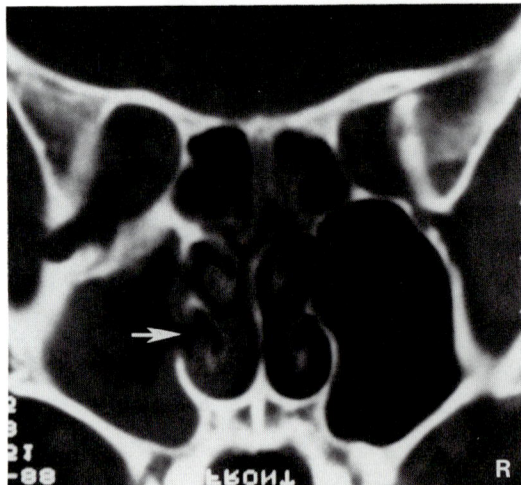

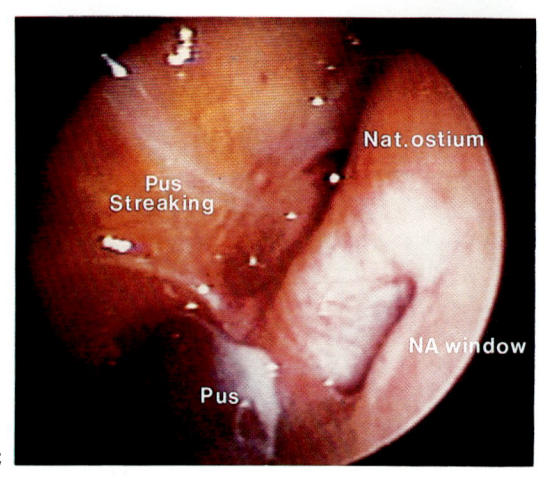

Figure 5–17. Endoscopic and CT findings in a patient with right suppurative maxillary sinusitis that failed to respond to Caldwell-Luc and nasal antral window surgery. **A**: Endoscopic view of right nasal cavity looking under inferior turbinate into inferior meatus. Note widely patent nasoantral (NA) window. **B**: Coronal CT scan shows patent right inferior meatal (arrow) nasoantral window and evidence of chronic right maxillary sinusitis. **C**: Transcanine fossa endoscopic view of right maxillary sinus shows a patent nasoantral (NA) window and retained pus pooling in floor of the maxillary sinus. Pus is streaking toward the natural (Nat.) ostium but not toward the nasoantral window. (Figure continued on next page.)

Endoscopic Sinus Surgery **123**

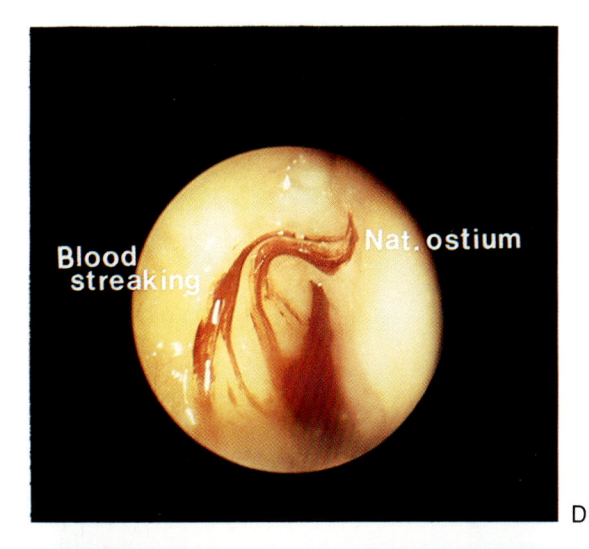

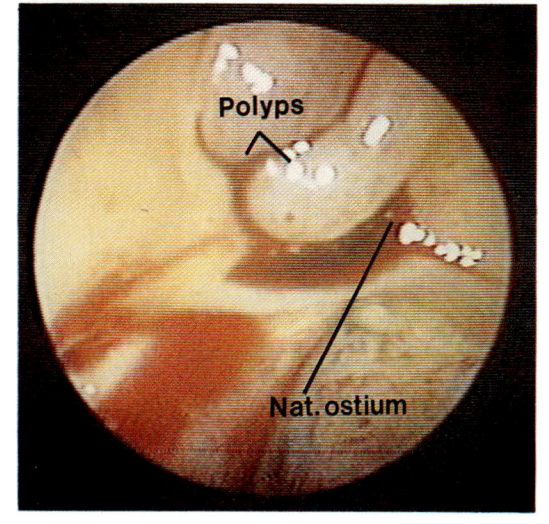

Figure 5–17. (*Continued*). **D**: Transcanine fossa endoscopic view of blood streaking toward the natural ostium. **E**: Close-up of **D** shows polyps blocking natural (Nat.) ostium. (Figure continued on next page.)

124 *Endoscopic Sinus Surgery*

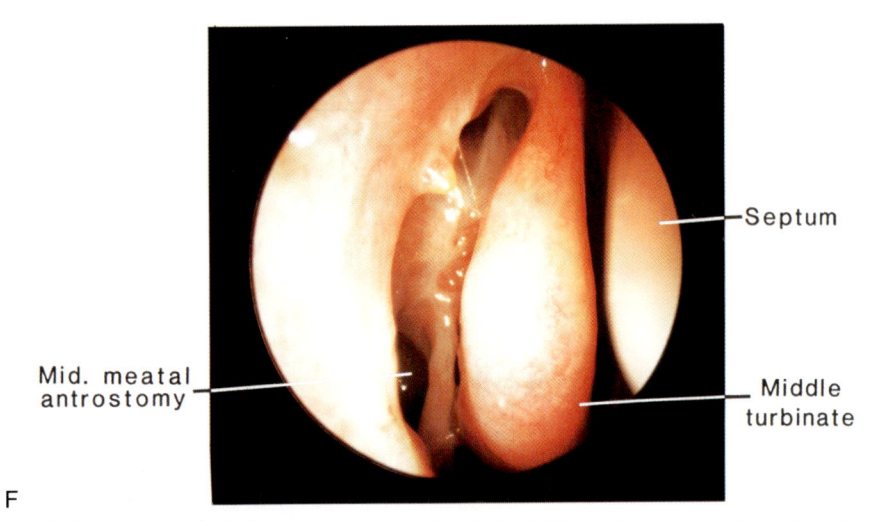

Figure 5–17. (*Continued*). **F**: Endoscopic view of right middle (Mid.) meatus 6 weeks after endoscopic sinus surgery shows mucosa in ethmoid cavity and large, patent middle meatal antrostomy created by connecting the accessory ostium in the posterior fontanelle with the natural ostium to restore normal pattern of mucociliary flow. Patient was freed of sinus symptoms.

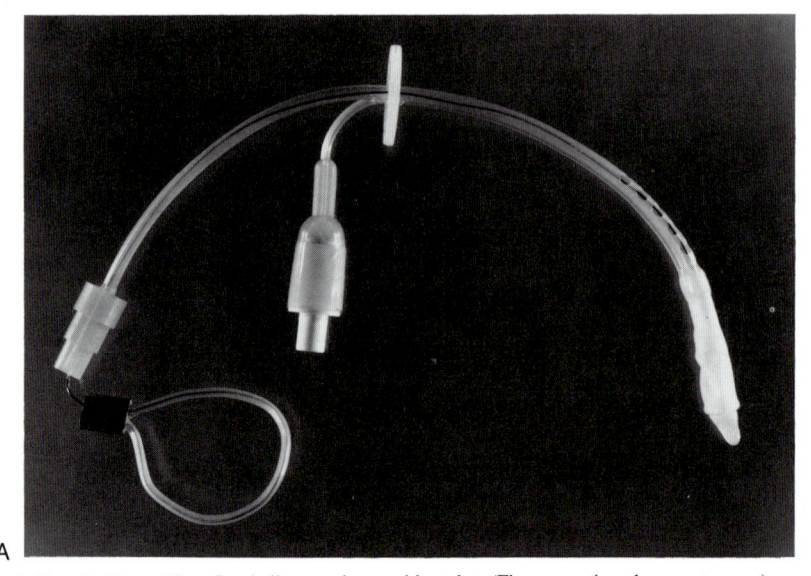

Figure 5–18. **A**: Xomed Post Pac balloon catheter with stylet. (Figure continued on next page.)

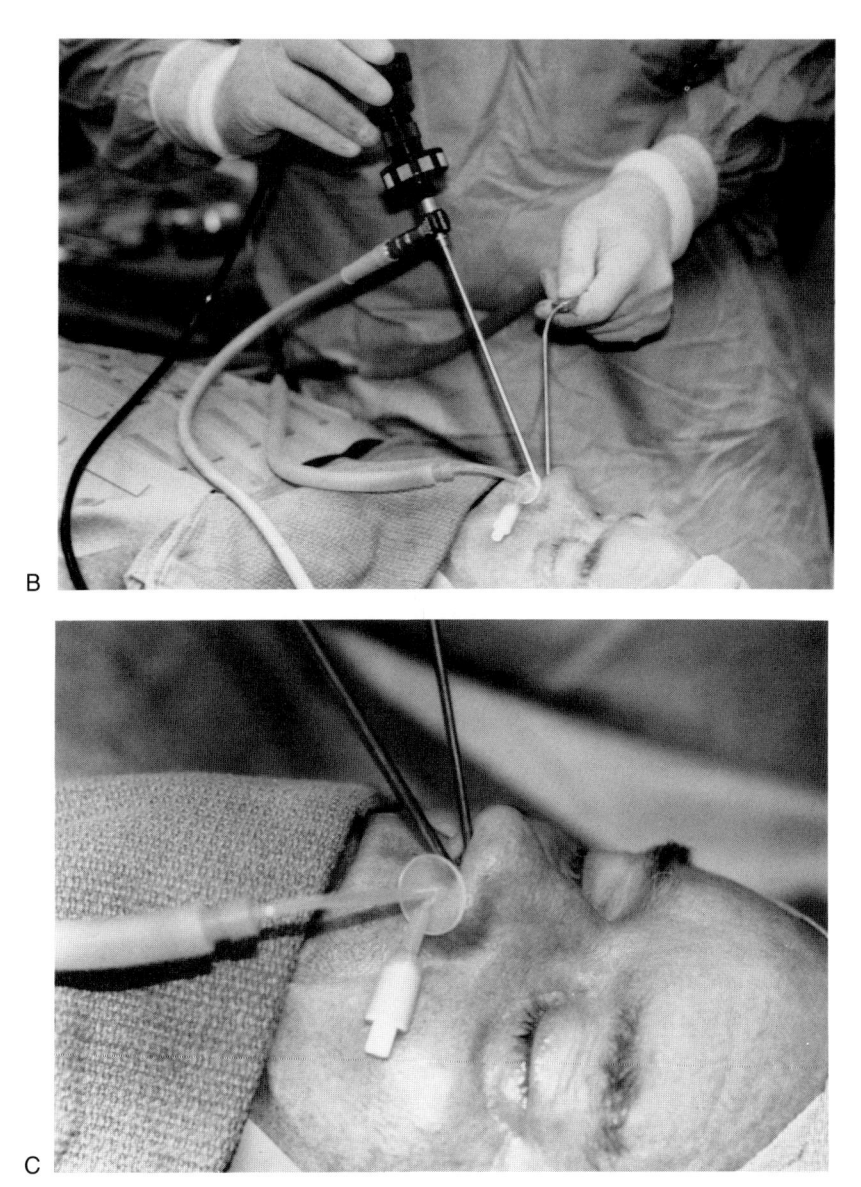

Figure 5–18. (*Continued*). **B**: Balloon catheter held in position by Silastic shroud abutted gently against the nostril in patient under local anesthesia. Catheter is connected to suction to keep patient's nasopharynx free of blood and irrigating solution that accumulate during ESS. **C**: Catheter and shroud can easily be moved aside to allow passage and manipulation of endoscopic surgery instruments. (Reprinted with permission from May et al.[8])

catheter is placed along the floor of the nose past the posterior choana and then inflated with no more than 5 cc saline (a greater amount may rupture the balloon). After inflation, the catheter is pulled back so that the balloon obstructs the posterior choana. The end of the catheter has perforations and is attached to suction to clear any secretions that pass by the balloon (Fig. 5–18B, C).

The Wigand Technique

Wigand[13] described an endonasal endoscopic approach that involves as a first step removing a portion of the middle turbinate to expose the ethmoid sphenoid complex. This approach is very similar to one described by Goldman[14] except that it is performed with endoscopes rather than headlight and speculum. The approach to the sinuses described by Kennedy et al[1,2] and Stammberger[3] leaves the middle turbinate undisturbed because visualization of the operative field is usually excellent with this technique, and the intact middle turbinate protects the cribriform plate from inadvertent injury from manipulation of instruments in this area.

In some patients, however, the middle turbinate may be absent, perhaps as a result of previous surgery, massive polyposis, or destruction by disease. Extensive disease may also obliterate surgical landmarks such as the uncinate process and bulla ethmoidalis. In such cases it may not be wise or effective to probe for the maxillary sinus ostium to establish the location of the orbit, and the Wigand approach may be safer. Because the ethmoid labyrinth widens posteriorly (see Chapter 1 for detailed anatomy), once the surgeon has removed the anterior portion of the middle turbinate he or she will have good visualization of a larger space, and thus will be able to manipulate instruments with less risk to vital neighboring structures.

To enter the posterior ethmoid cells safely in this circumstance, the surgeon should first identify key landmarks. The nasal septum, posterior nasal choana, and posterior attachment of the middle turbinate can be used to locate the anterior wall of the sphenoid sinus (Fig. 1–19B). This identification should be confirmed by penetrating the anterior wall of the sphenoid. Then, the surgeon knows that just anterior to the sphenoid sinus and at the level of the roof of the sphenoid sinus lies the roof of the ethmoid sinus. Thus oriented, the surgeon can locate and enter the posterior ethmoid cells.

Choice of Approach

No single approach to the paranasal sinuses will be appropriate in every case. For this reason, the endonasal sinus surgeon must be familiar with a variety of approaches so that he or she can use the one that will most effectively and safely result in removal of disease, reestablishment of sinus aeration, restoration of mucociliary flow, and, most importantly, relief of symptoms.

ANESTHESIA FROM THE SURGEON'S POINT OF VIEW

Anesthesia techniques and medications for local anesthesia with sedation (monitored anesthesia care [MAC]) and general anesthesia during sinus surgery were presented in

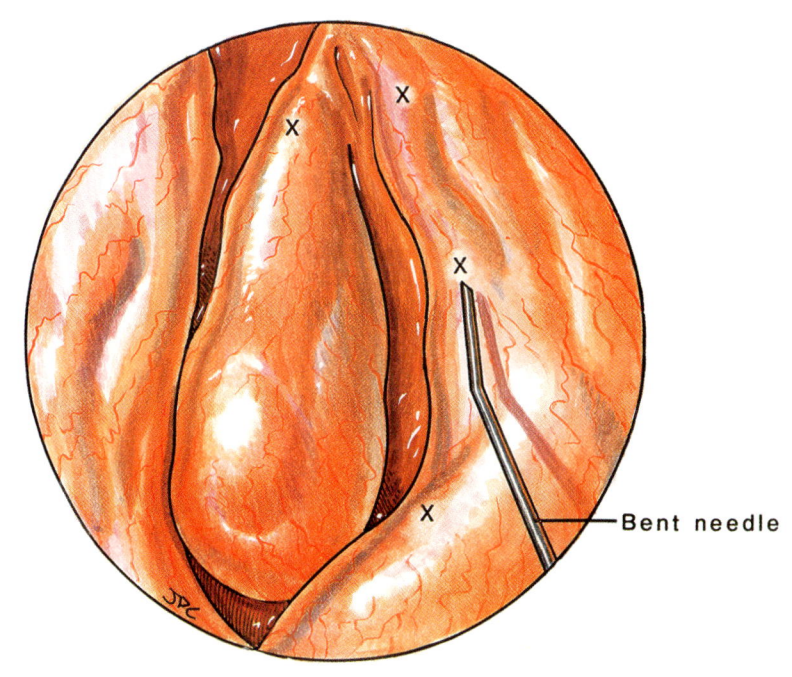

Figure 5–19. Endoscopic view of left lateral nasal wall showing sites for injection of 1% lidocaine and 1/100,000 epinephrine. Bending the tip of the needle is helpful in placing the injections where desired.

Chapter 4. This section presents considerations for the surgeon as he or she participates in the selection of anesthetic technique and the use of local anesthesia.

Choice of Anesthesia for Endoscopic Sinus Surgery

The decision to use MAC or general anesthesia for sinus surgery is based on the planned extent of surgery; the patient's medical, surgical, and anesthesia history; and the patient's preference for one or the other technique.

Most patients whose sinus disease is minimal are candidates for MAC. As mentioned in Chapter 4, MAC has two advantages over general anesthesia: (1) the patient can and will warn the surgeon by complaining of pain when dissection approaches the lamina papyracea, roof of the ethmoid sinus, or face of the sphenoid sinus; and (2) day-of-surgery discharge is more likely with local than with general anesthesia. For these reasons, local anesthesia with sedation is recommended for patients whose sinus disease is limited to the uncinate process, bulla ethmoidalis, and anterior ethmoid cells and for those who have not had previous sinus surgery.

Some patients who have undergone sinus surgery previously, however, request general rather than local anesthesia. In many cases these patients received inadequate anesthesia for a Caldwell-Luc procedure, creation of a nasal antral window, or polypectomy, and they do not want to repeat that painful experience. General anesthesia is also appropriate for (1) some patients with massive polyposis, (2) patients with suppurative sinusitis, (3) children, (4) patients with a great deal of scar tissue from previous surgery, (5) patients, such as those with extensive disease, whose surgery is expected to last longer than 2 hours, and (6) patients with reactive airway disease (asthma, ASA triad), to protect the airway from possible aspirated secretions that may lead to laryngobronchospasm (this complication occurs more often in such patients when sinus surgery is performed under local anesthesia; see Chapter 7).

Vasoconstriction and Local Anesthesia

The surgeon applies vasoconstrictive and local anesthetic agents for sinus surgery.

Vasoconstrictors

The 0.05% oxymetazoline spray applied before the patient was brought to the operating room provides sufficient decongestion of nasal mucosa when general anesthesia will be used. When MAC will be used for sinus surgery, cocaine is applied topically to promote vasoconstriction and for local anesthesia. For greater safety, the cocaine solution should be colored with methylene blue to prevent its confusion with one of the injectable agents, such as lidocaine, used during surgery.

Cocaine is applied by placing cotton pledgets (Neuropatties, Codman & Shurtleff, Randolph MA) in the cocaine solution, compressing them to drain excess solution, and placing two pledgets in each nasal cavity so that they cover and lie against the mucosa of the septum and turbinates. The pledgets should cover the area from the roof to the floor of the nose and extend posteriorly to the nasopharynx.

This area is innervated by the anterior ethmoid nerve and branches of the sphenopalatine nerve. The *anterior ethmoid nerve*, a terminal branch of the nasociliary branch of the ophthalmic division of the trigeminal nerve, courses with the anterior ethmoid artery through the orbit and into the anterior cranial fossa, runs along the olfactory groove, and, under cover of the nasofrontal bone, emerges just above the anterosuperior attachment of the middle turbinate to innervate the anterolateral nasal wall (see Chapter 1). Cocaine-soaked pledgets are usually effective in anesthetizing the area of the anterior ethmoid nerve.

The branches of the *sphenopalatine ganglion*, however, because they are located lateral to the posterior attachment of the middle turbinate, may not be as well anesthetized. This is particularly true when turbinoseptal variations prevent the pledgets from lying directly against the mucosa.

The cocaine-soaked pledgets are left in place for 5 minutes and then removed.

Local Anesthetic

A solution of 1% lidocaine with 1/100,000 epinephrine is used for local anesthesia. With a 21 gauge, 1.5 inch needle that has been slightly bent so that the tip can be placed just in front of the attachment of the uncinate process, four sites in the lateral wall of the nose on each side are injected with this solution, as indicated in Figure 5–19. A total of less than 1 cc should be injected on each side to cause blanching but not ballooning of tissues.

To block pain impulses from the increased concentration of pain fibers around the natural ostium of the maxillary sinus and face of the sphenoid sinus, anesthetic is injected into the second division of the trigeminal nerve. This injection is accomplished by passing the needle through the buccal sulcus into the pterygopalatine fossa or into the face of the sphenoid sinus just above the posterior nasal choana and lateral to the posterior attachment of the middle turbinate.

Ten minutes should be allowed for vasoconstrictor and anesthetic agents to promote maximal hemostasis and anesthesia.

Monitoring for Sinus Surgery

Regardless of the type of anesthesia provided, the patient's blood pressure, pulse, cardiac rhythm, and oxygen saturation (which should be kept above 90%) are monitored. The monitor that displays these variables should be in full view of the surgeon as well as the anesthesiologist (Fig. 5–3A) so that the surgeon can check the patient's blood pressure frequently.

ENDOSCOPIC SINUS SURGERY: STEP-BY-STEP

Management of each paranasal sinus structure will be discussed in the order that the structures are encountered during ESS. The terms "anterior OMC" and "posterior OMC" refer to anatomic compartments within the ethmoid complex. As described in Chapter 1, the anterior OMC is anterior and inferior to the basal lamella, whereas the posterior OMC is posterior and superior to the basal lamella. The term "OMC" refers to the entire ethmoid complex, both anterior and posterior OMC.

Nasal Septum

A nasal septoplasty is performed if the septum is deviated enough to interfere with the approach to the OMC on either or both sides. As a rule, septoplasty is performed if a 4 mm endoscope cannot be passed between the lateral wall of the nose and the septum in the region of the middle turbinate after the nasal mucosa has been decongested.

If bilateral OMC disease is present with a deviated septum, surgery may be performed on the open side before the septoplasty is performed and the obstructed OMC operated on. This is because, although septoplasty removes an anatomic obstacle to visibility, the mucosal edema and bleeding that may result from septoplasty can decrease visibility even more severely, especially when the video technique is used. If obstruction is such that the septoplasty must be performed first, blood that accumulates in the field should be washed away periodically with saline.

When septoplasty is performed to improve access to the OMC, bone and cartilage is removed from the bony-cartilaginous junction. This site is about 3 to 4 cm from the nostril and usually at the level of the anterior portion of the middle turbinate. The sharp edge of a Cottle elevator is used to separate bone from cartilage, and the perpendicular plate of the ethmoid is divided as high as possible with a heavy, angled, nasal septum scissors. Another cut is made with the scissors along the inferior border of the septum. Using scissors decreases the risk that the cribriform plate will be cracked and a cerebrospinal fluid (CSF) leak created. A Ferris-Smith forceps is used to remove the sectioned segment of septum.

If the septum continues to obstruct the view between the middle turbinate and lateral nasal wall, a long, wide nasal speculum is placed in the nasal cavity on the side where surgery will be performed (Fig. 5–5C). Either the assistant can hold the speculum or a self-retaining speculum holder may be used (Xomed). Use of the speculum is less than ideal because it decreases access for the endoscope and instruments.

Uncinate Process

The uncinate process and bulla ethmoidalis are exposed by using the back of a sinus sickle knife to retract the middle turbinate toward the nasal septum (Fig. 5–20). If the uncinate process is displaced medially and the infundibulum narrowed, as may occur in association with a concha bullosa, deviated septum, or hypoplastic maxillary sinus, there is risk of penetrating the orbit. This can be avoided by placing the double-ended maxillary sinus ostium seeker through the hiatus semilunaris into the infundibulum and displacing the uncinate medially toward the middle turbinate (Fig. 5–21A). Then the sickle knife is used to remove the uncinate process as close as possible to its attachment to the posterior edge of the lacrimal duct ridge. The knife is moved firmly, with sawing action, from anterosuperior to posteroinferior while care is taken not to lacerate or avulse the mucosa of the adjoining superior turbinate (Fig. 5–21B).

The cut is extended posteriorly along a line parallel to the lower border of the middle turbinate, and the uncinate process is displaced toward the middle turbinate. The uncinate process can be freed using the two-handed technique by using suction held in one hand to retract the middle turbinate toward the septum and with the other hand grasping the superior attachment of the uncinate with a small Blakesley ethmoid forceps and twisting the uncinate process while pushing it posteriorly and inferiorly (Fig. 5–22A, B). Note that the articulating arm of the Blakesley forceps is directed laterally.

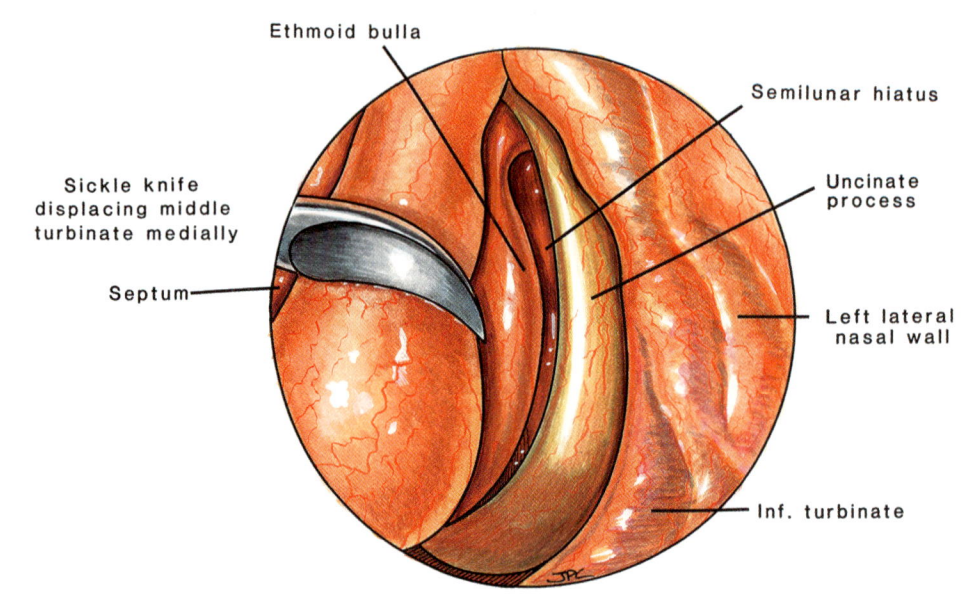

Figure 5–20. Left middle turbinate retracted with a sickle knife toward the septum to bring uncinate process and ethmoid bulla into view. Inf: inferior.

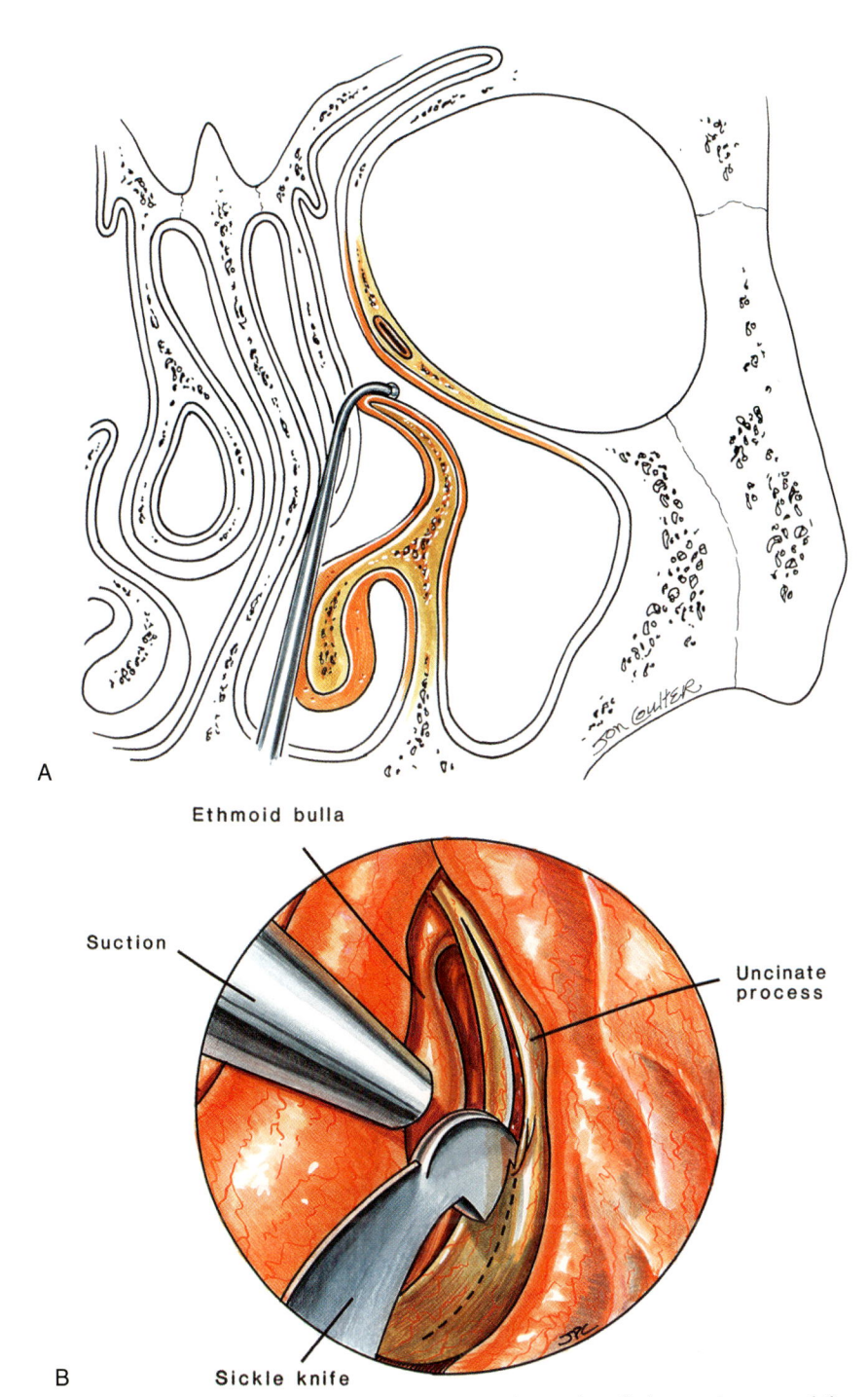

Figure 5–21. **A**: Double-ended maxillary sinus ostium seeker used to displace uncinate toward the middle turbinate. **B**: Left middle turbinate retracted with suction cannula held in surgeon's left hand and sickle knife held in surgeon's right hand to incise the uncinate process. The assistant is manipulating the endoscope.

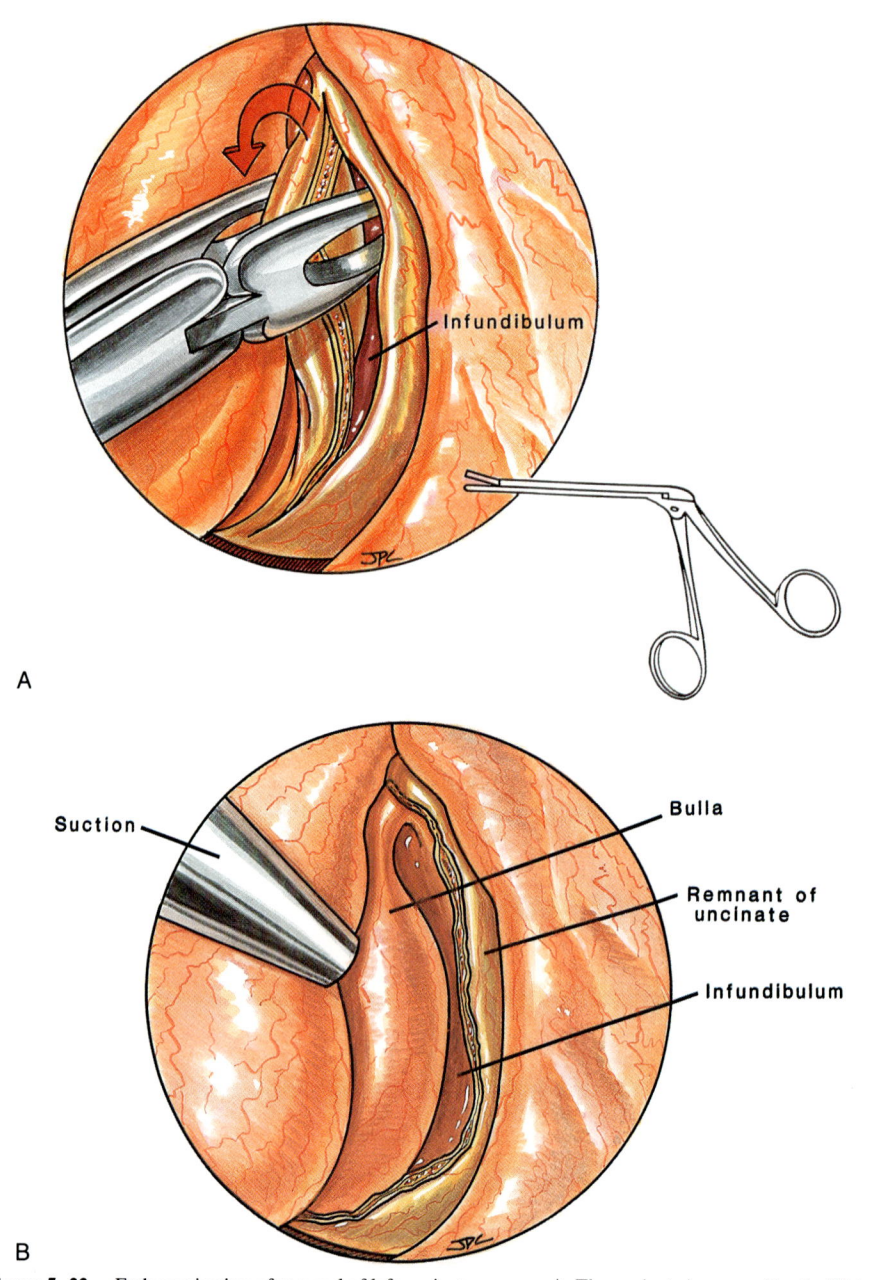

Figure 5–22. Endoscopic view of removal of left uncinate process. **A**: The uncinate is grasped by the Blakesley forceps, articulating blade toward the orbit, and as the forceps are closed the uncinate is twisted, pushed back, and turned out. **B**: Endoscopic view of uncinate process remnant. Bulla: Bulla ethmoidalis. (Figure continued on next page.)

Endoscopic Sinus Surgery 133

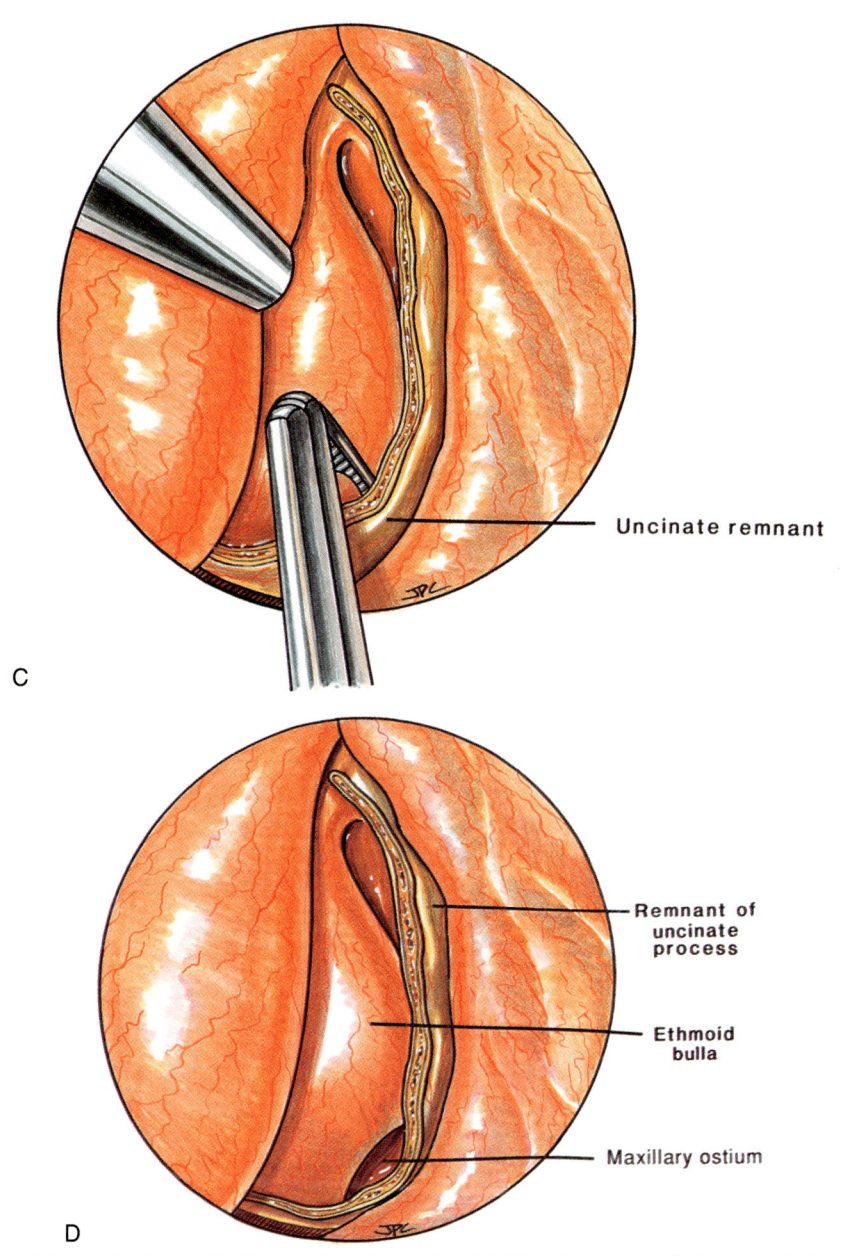

Figure 5-22. (*Continued*). **C**: The maxillary sinus ostium is hidden from view until the remnant of uncinate process overlying the ostium is removed with a Stammberger side-biting punch. **D**: Maxillary sinus ostium is visible once remnant of uncinate process has been removed.

If the maxillary sinus ostium cannot be visualized after removal of the uncinate process, it is usually because a remnant of the uncinate process is obstructing the view. This remnant can be removed with a side-cutting Stammberger antrum punch (Fig. 5–22C, D).

Maxillary Sinus Ostium

Kennedy et al[1,2] and Stammberger[3] recommend penetrating the bulla ethmoidalis after the uncinate process has been removed. We prefer to identify the maxillary sinus ostium first for two reasons, as noted previously: (1) assuring or reestablishing patency of the maxillary ostium and nasoantral canal is essential to the success of OMC surgery (Fig. 5–23A) and (2) the consistent and close relationship of the ostium to the orbit increases the likelihood that the orbit will be penetrated during surgery in this region (Figs. 1–4, 1–6, and 1–12).[9] An effective way to prevent this complication is to locate the ostium and then the orbit.

The maxillary sinus ostium can usually be visualized after the uncinate process has been removed. When the maxillary sinus ostium has been identified, it is cannulated with an olive-tip, 3 mm, short, curved Eicken antrum sinus cannula (Fig. 5–23B).

If the ostium is not readily identified, a double-ended maxillary sinus ostium seeker is inserted gently into the nose and directed inferoanteriorly, behind the uncinate process remnant and above the superior border of the inferior turbinate, while the orbit is palpated to detect movement. This maneuver permits the surgeon to insert the probe into the maxillary sinus ostium without injuring the orbit (Fig. 5–23C).

The maxillary sinus ostium may be enlarged by extending the posterior wall of the maxillary ostium to the posterior fontanelle. To prevent ostium stenosis, however, the surgeon should take care not to remove tissue circumferentially. Tissue also should be removed with care anterior to the ostium, especially with a side-cutting antrum punch, to avoid the possibility of injuring the lacrimal sac or nasolacrimal duct, which lie anterior to the ostium and the uncinate process.

Bulla Ethmoidalis

The safest way to enter the bulla ethmoidalis is to penetrate its inferomedial wall with a Blakesley ethmoid forceps. The 45° Struempel-Voss upturned ethmoid forceps (Fig. 5–24) can be used to remove the anterosuperior lip of bone on the bulla, an important landmark because just anterosuperior to this lamella is the anterior ethmoid artery (Fig. 5–25). The anterosuperior wall of the bulla ethmoidalis also marks the junction between the roof of the ethmoid sinus and the nasofrontal recess. This landmark is so useful that in cases where exploration of the nasofrontal recess is planned it is preserved until after the nasofrontal recess and frontal sinus isthmus are entirely exposed.

Basal Lamella

Because disease often appears to be less severe and extensive on CT than becomes apparent at surgery, surgery generally extends one lamella beyond the area involved on CT scans.

Endoscopic Sinus Surgery   135

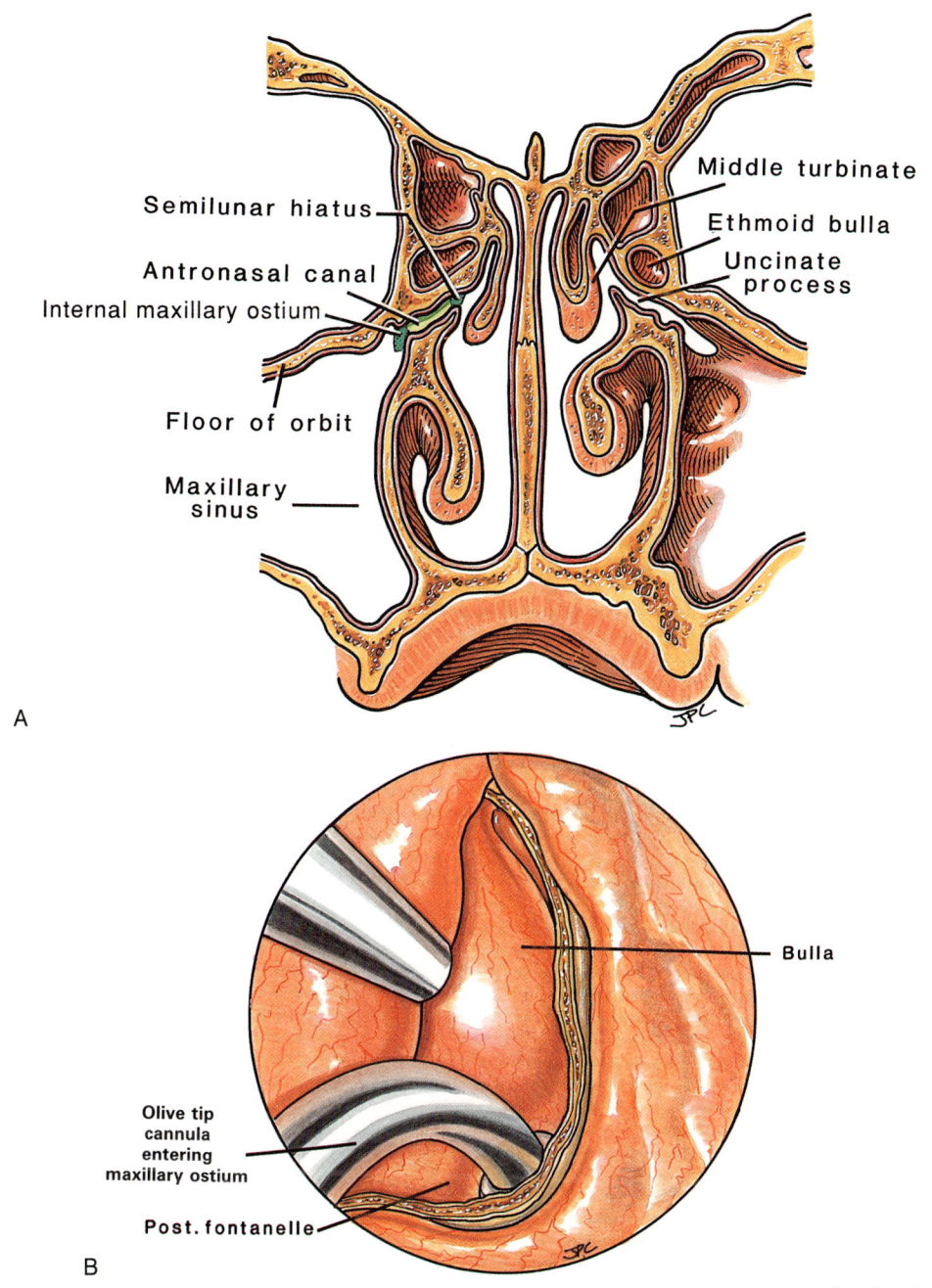

Figure 5–23. **A**: Relationships of structures in ostiomeatal complex to nasoantral canal and orbit. **B**: Olive-tip cannula in left maxillary sinus ostium (uncinate process has been removed). Post.: posterior. (Figure continued on next page.)

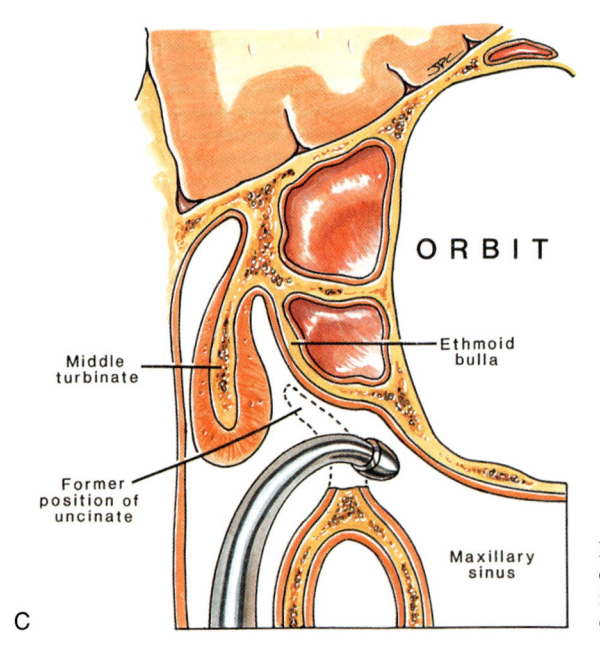

Figure 5–23. (*Continued*). **C**: Double-ended maxillary ostium sinus seeker inserted into nasoantral canal to reach maxillary sinus ostium.

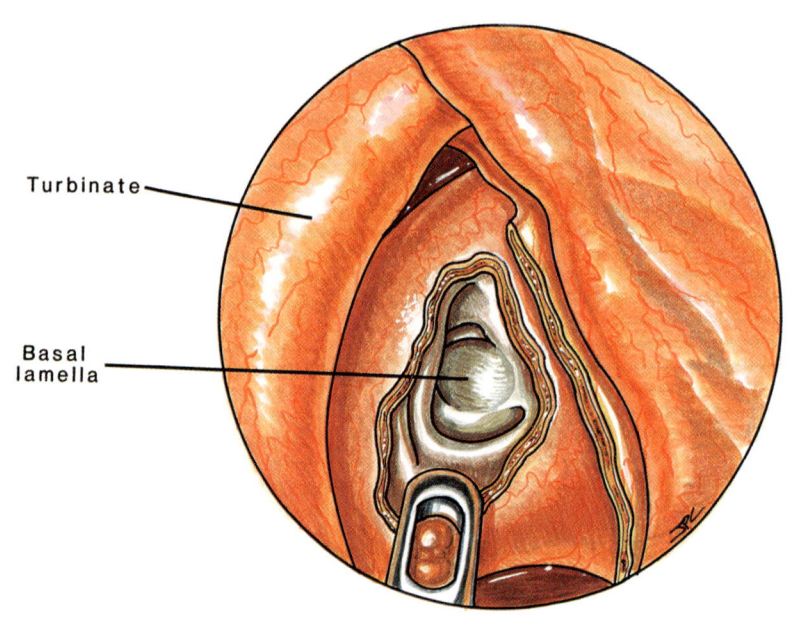

Figure 5–24. Left bulla ethmoidalis opened wide.

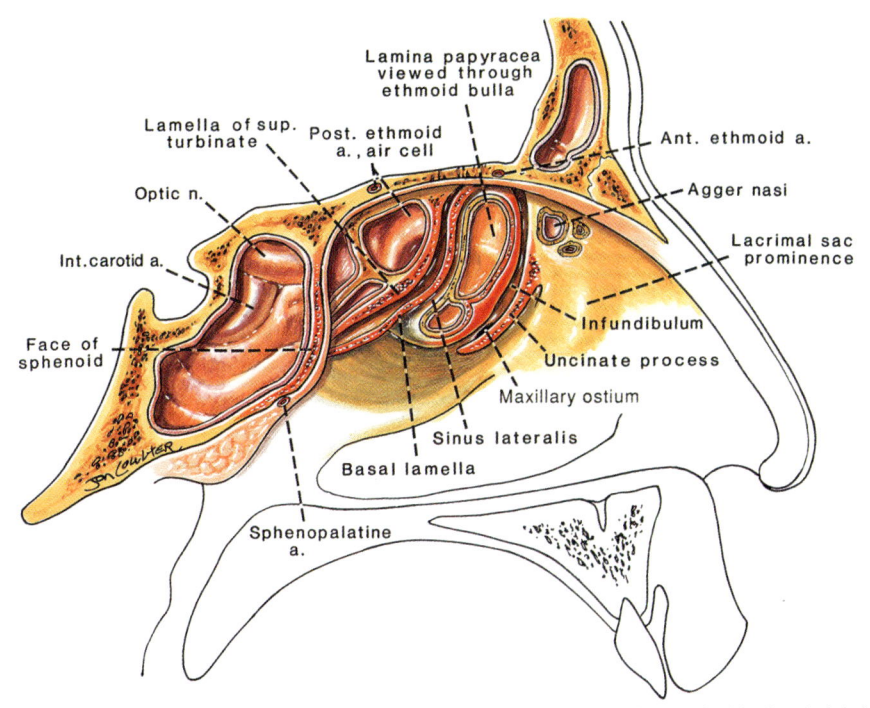

Figure 5–25. Left lateral nasal wall after completion of surgical dissection with key surgical landmarks labeled.

Thus, if diffuse disease is evident in the anterior ethmoid cells on CT, the surgeon may plan to extend surgery into the posterior ethmoid cells by penetrating the basal lamella.

When the contents of the bulla ethmoidalis have been removed, the basal lamella may be identified (Figs. 5–24 through 5–26) as a bluish gray, sloping, thin, on occasion transparent, bony septum between the roof of the bulla ethmoidalis and the posterior ethmoid cells that lie superior and posterior to the bulla ethmoidalis.

The basal lamella is penetrated posteriorly and inferiorly through the strut between the middle turbinate and the lamina papyracea (Fig. 5–26), and the posterior ethmoid cells are cleared of diseased mucosa.

Roof of the Ethmoid Sinus

After diseased mucosa has been removed from the posterior ethmoid cells, the roof of the ethmoid sinus is viewed and palpated (Fig. 5–27).

To warn the surgeon of the depth of surgical exposure in this area, each straight instrument is marked with a green, a yellow, and a red band placed 5, 7, and 9 cm, respectively, from its tip (Fig. 5–28).[15] By referring to measurements made on the preoperative lateral sinus roentgenograph (Figs. 5–1 and 5–29)[5] and noting what colored bands on the instruments are still visible outside the nares, the endoscopic sinus surgeon can remain aware of the depth of penetration.

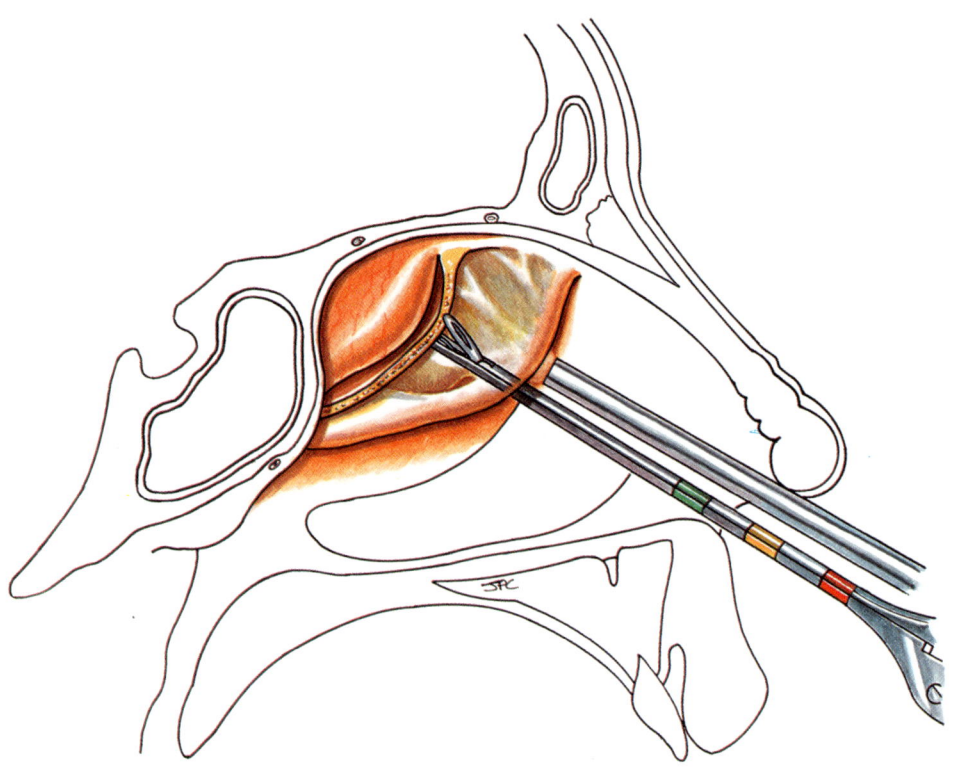

Figure 5-26. Basal lamella is identified and palpated.

Endoscopic Sinus Surgery **139**

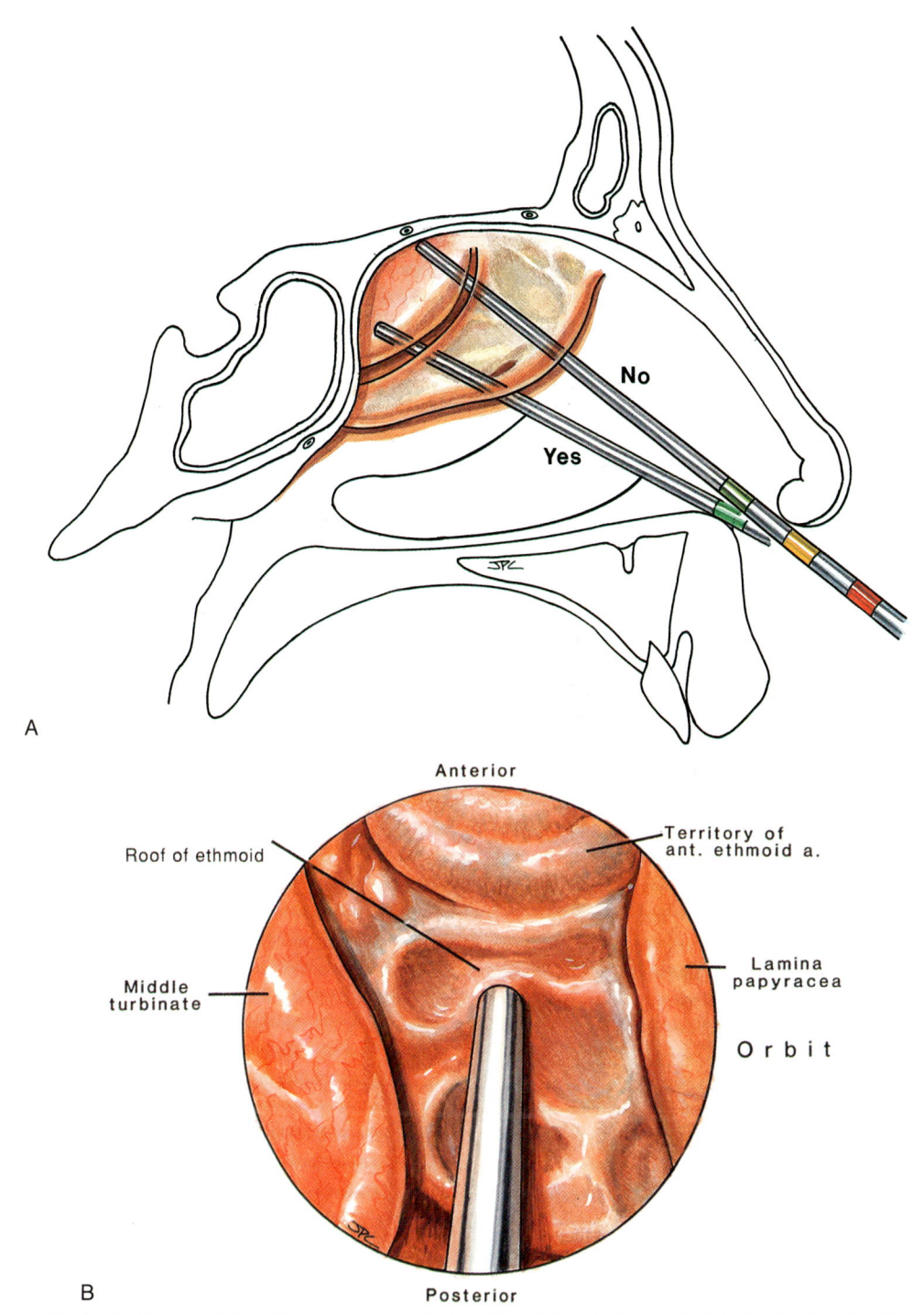

Figure 5–27. **A**: Safe ("yes") way to penetrate the basal lamella is posteriorly and inferiorly rather than ("no") anteriorly and superiorly. This is shown by the endoscopes passed through the opening made safely ("yes") and at high risk for penetrating the skull base ("no"). Note that the distance between the basal lamella and skull base is greater with the safer route. **B**: Roof of the ethmoid sinus is visible after basal lamella and posterior ethmoid cells have been removed. ant.: anterior; a.: artery.

140   *Endoscopic Sinus Surgery*

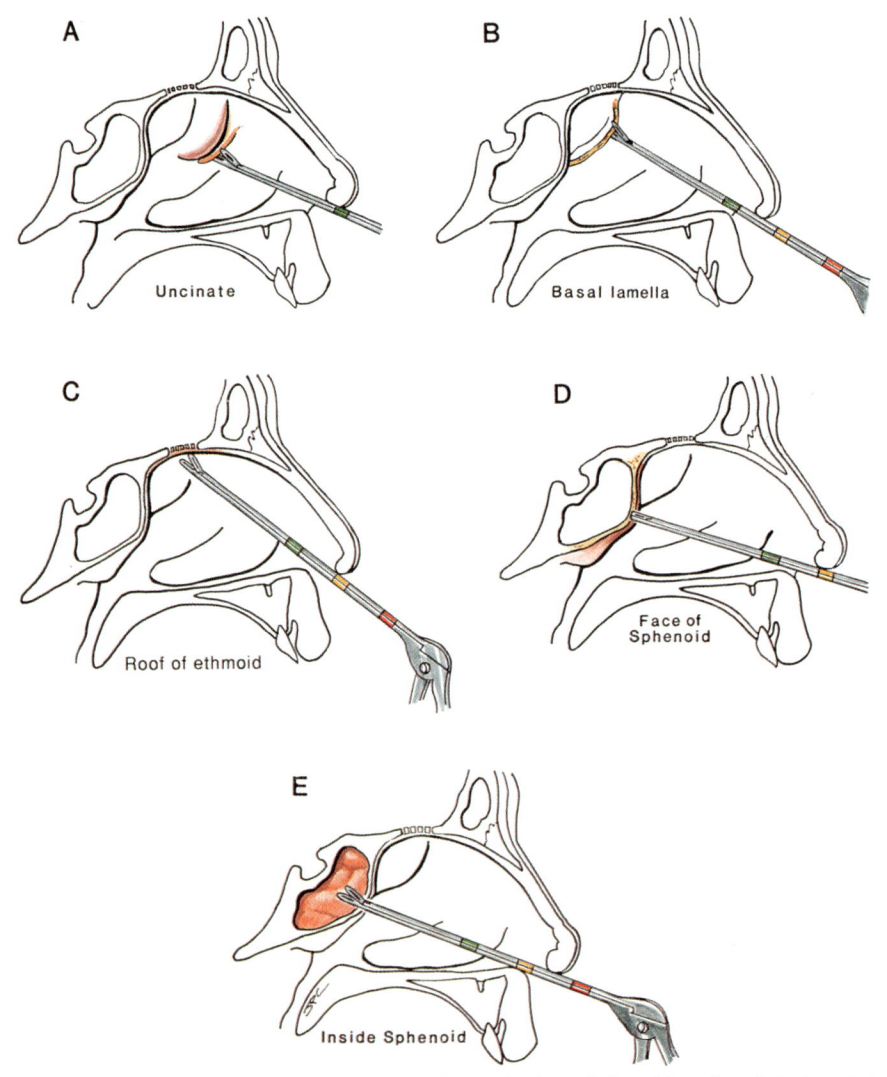

Figure 5–28. Instruments are marked with green, yellow, and red tape 5, 7, and 9 cm from their tips to help the surgeon locate key structures during endoscopic sinus surgery. **A**: When the instrument is inserted to the depth of the green tape, its tip is at the uncinate process. **B**: When the instrument is inserted to between the green and yellow tapes, its tip is at the basal lamella. **C**: When the yellow tape is at the nares, the tip of the instrument is at the roof of the ethmoid sinus and at the face of the sphenoid sinus (**D**). **E**: When the instrument is inserted to between the yellow and red tapes and held at an angle of 30° from the floor of the nose, its tip is in the sphenoid sinus.

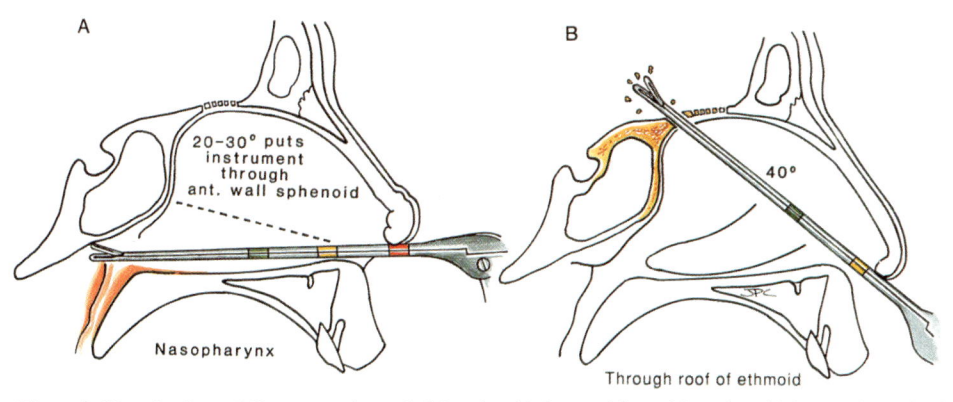

Figure 5–29. Angles and distances to the roof of the ethmoid sinus and face of the sphenoid sinus as determined on a preoperative plain lateral radiograph are used during surgery to prevent penetration of the roof of the ethmoid sinus. The face of the sphenoid sinus is between 25° and 35° from the floor of the nose. **A**: If the red tape on the forceps is at the nares and the angle of the forceps from the floor of the nose is less than 25°, the tip of the forceps is probably in the nasopharynx. **B**: If the red tape on the forceps is at the nares and the angle of the forceps from the floor of the nose is 40° or greater, the tip of the forceps has most likely penetrated the roof of the ethmoid sinus.

The green (5 cm) or yellow (7 cm) band should always be visible until surgery reaches the roof of the ethmoid sinus or the face of the sphenoid sinus is approached. If the yellow band is just visible outside the nares and the instrument makes an angle of greater than 40° with the floor of the nose, the tip of the instrument is at the roof of the ethmoid sinus (Fig. 5–29B).

An upbiting Kerrison forceps is used to extend dissection from the posterior ethmoid cells anteriorly along the roof of the ethmoid sinus to the nasofrontal recess (Fig. 5–30). Next, a downbiting Kerrison forceps is used to extend the dissection along the roof of the ethmoid sinus, from anterior to posterior, until the face of the sphenoid sinus is reached. The Kerrison forceps are safer than ethmoid forceps for this step in the procedure because the flat end of the forceps is used to palpate the roof of the ethmoid sinus; this blunt end presents less risk of penetrating the dura while the jaws are manipulated to nip off ridges of bone. A special effort is made to stay close to the orbital side and away from the superior attachment of the middle turbinate, because the bone over the roof of the ethmoid is thicker close to the orbit as a result of fusion of the frontal bone in this area. In contrast, the bone toward the middle turbinate may be paper thin and vulnerable to penetration and CSF leakage.

Lamina Papyracea

When the roof of the ethmoid sinus has been cleared of diseased mucosa or polyps, upturned ethmoid forceps are used to expose the lateral wall of the ethmoid complex, the lamina papyracea. The lamina papyracea appears yellow because that is the color of the orbital fat that shows through this thin, transparent bony membrane separating the orbit from the ethmoid sinus. If the lamina papyracea is abraded by an instrument, vibrations may be felt by the surgeon's finger placed on the globe; dehiscence or inadvertent breaching of the lamina papyracea may be noted by looking at the area through the endoscope while putting light pressure on the globe (the Stankiewicz maneuver).[16]

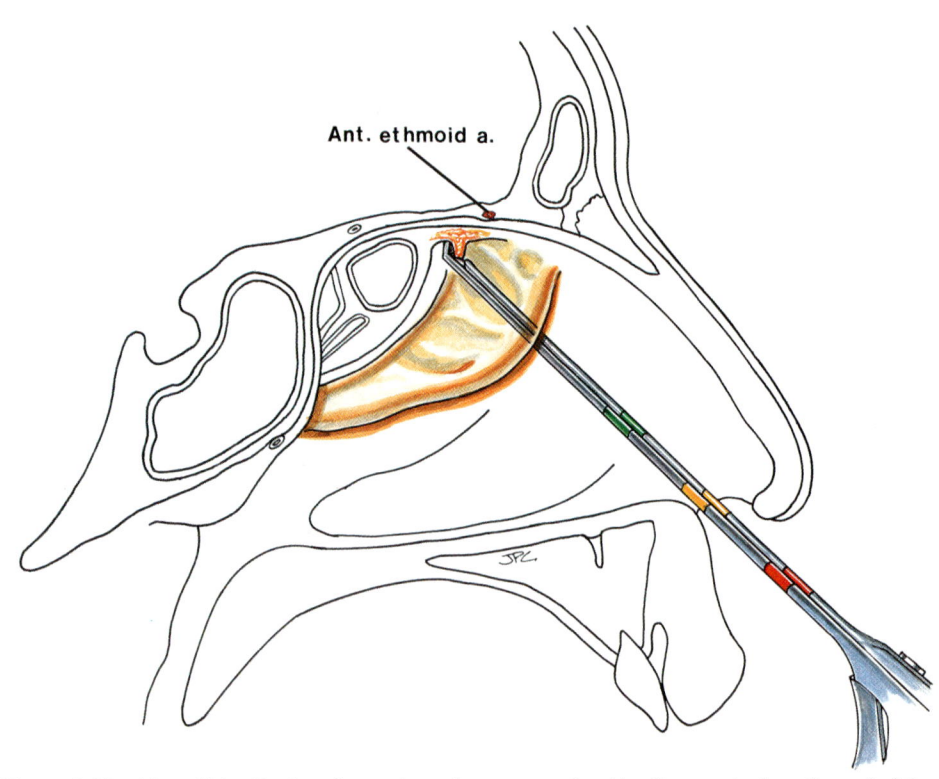

Figure 5–30. The upbiting Kerrison forceps is used to remove ethmoid cell remnants along the roof of the ethmoid sinus. The surgeon is removing the anterosuperior remnant of the bulla ethmoidalis. Note the relationship of the remnant to the anterior (Ant.) ethmoid artery (a.).

Sphenoidotomy

The face of the sphenoid sinus is located during surgery by identifying the posterior attachment of the middle turbinate, the arch of the posterior choana, and the posterior aspect of the nasal septum (Fig. 5–31).

Sphenoidotomy is associated with significant risks, including leakage of CSF or penetration injury to the brain (Fig. 5–29B). The optic nerve and carotid artery are also at risk during surgery involving the sphenoid sinus (Fig. 5–32).

Preventing Complications

The first step in preventing these complications is careful assessment of axial CT scans as well as coronal CT scans and lateral and base x-ray views of the paranasal sinuses to determine the size and symmetry of the sphenoid sinuses and their relationship to the optic nerve and carotid artery.

Next, the angles and distances from surgical landmarks to the sphenoid sinuses should be determined on preoperative images and in the operating room. Angles and distances will

Endoscopic Sinus Surgery   143

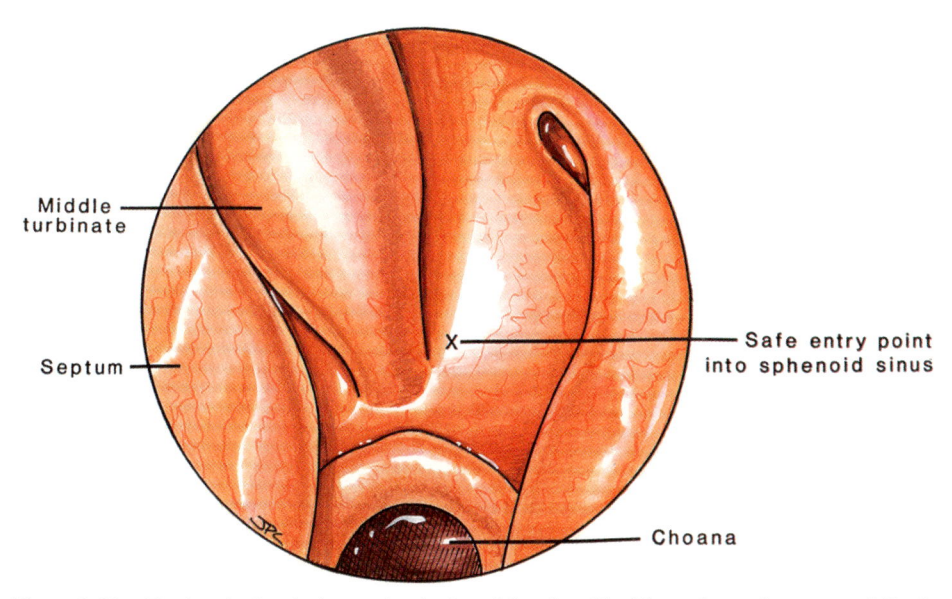

Figure 5–31. The three landmarks for entering the face of the sphenoid safely are the nasal septum medially, the posterior nasal choana inferiorly, and the posterior attachment of the middle turbinate.

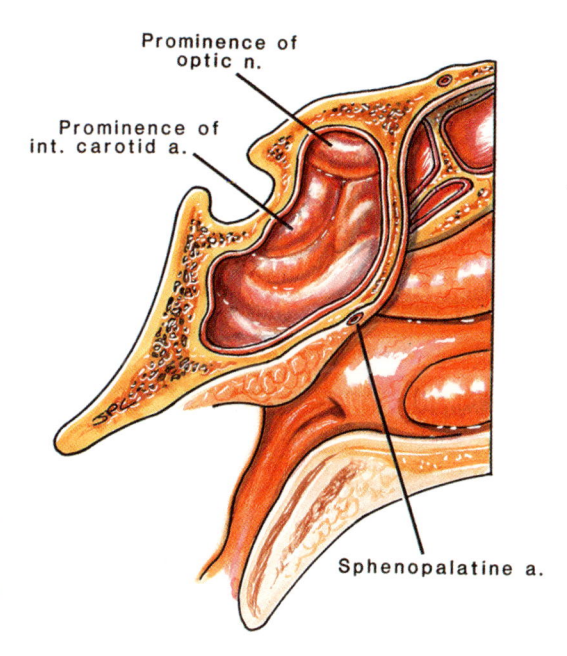

Figure 5–32. The internal (int.) carotid artery (a.) and optic nerve (n.) are prominent vital structures in the lateral wall of the sphenoid sinus. Note the relationship of the sphenopalatine artery at the inferior aspect of the front face of the sphenoid sinus.

vary among individuals, as well as by age and sex, and so these must be measured for each surgical candidate.[5] As a guide, however, the front face of the sphenoid sinus in adults is usually at a 30° angle from the hard palate and 7 cm posterior to the anterior nasal spine (Fig. 5–28E). If these measurements are not adequate to identify the anterior face of the sphenoid during surgery, C-arm fluoroscopy may be used to locate this landmark with certainty.

Procedure for Sphenoidotomy

The face of the sphenoid sinus is entered with a straight Blakesley forceps (Fig. 5–33) and the anterior wall is removed with downbiting and upbiting Kerrison forceps (Fig. 5–34). Bone can be removed safely from the superomedial and inferior walls of the sphenoid sinus; the superior portion of the lateral sphenoid wall is avoided, however, because the optic nerve and carotid artery are located there.

Extreme caution must be used when inserting instruments into the sphenoid sinus or removing material from the sinus. Suction may be used to remove polyps or debris from the sinus; only material removed in this way is grasped with a forceps. Fungal concretions within the sphenoid cavity can be extracted by first mobilizing them with an Eicken antrum cannula (Fig. 5–12) or a blunt Dandy nerve hook (3 mm, Codman & Shurtleff, item 38-1080) and then removing the debris with irrigation and suction.

The territory of the sphenopalatine artery lies inferior to the front face of the sphenoid sinus (Fig. 5–32), and this vessel can usually be protected by elevating mucosa from bone inferiorly, between the opening in the face of the sphenoid sinus and the posterior nasal choana. Active bleeding from the sphenopalatine artery can be controlled with a suction coagulator (Fig. 5–13).

Agger Nasi and Nasofrontal Recess

When the maxillary, anterior and posterior ethmoid, and sphenoid sinuses have been marsupialized, the surgeon's attention may be directed to the anterior attachment of the middle turbinate. This landmark identifies a safe entry point into the anterior extent of the nasofrontal recess. The agger nasi cells and lacrimal sac and duct are anterior to the anterior attachment of the middle turbinate (Fig. 5–35). Schaefer and Close[17] recommend using an upbiting Kerrison forceps to remove the anterolateral attachment of the middle turbinate to expose the agger nasi and nasofrontal recess. Because this technique may result in formation of adhesions between the anterior edge of the middle turbinate and the lateral nasal wall, with secondary obstruction of the nasofrontal recess, every effort is made to preserve the integrity of the mucosa over the arch found between the anterior attachment of the middle turbinate and the lateral nasal wall (Fig. 5–36).

The agger nasi may be seen as a bulge in the lateral nasal wall just anterior to the anterior attachment of the middle turbinate. These cells are opened and abnormal mucosa removed carefully (Fig. 5–37). The lacrimal sac, orbit, and anterior cranial fossa are protected from injury during surgery in the agger nasi by keeping the tips of the 45° or 90° ethmoid forceps in a vertical position rather than directing them medially or laterally (Fig. 5–37).

The nasofrontal recess can be viewed with a 0° or 30° endoscope (Fig. 5–38A). Enough polypoid tissue may be removed from this space to visualize the opening into the

Endoscopic Sinus Surgery **145**

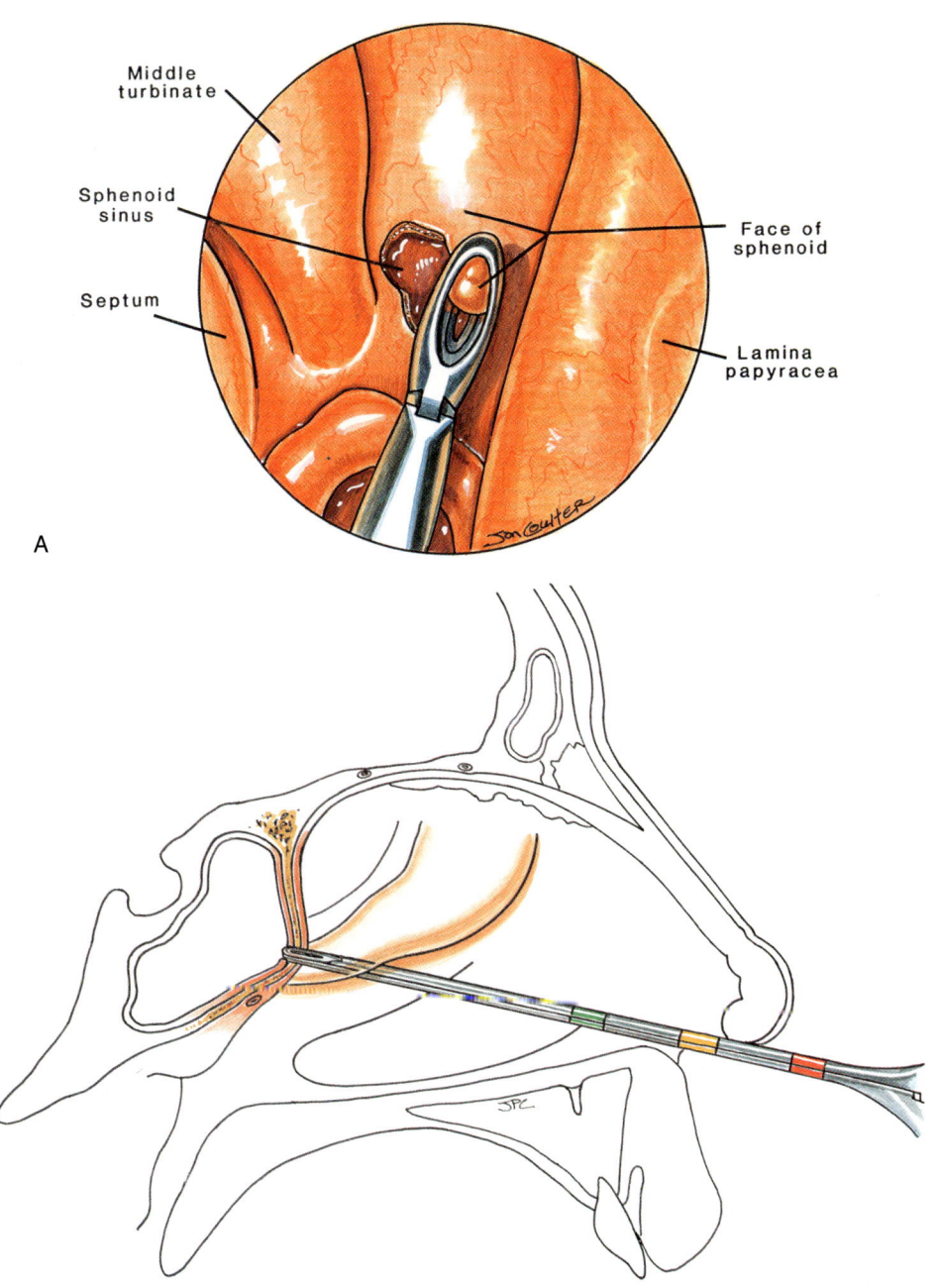

Figure 5–33. Penetrating the anterior face of the left sphenoid with Blakesley forceps. **A**: Endoscopic view at surgery. **B**: Sagittal view.

146   *Endoscopic Sinus Surgery*

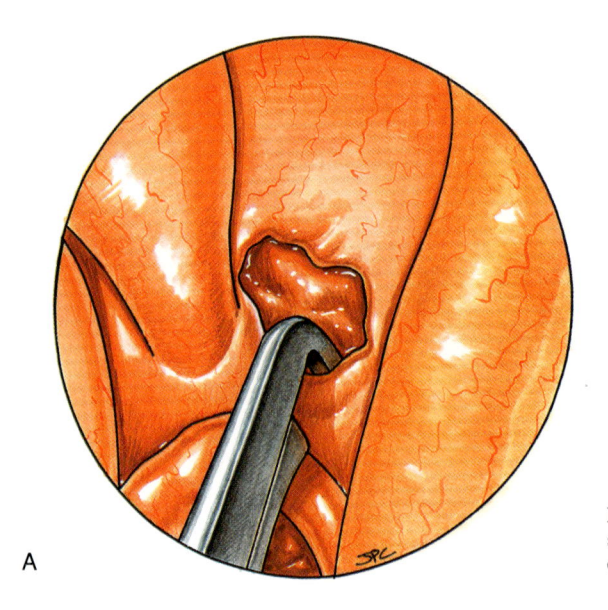

Figure 5–34. Front wall of left sphenoid sinus removed with Kerrison forceps. **A**: Endoscopic view at surgery. **B**: Sagittal view.

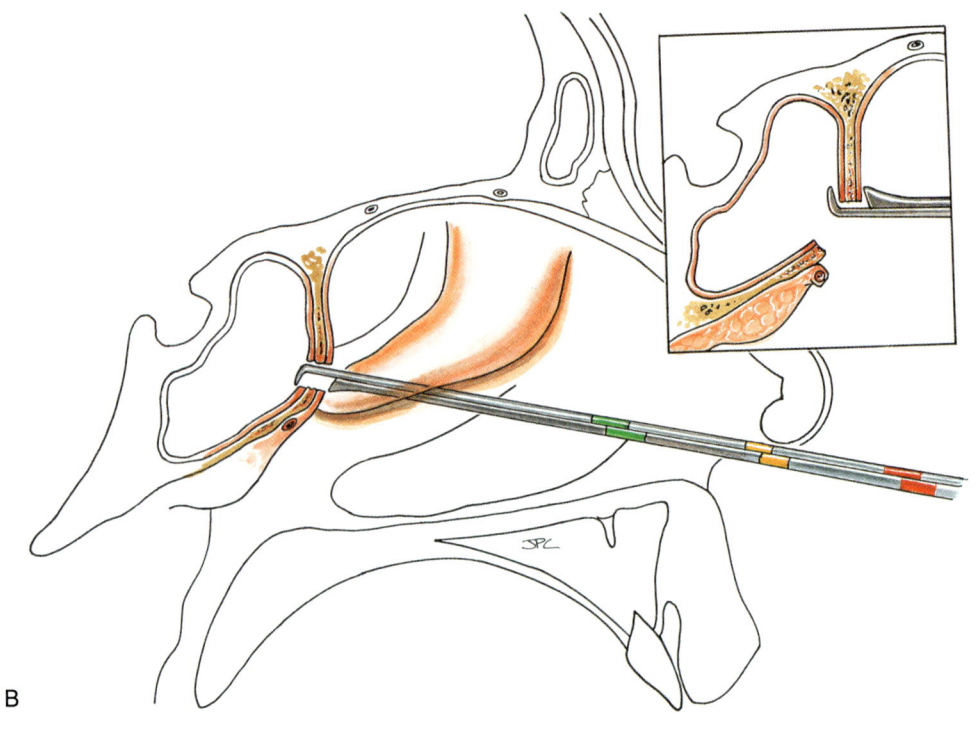

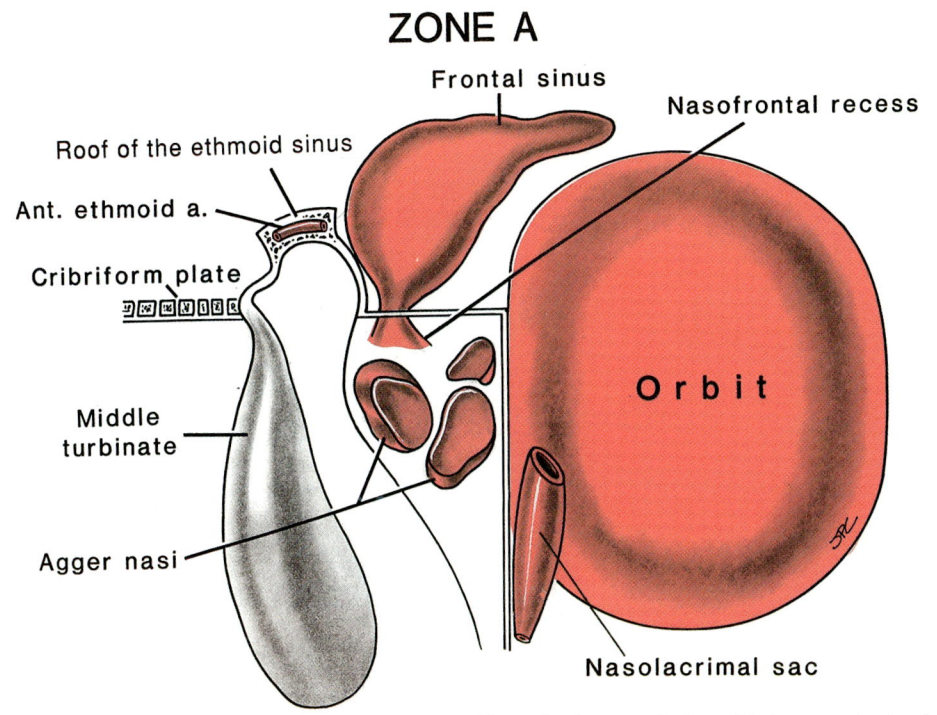

Figure 5–35. Anterior attachment of the middle turbinate. In the coronal plane this important landmark indicates the anterior extent of the cribriform plate, agger nasi, nasofrontal recess, and nasal lacrimal sac and duct. a.: artery; Ant.: anterior.

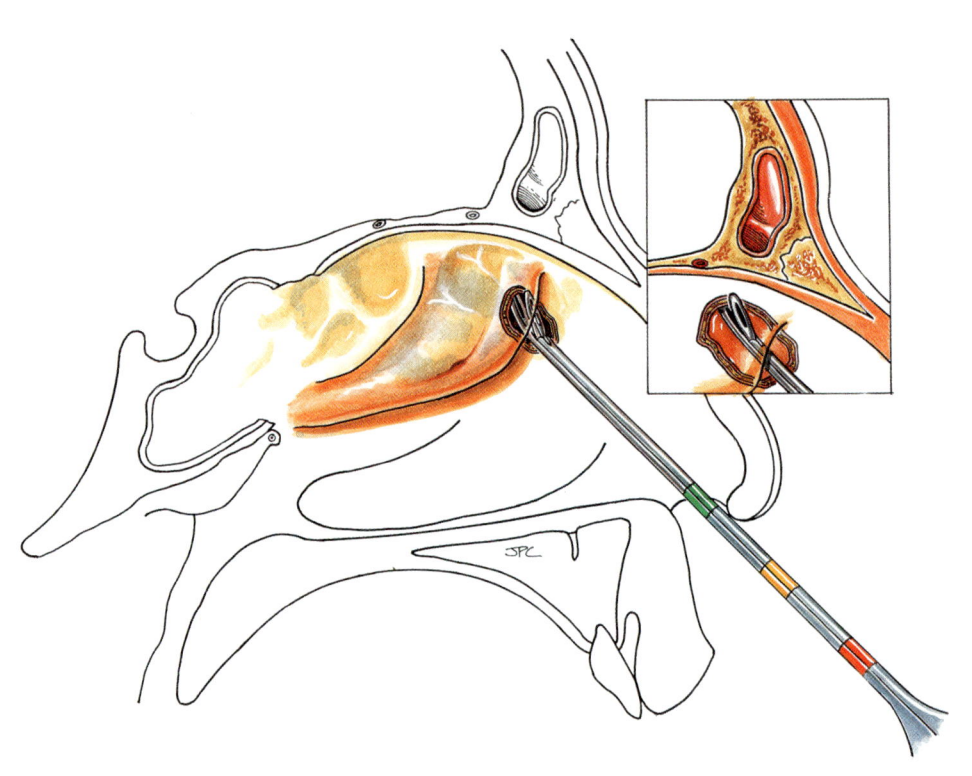

Figure 5–36. Left agger nasi cells opened with an angled Blakesley forceps placed under the anterolateral attachment of the middle turbinate. To decrease the likelihood of adhesions, the mucosal bridge between the middle turbinate and the lateral nasal wall should be preserved.

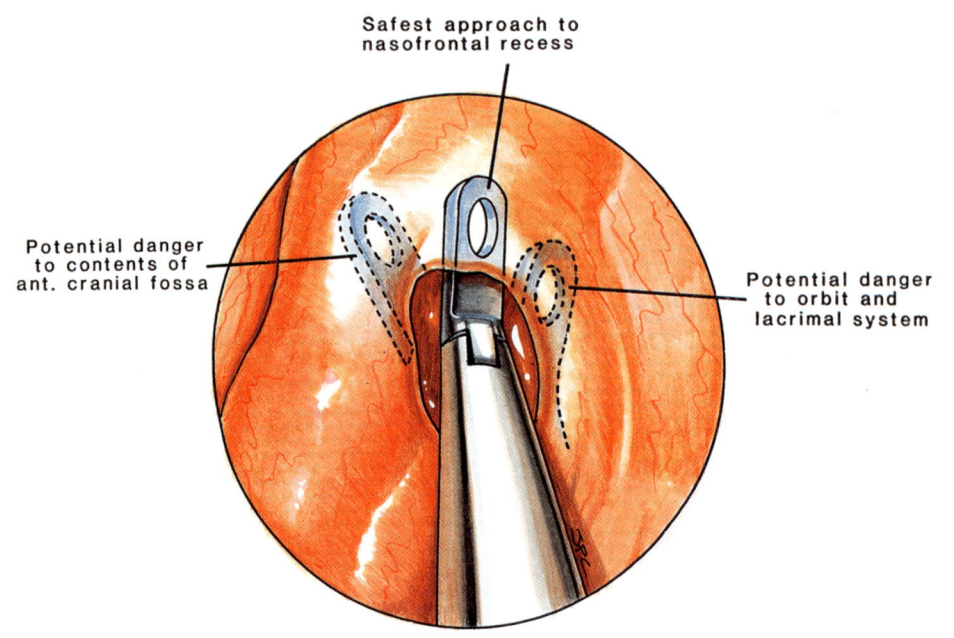

Figure 5–37. The angled forceps must be used with caution in the nasofrontal area because of the danger of penetrating the orbit laterally or the anterior (ant.) cranial fossa medially.

Endoscopic Sinus Surgery **149**

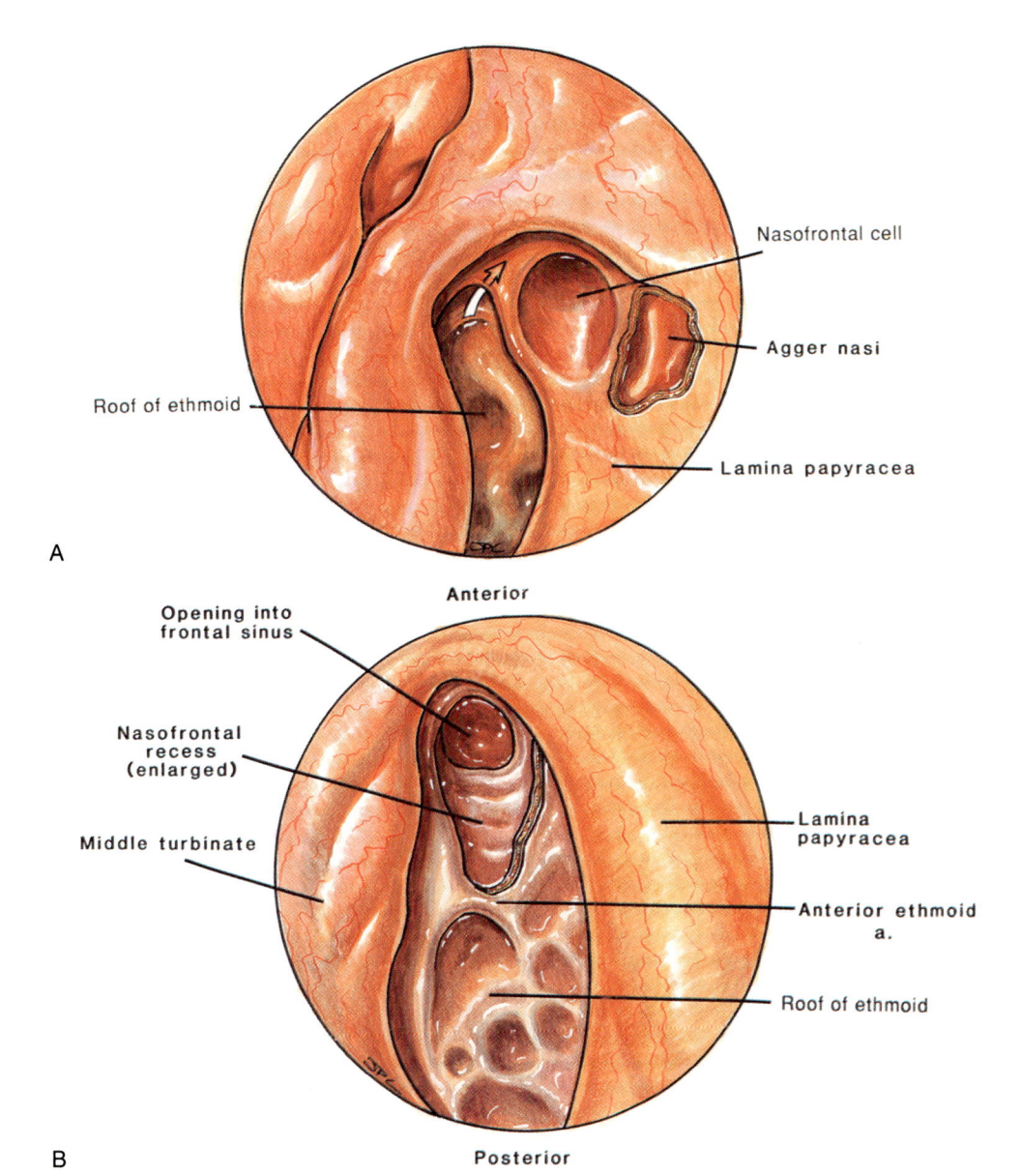

Figure 5–38. Endoscopic views of left nasofrontal recess after agger nasi and nasofrontal cells have been opened. **A**: A 0° endoscopic view. Note the nasofrontal channel (arrow) that runs above the roof of a nasofrontal cell. This channel leads to the frontal sinus isthmus and opening into the frontal sinus. **B**: A 30° endoscopic view. Opening into the frontal sinus (nasofrontal isthmus) is visible in most anterior aspect of the nasofrontal recess, next to the lamina papyracea. a.: artery.

frontal sinus or the nasofrontal isthmus (Fig. 5–38B), but to prevent secondary stenosis the mucous membrane in the region of the nasofrontal isthmus, especially that on the posterior wall, should not be disturbed. If the frontal sinus appears opaque on roentgenographic images, an effort should be made to cannulate and irrigate the frontal sinus with a 3 mm, long, olive-tipped, curved Eicken antrum cannula.

SPECIAL SURGICAL SITUATIONS

The presence of certain circumstances may lead the surgeon to alter the procedure for ESS or to perform an external surgical procedure rather than endoscopic surgery.

Endoscopic Sinus Surgery

Special situations that may need to be managed during ESS include obstruction by the middle turbinate, adhesions, and stenosis of the maxillary sinus ostium or nasofrontal recess.

Middle Turbinate

The goal of the typical ESS procedure is to remove disease in the anterior OMC without removing the middle turbinate. This structure may need to be removed partially, however: (1) if it has been replaced by polyps, (2) if there is a large concha bullosa, (3) if it is thinned and floppy as a result of compression by the nasal septum or is without support after surgery of the OMC (because such a turbinate may adhere to the lateral nasal wall and obstruct the maxillary sinus ostium after ESS), (4) if it contributes to nasal obstruction, or (5) if it is so enlarged or severely lateralized that it interferes with surgical exposure of the lateral nasal wall or the approach to the sphenoid sinus.

In such cases, the middle turbinate is crushed with a straight forceps along its superior attachment (Fig. 5–39A) and sectioned with a sinus scissors (Fig. 5–39B). The antero-inferior third is removed (Fig. 5–39C), leaving a remnant of the anterior and the posterior attachments as landmarks (Fig. 5–39D).

Adhesions and Stenosis

Adhesions or stenosis can be prevented or treated with Silastic sheeting stents. To prevent adhesions to the nasal septum, 0.02 inch thick Silastic sheeting may be cut to fit against the nasal septum on each side and held in place with a 4-0 Prolene suture through the sheeting and septum. To prevent or treat adhesions or stenosis of the maxillary ostium or nasofrontal recess, a piece of Silastic sheeting may be fashioned, inserted where appropriate, and tied with 4-0 Prolene with a long enough end that it can be used to pull the stent out.

Stents are left in place for up to 3 weeks, depending on the patient's tolerance of the stent and the degree to which granulation tissue or crusts form.

Stenosis of the Nasofrontal Recess or Isthmus

Stenosis of the nasofrontal recess or isthmus can be managed by endoscopic endonasal surgery. When the nasofrontal recess has been opened and the opening into the frontal sinus identified (Fig. 5–40A), an indwelling catheter is placed to keep the passage open and

Endoscopic Sinus Surgery **151**

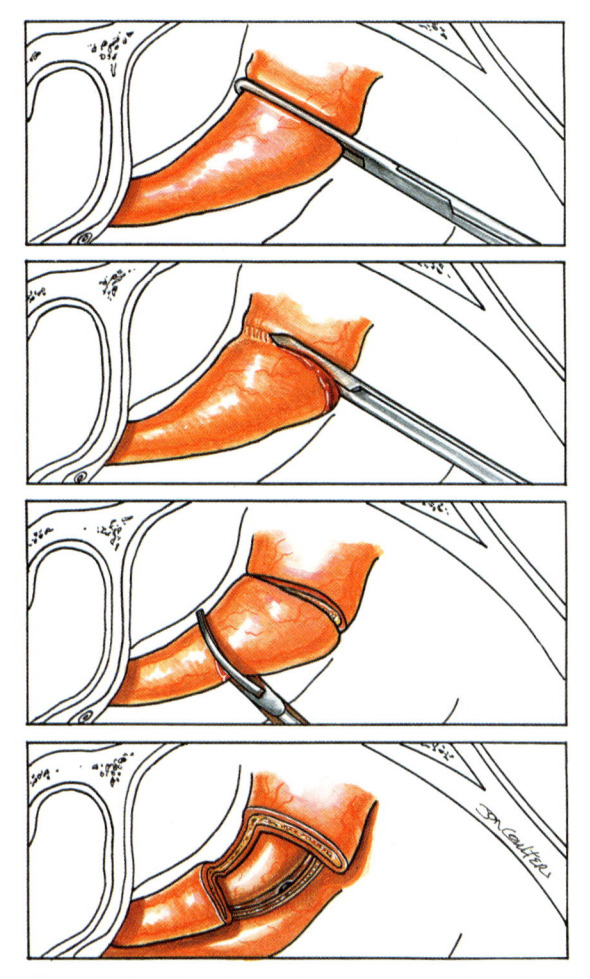

Figure 5–39. Top to bottom: Removing the middle turbinate.

152   Endoscopic Sinus Surgery

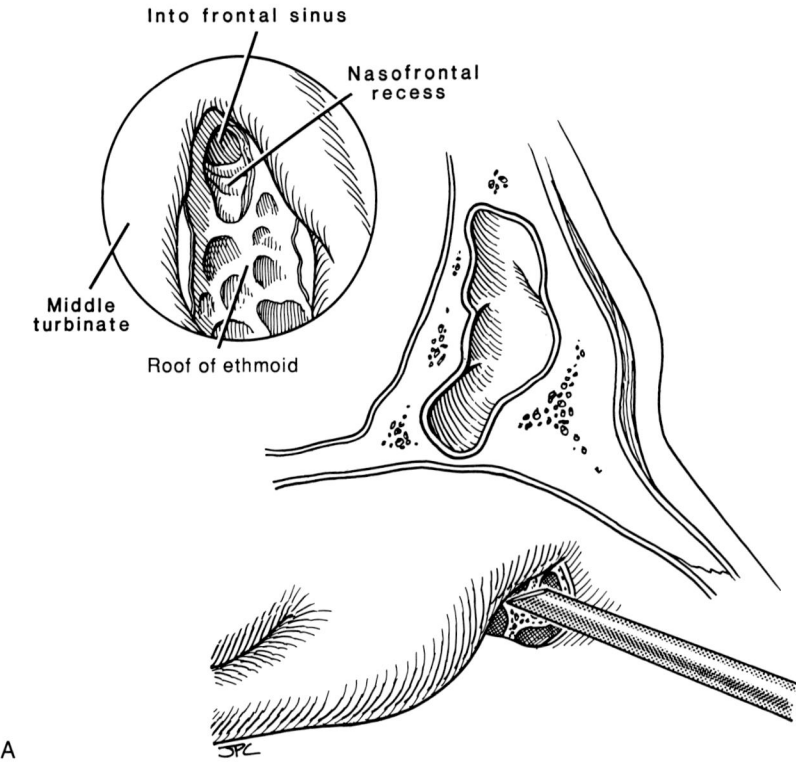

Figure 5–40. Steps involved in cannulating the frontal sinus. **A**: A 30° endoscope is placed under left middle turbinate to visualize the opened nasofrontal recess and opening into the frontal sinus. (Figure continued on next page.)

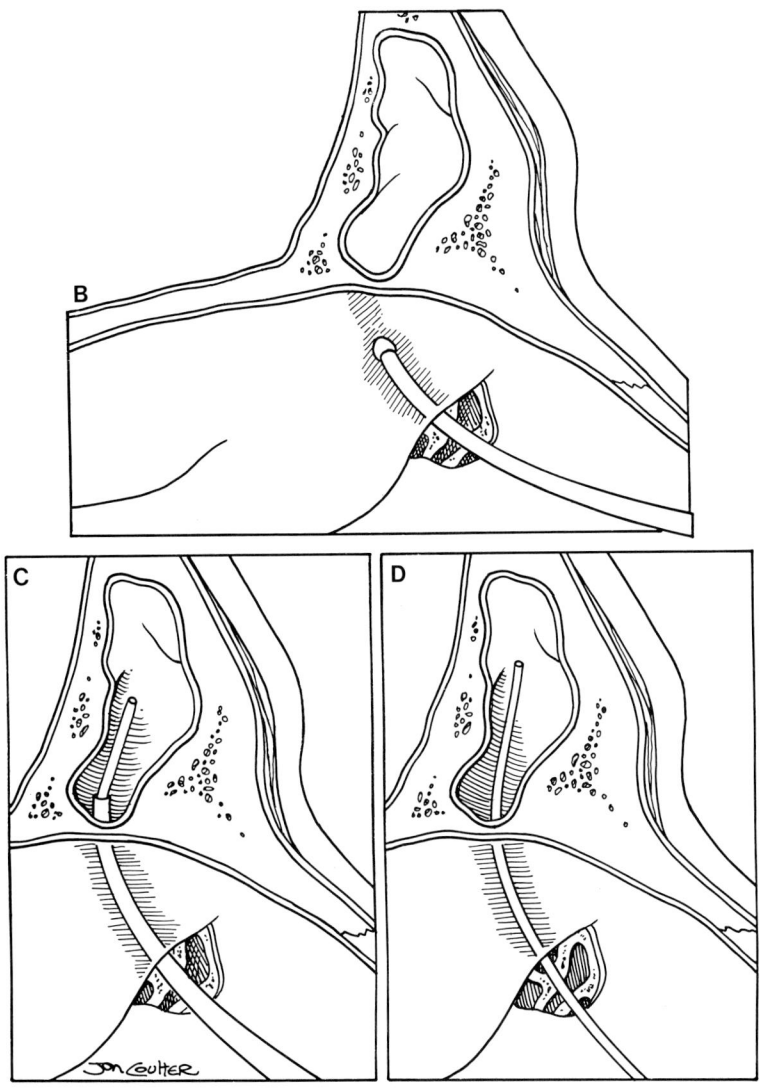

Figure 5–40. (*Continued*). **B**: Curved Eicken antral cannula is used to probe and cannulate the nasofrontal isthmus. **C**: Malleable suction tip is placed into the frontal sinus and a catheter is threaded through the cannula into the frontal sinus. **D**: The cannula is removed, leaving the catheter in place. (Figure continued on next page.)

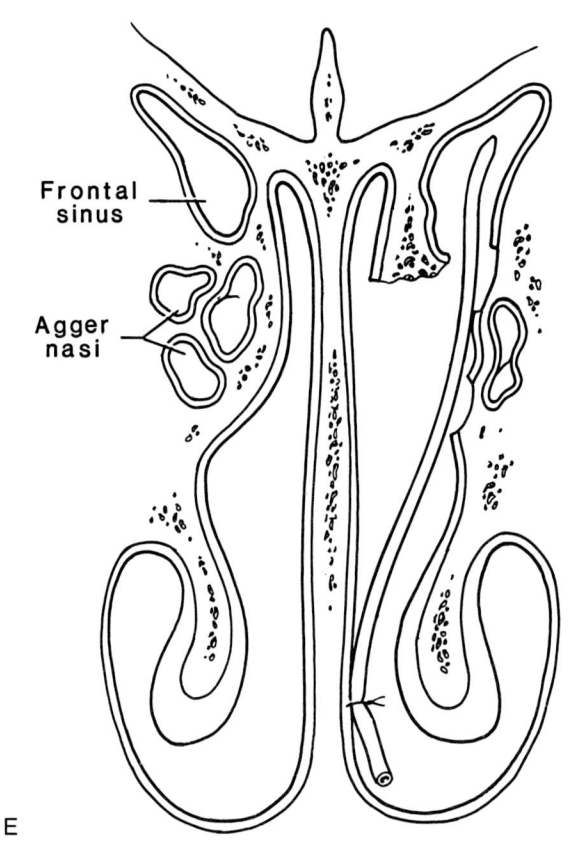

Figure 5–40. (*Continued*). **E**: The catheter is trimmed and sutured to the nasal septum with 4-0 Prolene.

promote reestablishment of the mucosal lining of the isthmus. A 23 cm malleable suction tip (Fig. 5–12) is bent to conform to the curve of a no. 3 long, curved Eicken antrum cannula (Fig. 5–40B) and placed into the frontal sinus (Fig. 5–40C). The position of the suction tip can be confirmed by a cross-table lateral radiograph, or the suction tip can be inserted into the frontal sinus with the guidance of biplane fluoroscopy. A catheter (Fig. 5–12) is then threaded through the suction tip and into the frontal sinus (Fig. 5–40C). The suction tip is removed as the catheter is advanced into the frontal sinus (Fig. 5–40D). Finally, the catheter is trimmed and sutured to the nasal septum with 4-0 Prolene (Fig. 5–40E).

The catheter is left in the isthmus for 3 weeks.

If the frontal sinus ostium cannot be identified with an angled endoscope placed endonasally, a Lynch approach with trephination may be used (Fig. 5–41, A–D); when the frontal sinus is entered by this means, purulent material will drain from the wound or sinus trocar cannula (Fig. 5–41E). An endoscope can be placed through the trocar cannula into the frontal sinus to inspect its contents directly (Fig. 5–41F) and to search for the ostium. If the ostium still cannot be visualized, the frontal sinus can be irrigated through the trephine with saline solution or fluorescein, and the outflow from the ostium watched for through an endoscope directed toward the nasofrontal recess.[18,19]

Endoscopic Sinus Surgery   155

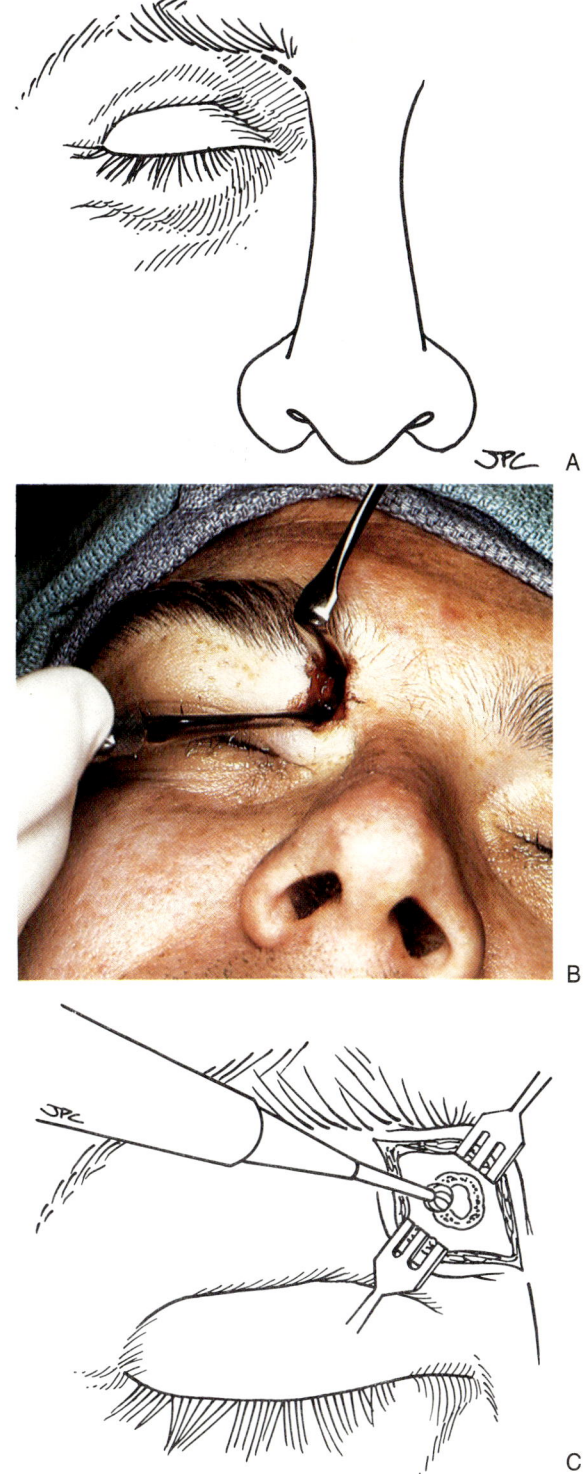

Figure 5–41. Technique for finding the endonasal site of frontal sinus drainage. **A**, **B**: Lynch incision. **C**: Trephination. (Figure continued on next page.)

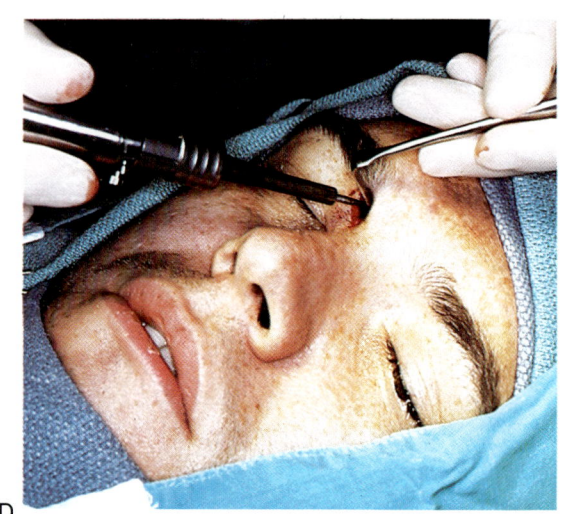

Figure 5–41. (*Continued*). **D**: Trephination. **E**: Pus released upon entering frontal sinus. **F**: Endoscope placed through trocar sleeve into frontal sinus allows direct inspection of the frontal sinus and instillation of methylene blue or fluorescein to identify the endonasal drainage site.

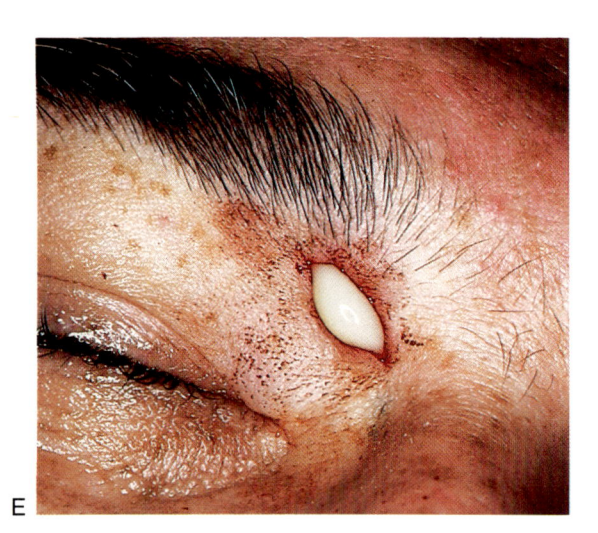

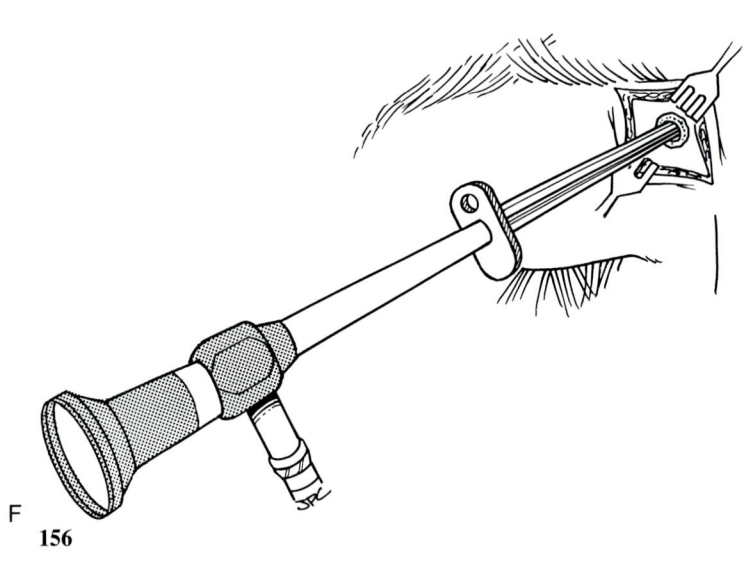

Frontal Sinus Ostioplasty

Frontal sinus ostioplasty is an endonasal procedure to open the nasofrontal isthmus to promote drainage from the frontal sinus.[20] This procedure is to be distinguished from a frontal sinus osteoplasty, which is an external procedure in which the anterior table of the frontal sinus is opened, the mucosal lining removed, and the frontal sinus cavity obliterated with fat.

Indications and Contraindications

Candidates for frontal sinus ostioplasty include: (1) those with persistent symptoms of nasofrontal recess obstruction after intensive medical management and ESS; (2) those with extensively pneumatized frontal sinuses (because it is difficult with an external procedure to ensure that all mucosa has been removed); (3) those with disease limited to the nasofrontal recess; and (4) those who object strongly to an external incision.

Contraindications to endonasal ostioplasty include: (1) presence of a frontal sinus osteoma or tumor; (2) disease that is limited to the lateral-most recesses of the frontal sinus and cannot be reached endonasally; (3) most cases of displaced fractures of the anterior or posterior table of the frontal sinus; (4) CSF leaks through the posterior table of the frontal sinus; and (5) osteomyelitis involving the anterior or posterior wall that requires extensive removal of bone.

The Technique

Before frontal sinus ostioplasty, the dimensions and anatomic relationships of the frontal sinus, nasofrontal recess, and isthmus should be determined from axial (Fig. 5–42A) and coronal (Fig. 5–42B) CT scans of the frontal sinuses. These relationships are demonstrated in Figure 5–42C and D, in which red, blue, and brown indicate the Draf[21] modifications used to enlarge the frontal sinus opening into the nasofrontal recess.[20]

The frontal sinus ostioplasty technique described is based on a similar approach with a binocular operating microscope reported by Draf[21] and the endoscopic technique reported by Wigand and Hosemann.[22] Figure 5–43 shows the steps of the procedure, which is performed with C-arm fluoroscopic and endoscopic guidance and the usual ESS instrument set plus the double-ended maxillary sinus ostium seeker, Kerrison forceps, and drill (Xomed) (Fig. 5–43). (The Skeeter drill is shown in Figure 5–43, but Xomed has developed an improved Micro-Slim drill for endonasal endoscopic surgery because the Skeeter drill burr is too small and the drill motor lacks sufficient torque for ESS). The procedure and its results in one patient are shown in Figure 5–44.

The opening into the nose from the frontal sinus can be enlarged significantly with the frontal sinus ostioplasty technique because dissection can extend as far medially as the septum. And in cases of bilateral disease the intrasinus septum, nasofrontal "beak," and bone of the anterior floor of the frontal sinus on the opposite side can be removed to the lamina papyracea. Endonasal ostioplasty has become our surgical approach of choice over an external frontal osteoplasty for the following reasons: (1) the wide exposure; (2) lower morbidity with endonasal versus an external procedure; and (3) the fact that the frontal sinus ostioplasty technique leaves the isthmus lined with mucosa.

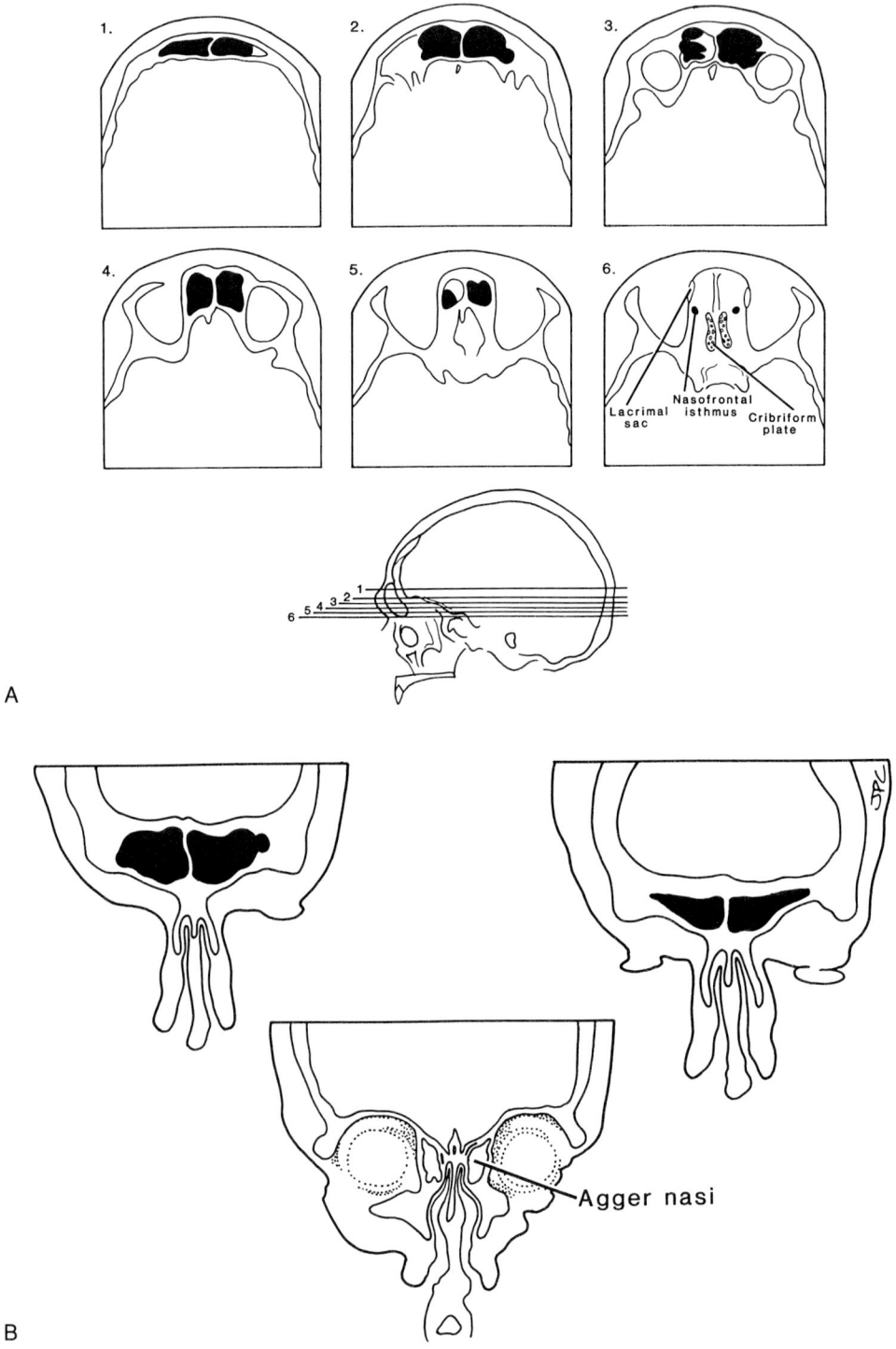

Figure 5–42. Survey CT of the frontal sinus used to determine dimensions of the sinus and anatomical relationships to nasofrontal recess and isthmus. **A**: Axial CT scan, cuts 1 through 6. Frontal sinus narrows to a small isthmus as it drains into the nasofrontal recess. **B**: Coronal CT scans show relationship of the frontal sinus to the orbit and agger nasi cells. **C, D**: Demonstration of these relationships and the Draf[21] approach (boxes labeled 1, 2, and 3 correspond to Draf I, II, and III procedures) to enlarge the frontal sinus drainage into the nasofrontal recess.[20] a.: artery; Ant.: anterior; Sup.: Superior; turb.: turbinate.

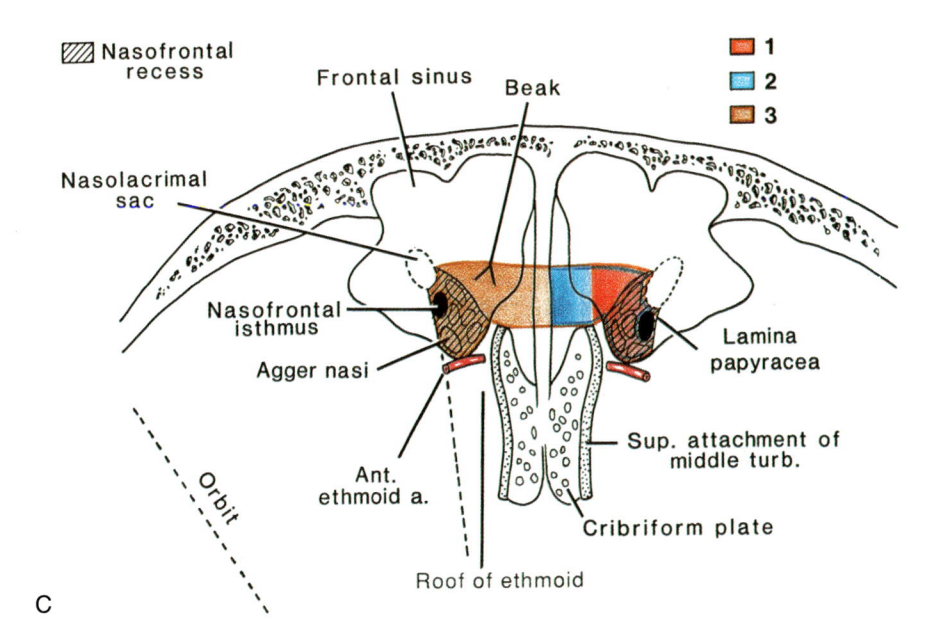

Endoscopic Sinus Surgery 159

- Nasofrontal recess
- Frontal sinus
- Beak
- ■ 1
- ■ 2
- ■ 3
- Nasolacrimal sac
- Nasofrontal isthmus
- Agger nasi
- Lamina papyracea
- Ant. ethmoid a.
- Sup. attachment of middle turb.
- Cribriform plate
- Roof of ethmoid
- Orbit

C

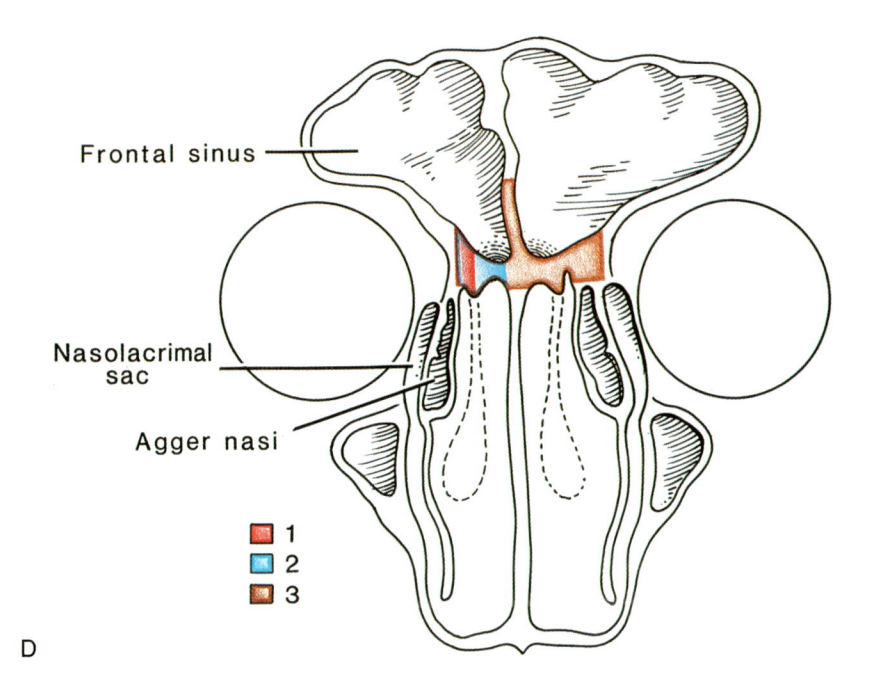

- Frontal sinus
- Nasolacrimal sac
- Agger nasi
- ■ 1
- ■ 2
- ■ 3

D

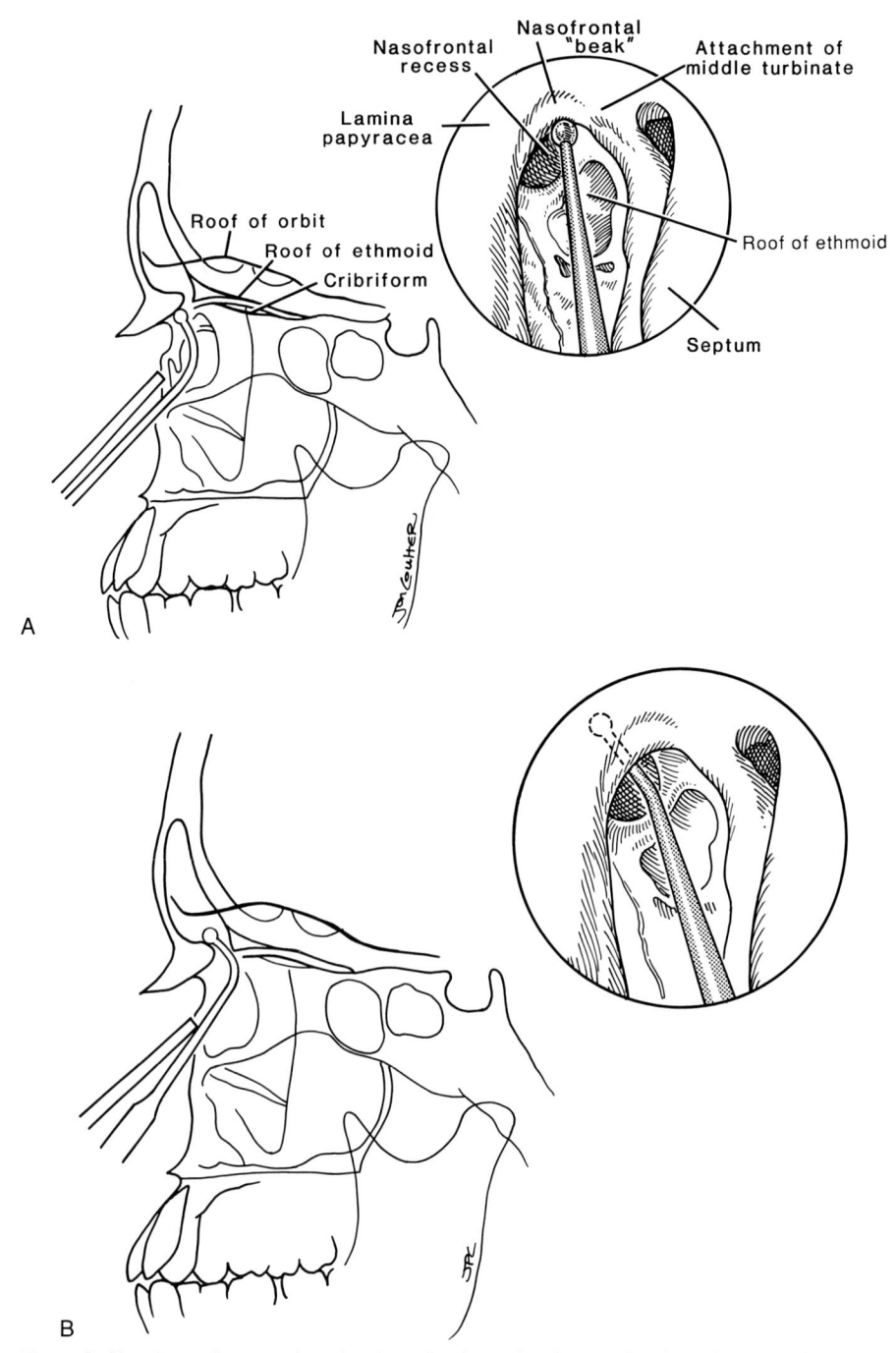

Figure 5–43. C-arm fluoroscopic and endoscopic views of each step of endonasal endoscopic frontal sinus ostioplasty procedure. **A**: Nasofrontal recess is probed with a double-ended maxillary sinus ostium seeker. Note probe against nasofrontal "beak." **B**: Probe inserted into frontal sinus through nasofrontal isthmus. (Figure continued on next page.)

Endoscopic Sinus Surgery   **161**

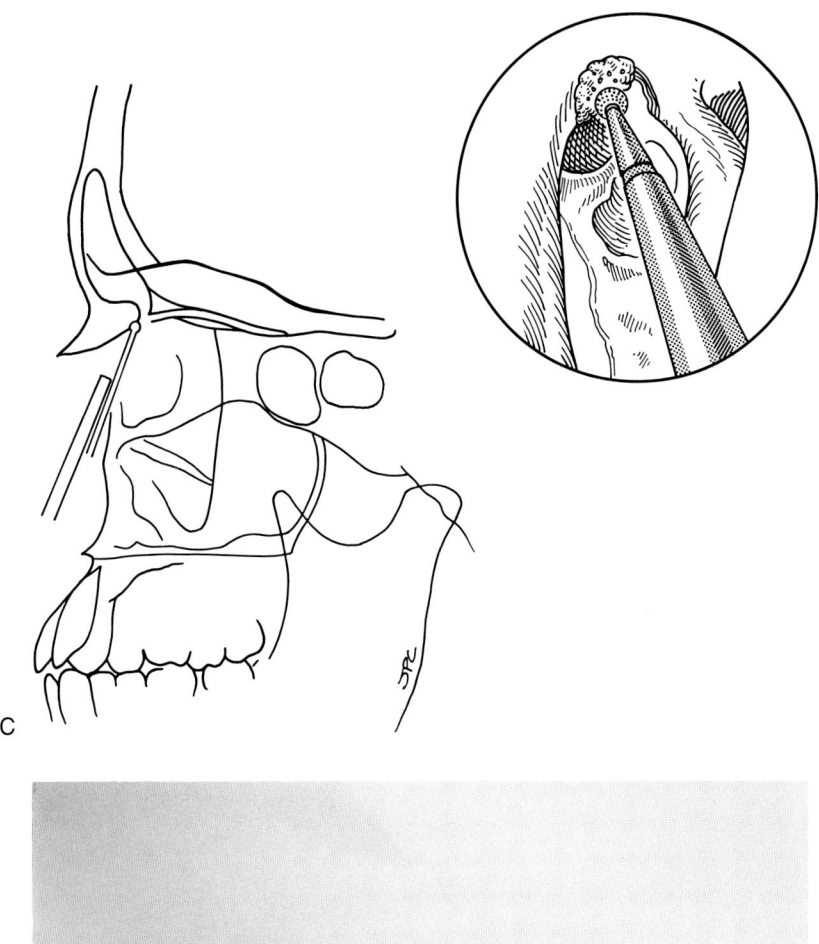

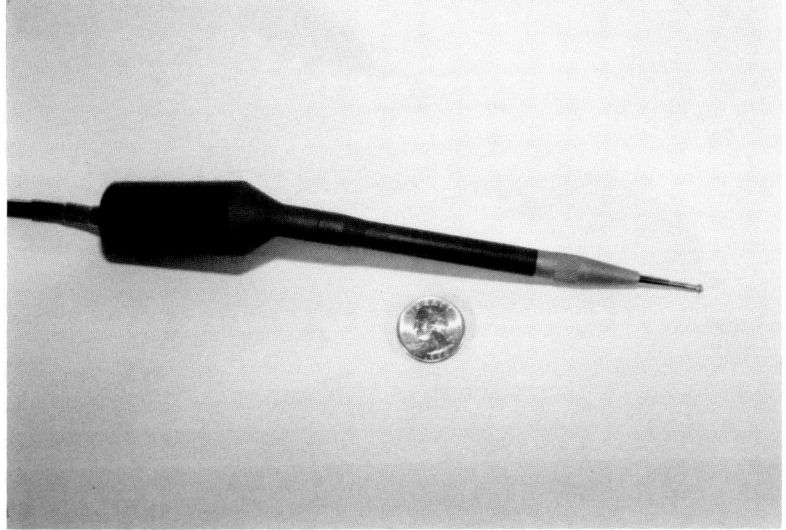

Figure 5–43. (*Continued*). **C**: Drill is used to thin nasofrontal "beak." (Skeeter drill shown is less than ideal because the largest burr [inset] is only 2 mm and because the motor has inadequate torque for ESS. The advantages of this drill are that it is lightweight and only the tip of the rotating shaft and burr are exposed to surrounding tissues.) **D**: An improved drill for ESS, the Xomed-Treace MPS2000 Micro-Craft drill with MicroSlim handpiece. (Figure continued on next page.)

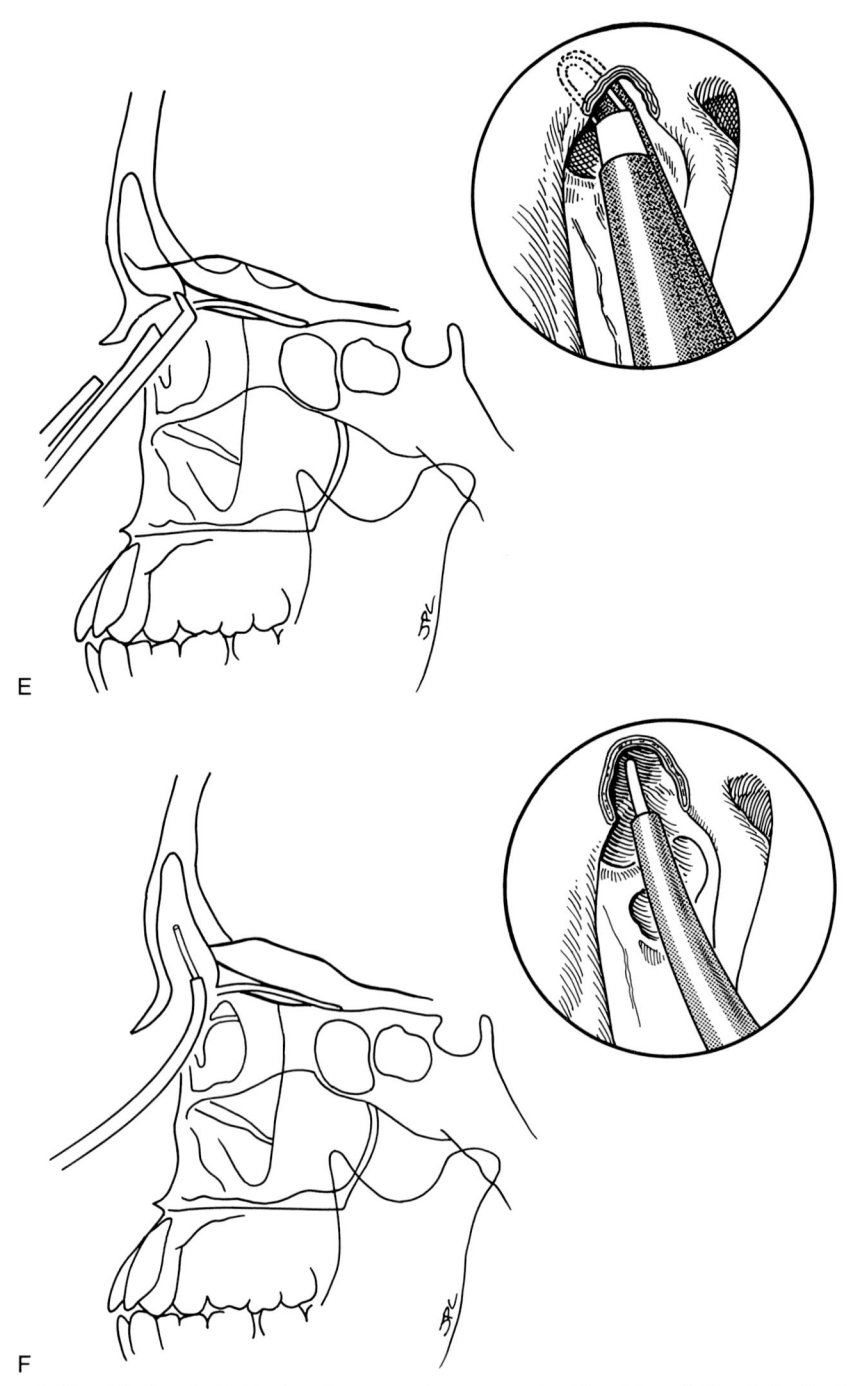

Figure 5–43. *(Continued).* **E:** Kerrison forceps used to remove the thinned bony ledge of the "beak." **F:** Widened nasofrontal isthmus permits passage of a large catheter, although with this technique the opening into the nose is so large that the catheter is rarely needed.

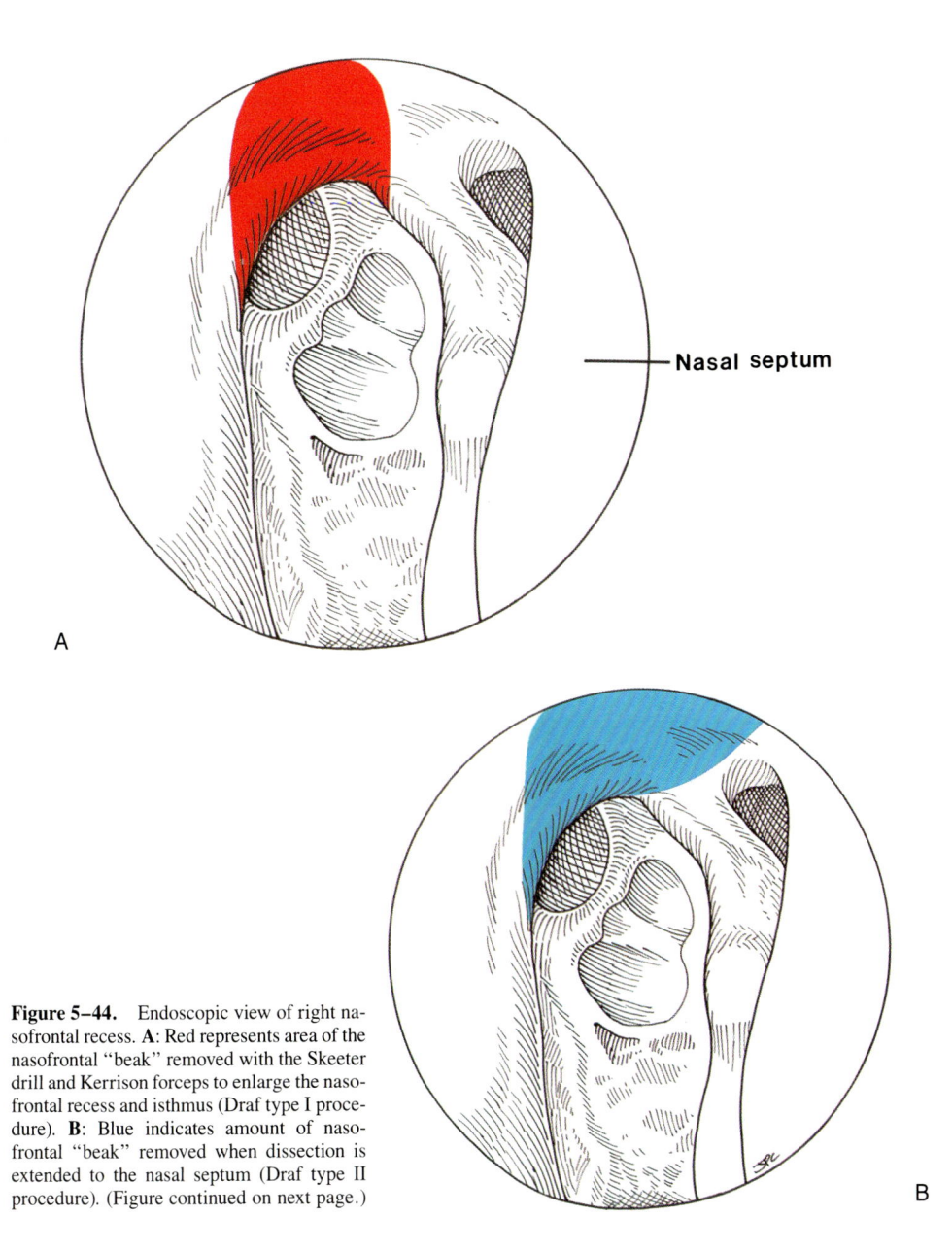

Figure 5-44. Endoscopic view of right nasofrontal recess. **A**: Red represents area of the nasofrontal "beak" removed with the Skeeter drill and Kerrison forceps to enlarge the nasofrontal recess and isthmus (Draf type I procedure). **B**: Blue indicates amount of nasofrontal "beak" removed when dissection is extended to the nasal septum (Draf type II procedure). (Figure continued on next page.)

164   *Endoscopic Sinus Surgery*

Nasofrontal isthmus
Ant. ethmoid a.
Lamina papyracea

Roof of ethmoid

C

Nasofrontal isthmus

Nasofrontal recess
Lamina papyracea
Ant. ethmoid a.

Roof of ethmoid

D

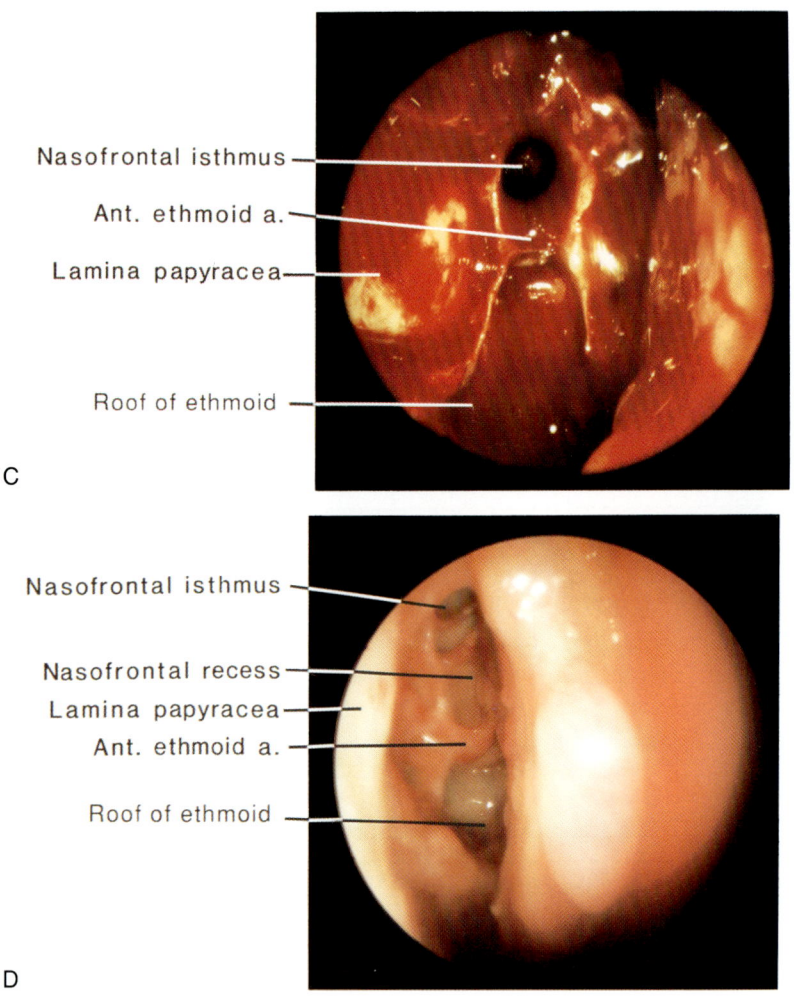

Figure 5–44. (*Continued*). **C**: A 30° endoscopic view of left nasofrontal isthmus after Draf II procedure. Note that right nasofrontal isthmus is enlarged widely to the lamina papyracea laterally, roof of the ethmoid sinus posteriorly, and, by removal of the nasofrontal "beak," to the anterior attachment of the middle turbinate anteriorly. **D**: Six weeks postoperatively the nasofrontal recess is widely patent and covered with mucosa. The patient's preoperative symptoms were relieved. Ant.: anterior; a.: artery.

Maxillary Sinus Disease

Disease in a maxillary sinus usually can be managed by endonasal ESS. In some cases, however, a transcanine approach may need to be added or a modified or full Caldwell-Luc procedure with stripping of the mucosal lining and creation of an inferior meatal nasoantral window may be needed. One or more of these approaches may be indicated to treat patients with the following disorders: foreign body, fungal sinusitis, recurrent massive polyposis, Samter's syndrome, reactive nasosinus mucosal disease, dysmotility, or irreversible mucosal changes suggested by persistent suppurative sinusitis in spite of adequate medical and surgical treatment.

Endonasal Endoscopic Management

The maxillary sinus may be visualized by inserting a 30° endoscope through an enlarged middle meatal antrostomy, and diseased mucosa may be removed with an angled forceps or a giraffe forceps (3 mm, 70°, vertical-cutting, double-action sinus forceps) (Fig. 5–11).

Transcanine Approach

If the maxillary sinus cannot be viewed directly by the endonasal endoscopic route, even after the middle meatal maxillary antrostomy has been enlarged maximally by removing the membrane of the posterior fontanelle, then an endoscope is inserted through a trocar cannula placed in the canine fossa (Fig. 5–45).

Fluid can be instilled and debris, even fungal debris (which may have the consistency of clay), can be evacuated from the maxillary sinus either through the enlarged middle meatal antrostomy route or through the trocar cannula in the canine fossa. The maxillary sinus mucosal lining is biopsied if fungus or a malignancy is suspected.

Modified Caldwell-Luc Procedure

When greater exposure is required in the maxillary sinus, a modified Caldwell-Luc procedure may be performed. The traditional Caldwell-Luc procedure, developed at the turn of the century, involves making a buccal-labial incision, removing bone over the canine fossa, stripping the maxillary sinus mucosa, and creating a nasoantral window through the inferior meatus. For the modified procedure, the canine fossa puncture is enlarged with a Kerrison forceps to permit passage of a second trocar cannula (Fig. 5–46). By passing the endoscope through one cannula and a catheter for irrigation and suction through the other, irrigation and suction can be performed under direct visualization (Fig. 5–47).

If the maxillary sinus cannot be visualized adequately through the endoscope, enough tissue and bone may be removed from the borders of the trocar puncture wound to permit direct viewing, with a headlight, of the maxillary sinus. When diseased mucosa, cysts, polyps, or debris filling the maxillary sinus have been removed, this transantral route can be used for a traditional approach to the ethmoid and sphenoid sinuses.

This modified Caldwell-Luc approach with its limited mucosal incision and bone removal carries less risk of injury to the infraorbital nerve and the anterosuperior and posterosuperior alveolar nerves. The risk of injuring the infraorbital nerve can be decreased further by not retracting soft tissue in the territory of the infraorbital nerve and not removing bone posterolaterally. Observing this latter caution also decreases the likelihood of injuring the anterosuperior and posterosuperior alveolar nerves.

Traditional External Sinus Surgery

The traditional external approach to the maxillary sinus, a Caldwell-Luc procedure, is associated with postoperative pain, swelling, and ecchymosis in the cheek and gingival area, and not uncommonly with prolonged infraorbital pain and numbness.[23] Endonasal ESS, in contrast, is often successful in reestablishing maxillary sinus mucociliary flow with preservation of sinus mucosa and without the need for an inferior meatus nasoantral window. The lower morbidity associated with endoscopic versus external maxillary sinus

166 *Endoscopic Sinus Surgery*

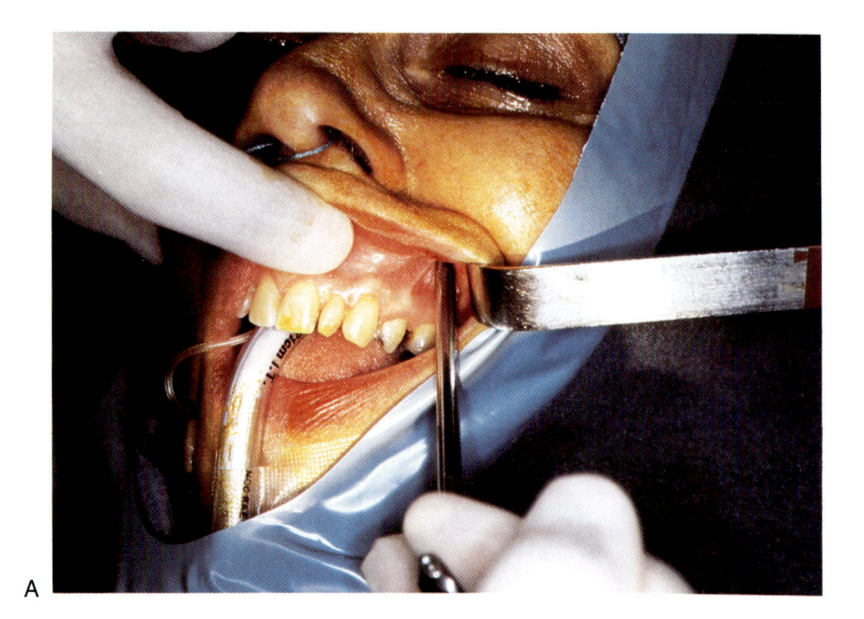

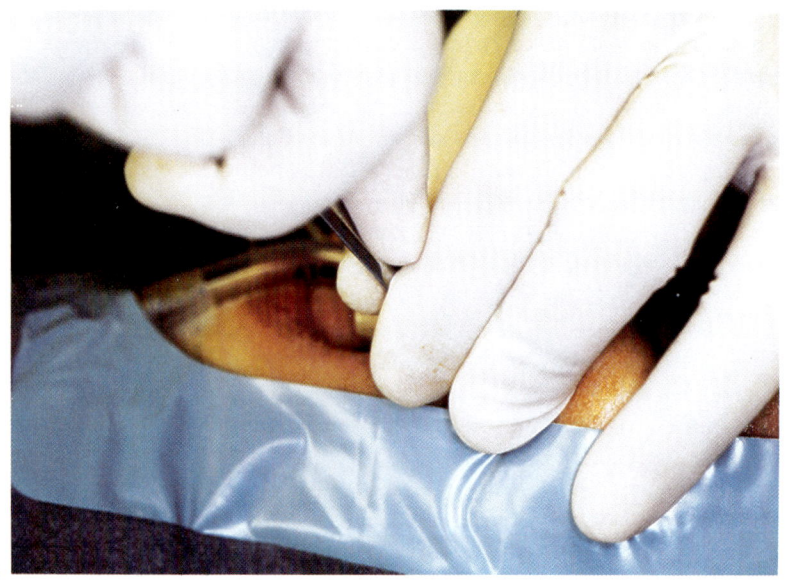

Figure 5–45. Canine fossa puncture technique. **A**: Trocar and cannula (Fig. 5–10) are placed perpendicular to the face of the maxilla in the canine fossa and directed posteriorly, laterally, and superiorly toward the malar eminence. **B**: To ensure that the trocar penetrates only the anterior wall of the maxillary sinus, it is rotated back and forth with pressure until it begins to penetrate the anterior wall, and then the surgeon places a finger of the other hand in front of the hand holding the trocar so that when further pressure is applied and the trocar penetrates the anterior wall this finger will keep the trocar from moving too much farther into the sinus.

Endoscopic Sinus Surgery   **167**

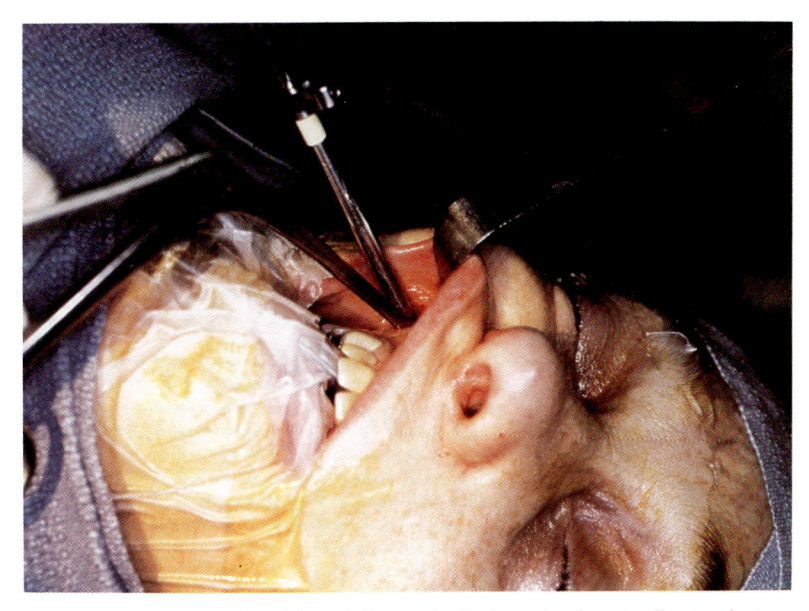

Figure 5–46.   A second trocar is placed through the opening in the canine fossa to allow two instruments to be used together in this modified (or mini-) Caldwell-Luc procedure.

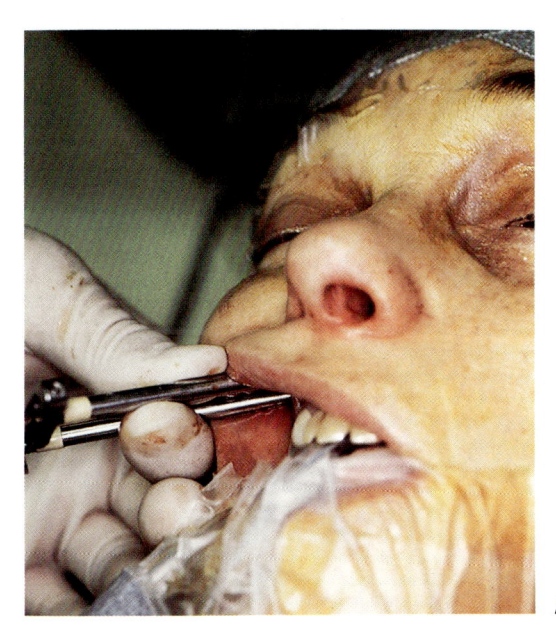

Figure 5–47.   **A**: Inserting two trocar cannulas into the maxillary sinus allows the surgeon to irrigate and suction under endoscopic visualization. (Figure continued on next page.)

168 *Endoscopic Sinus Surgery*

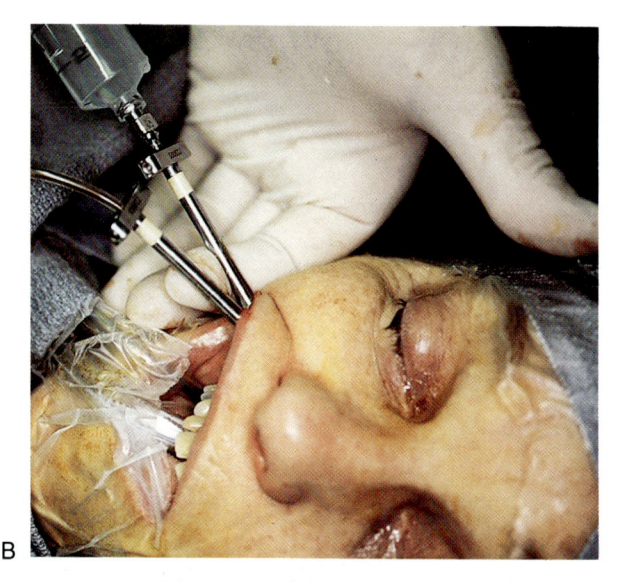

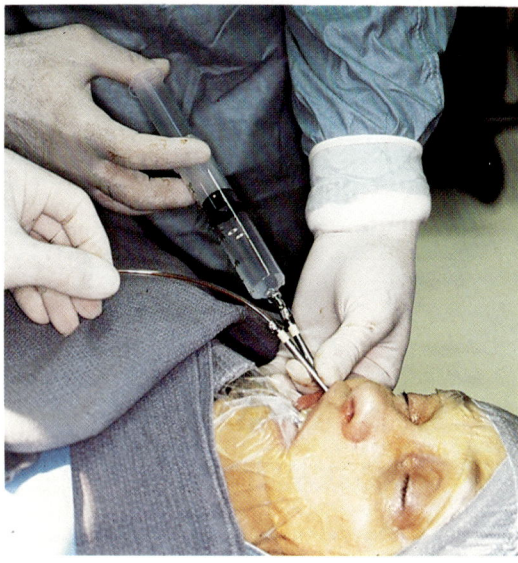

Figure 5–47. (*Continued*). **B**, **C**: Technique for irrigating through one trocar cannula and suctioning through the other.

surgery has led to the Caldwell-Luc procedure being reserved for patients with diseases involving the maxillary sinus that cannot be managed endoscopically, as has been previously mentioned.

PREVENTION AND MANAGEMENT OF BLEEDING

The typical blood loss during ESS, whether performed with local or general anesthesia, is about 75 cc, much less than with a traditional external approach. Some patients lose significantly more blood than the average. In most cases this occurs because of factors related to their disease. Patients whose sinus mucosa is hyperplastic, leathery, and friable as a result of previous surgery tend to bleed more than others. Once mucosa is removed in any patient, however, significant bleeding from the mucosa usually stops.

Bleeding from the nasosinus mucosa is minimized by the topical application of a decongestant, the injection of a vasoconstrictor medication, and anesthesia techniques that keep the patient hypotensive. General techniques to manage bleeding during ESS include hemostasis and cautery.

Hemostasis

Oozing of blood during ESS can be controlled effectively by periodic applications of an oxymetazoline- or epinephrine (1:1000)–moistened cotton pledget. The pledget is removed after a few seconds; if oozing persists, the pledget is replaced in the sinus cavity and surgery is continued elsewhere for a few minutes.

Anterior Ethmoid Artery

The anterior ethmoid artery is usually well protected by a bony canal as it crosses the anterior aspect of the roof of the ethmoid sinus at the level of the anterior face of the bulla ethmoidalis, just behind the nasofrontal recess. When bleeding from this artery does occur, it usually is easily controlled by applying an oxymetazoline- or epinephrine (1:1000)–moistened cotton pledget. If the injured portion of this artery retracts into the orbit, however, intraorbital bleeding can occur; to control this bleeding the vessel may need to be exposed via an external ethmoid sinus approach and cauterized with a wet-field bayonet bipolar forceps (refer to Chapter 7 for details). A suction cautery is usually effective in controlling bleeding from the territory of the anterior ethmoid artery along the ethmoid cavity roof.

Sphenopalatine Artery

Pulsatile bleeding that begins when the surgeon is operating at the inferior aspect of the face of the sphenoid is usually from the sphenopalatine artery, which runs from lateral to medial just above the arch of the posterior choana. Injury to this artery usually occurs when the posterior attachment of the middle turbinate is avulsed or when the inferior aspect of the face of the sphenoid is entered. Injury to this artery can be avoided by sharply cutting the middle turbinate rather than avulsing it, not disturbing the posterior attachment of the middle turbinate, and displacing the mucosa from the face of the sphenoid inferiorly toward the arch of the posterior choana before penetrating the face of the sphenoid.

Bleeding from the sphenopalatine artery can be controlled by bipolar or suction cautery. If suction cautery is used, it should be applied in short bursts interspersed with saline irrigation to prevent heat buildup and possible injury to the adjacent orbit, dura, and optic nerve.

Injury to the carotid artery is discussed in Chapter 7.

Postoperative Dressings

Postoperative oozing can be controlled by placing a dressing made with cotton pledgets (Neuropatties) between the middle turbinate and lateral wall of the nose. To make this dressing, three pledgets are sutured with 2-0 silk to the finger of a non-Latex (to eliminate the possibility of an allergic reaction to Latex) surgical glove, leaving the sutures long. The dressing is coated with mupirocin (Bactroban), rather than a product containing petrolatum, to decrease the possibility of myospherulosis (a granulomatous foreign body reaction to petrolatum particles;[24] see Chapter 7) (Fig. 5–14). One dressing is placed in each nasal passage and the excess suture lengths are then tied together over the columella to prevent the dressing from sliding into the nasopharynx.

If a septoplasty has been performed, another like dressing may be placed between the inferior turbinate and the nasal septum. A Merocel sponge (Americal, Mystic, CT) may also be placed in the sinus cavity as a pressure dressing to prevent bleeding and hold the middle turbinate against the lateral nasal wall.

Dressings are left in place several hours or overnight, depending on the amount of bleeding. Patients discharged the day of surgery with the dressing in place return the following day for dressing removal.

POSTOPERATIVE CARE

Planning for postoperative care begins when the decision for surgery is made.

Outpatient Versus Inpatient Postoperative Care

Some patients can be discharged the day of ESS, but others are more appropriately admitted overnight to the hospital: those who would be more comfortable in the hospital setting;[25] those with medical problems such as cardiovascular disease, reactive airway disease, or insulin-dependent diabetes; those who were operated on late in the day and have not fully recovered from anesthetic agents; those with inadequately controlled nausea and vomiting or pain; and patients who have persistent bleeding.

Patients with persistent anterior or posterior nasal bleeding are not discharged until this is controlled. Removing the dressing, suctioning clots, spraying oxymetazoline on the mucosa, and replacing the dressing may be effective in stopping bleeding. However, if bleeding persists, a balloon catheter is positioned to prevent blood entering the pharynx, and the nasal cavity is packed as described in the previous section. Patients who have had this treatment remain overnight in the hospital. The balloon and packing are removed the next day, and if no bleeding occurs during a 2-hour observation period, the patient is discharged.

Hospitalization overnight for observation after ESS is also appropriate for patients who will be returning home by air or an extended automobile trip.

Routine Postoperative Orders

Routine postoperative orders for the care of patients who have undergone ESS are listed in Table 5–2.

Patients are offered clear liquids when they are fully alert and are free of nausea. For those operated on under local anesthesia with sedation, this is usually soon after surgery

Table 5–2 Routine Orders for Care of Patients After Endoscopic Sinus Surgery

COMPONENT OF CARE	MANAGEMENT
Admission	Admit to Otolaryngology-Head and Neck Unit
Positioning	Elevate head of bed 30° for first 12 hours
Dressing	Change moustache dressing PRN
Respiratory support	Face tent to supply 30% oxygen in warmed, humidified air
Hydration	5% dextrose in Ringer's lactate solution, 100 cc/hour
	Discontinue IV when taking fluids well PO
Nutrition	Begin clear liquid diet when awake and fully alert
	Advance diet as tolerated
Antibiotic therapy	Until tolerating fluids PO: cefapirin sodium 1 g IV q 6 hours
	When tolerating fluids PO:
	cefuroxime axetil 500 mg PO BID
	or
	amoxicillin 500 mg with clavulanate 125 mg PO TID
Pain relief	If tolerating fluids PO:
	acetaminophen 300 mg with codeine phosphate 30 mg (Tylenol No. 3), 1 or 2 tablets PO q 3–4 hours PRN
	or
	acetaminophen 325 mg with propoxyphene napsylate 50 mg (Darvocet-N-50), 1 or 2 tablets PO q 3–4 hours PRN
	If not tolerating fluids PO: meperidine HCl 50–75 mg with hydroxyzine HCl 25–50 mg IM q 3–4 hours PRN
Antiemetic	ONE of the following:
	Per rectum: prochlorperazine 25 mg BID PRN
	promethazine HCl 25 mg q 4–6 hours PRN
	trimethobenzamide HCl 200 mg q 6 hours PRN
	Intramuscularly: prochlorperazine 10 mg IM q 2–4 hours PRN
	promethazine HCl 25 mg IM q 4–6 hours PRN
	trimethobenzamide HCl 200 mg IM q 6 hours PRN
Activity	Up ad lib

*BID: twice daily; IM: intramuscularly; PO: orally; PRN: as needed; q: every; TID: three times daily.

and by 4 hours after surgery they are able to tolerate a full regular diet. Patients who have had general anesthesia may not be able to tolerate clear fluids until the morning after surgery.

Patients with limited sinus disease and no evidence of suppurative infection are not prescribed antibiotic medications. Those with acute or chronic suppurative sinusitis are prescribed antibiotic therapy for 7 days postoperatively.

Many patients complain of headache and a feeling of pressure in the paranasal region after ESS, but only rarely do patients complain of significant pain after this procedure. This is in contrast to the pain patients experience after surgery via a traditional Caldwell-Luc approach.

It is usual for blood to begin oozing from the operative area when the intranasal dressing is removed the morning after surgery. This oozing usually stops spontaneously after 20 to 60 minutes. At this time excess blood is suctioned from the nose, oxymetazoline is sprayed into the nose, and a moustache dressing is applied (Fig. 5–14). The patient is kept on bed rest for 2 hours after removal of the dressing and told to sniff rather than blow the nose and to sneeze, if necessary, with the mouth open.

Postoperative Medications

Medications may be prescribed to manage infection or for relief of symptoms after ESS.

Antibiotics

If an infection develops in the immediate postoperative period and the patient is not already receiving an antibiotic, amoxicillin is prescribed and is effective in most cases. Augmented penicillin is prescribed if there is a suspicion that the causative organism is resistant to beta lactamase, and if one of these agents is not effective a cephalosporin or quinolone (particularly for *Pseudomonas*) is prescribed. Patients who are allergic to penicillin and cephalosporins are prescribed trimethoprim with sulfamethoxazole (Bactrim or Septra), clarithromycin (Biaxin), or azithromycin (Zithromax).

Antihistamines

Postoperative allergy-like symptoms have been treated effectively with antihistamines such as terfenadine (Seldane) and astemizole (Hismanal) that have long half-lives and few side effects, especially drowsiness. Antihistamines may, however, cause excessive nasal and sinus dryness.

Mucolytics

Patients who have thick mucous secretions postoperatively may be prescribed a mucolytic agent (Humibid L.A.) or expectorant with cough suppressant such as guaifenesin with dextromethorphin (Humibid DM).

Decongestants

Various preparations containing decongestants such as pseudoephedrine or phenylpropanolamine are available in a variety of strengths and combinations with mucolytic or other agents.

Steroids

As previously discussed, patients who have polyposis are given a bolus of prednisone preoperatively and tapering doses for several days afterward on the following schedule: 80 mg/day for preoperative days 5 and 4; 60 mg/day for preoperative days 3 and 2; 40 mg/day for preoperative day 1 and postoperative day 1; and 30, 20, and 10 mg/day, respectively, on postoperative days 2, 3, and 4.

Beclomethasone aqueous nasal spray is also prescribed, two applications to each side of the nose four times each day for 1 week, three times per day for 1 week, and twice a day thereafter.

Recurrent polyps are treated by injecting them with 0.5 ml betamethasone sodium phosphate 4 mg/ml every 6 weeks as necessary.

Discharge Instructions to the Patient

Patients are given instructions for nasal irrigations or douching, prescriptions and instructions for use of postoperative medications, and activity instructions.

Nasal Irrigations

Starting 1 week after surgery, the patient should irrigate the nasal cavity twice a day for 3 to 6 weeks if crusts are present or secretions are thick or sticky. A Water Pik (Model WP 20W, Teledyne Water Pik, Fort Collins, CO) with a Gossan Nasal Irrigator Tip (item AGNI, Anthony Products, Indianapolis, IN) should be used to direct 240 cc (1 cup) of solution (saline, Alkalol, or salt/soda/syrup) into each side of the nose.

Saline solution may be prepared by measuring out 1 cup (240 cc) of boiled water into a clean container, adding 1/3 teaspoon of table salt to the cup of water, and allowing the solution to cool to body temperature.

Alkalol (Alkalol Co., Taunton, MA) and water in a ratio of 1:1 is advised for patients whose nasal secretions are thick and who have large crusts in the nose.

Salt/soda/syrup solution is advised for patients with chronic mucositis, as may accompany ASA triad. This solution is prepared the same way as saline solution but with the addition of 1/3 teaspoon of baking soda and 1/3 teaspoon of pancake syrup, honey, or molasses. (The syrup makes this hypertonic solution more pleasant to use.)

Activity

Patients whose occupations are not physically demanding are told they may return to work within 2 days of surgery; those whose occupations require physical exertion are told they should not return to work for 7 to 10 days after surgery. Patients may swim by 3 weeks after surgery, but they are advised against diving for 6 weeks after surgery.

Postoperative Office Visits

The patient should be seen within the first week after surgery for follow-up care; additional visits are scheduled as needed.

First Week

At the first postoperative visit, the patient's nose is decongested and anesthetized by placing pledgets containing a solution of 2% tetracaine and 1% phenylephrine in the nose. The pledgets are removed after 10 minutes and clots are removed by gentle suctioning. Any *adhesions* present between the septum and the middle turbinate or between the middle turbinate and the lateral wall are lysed with a knife or scissors, such as Belluci scissors. If adhesions are extensive, a stent made of x-ray film is sutured in place and removed in 1 week. *Crusts* that are not removed by gentle suctioning are not disturbed, although forceps may be used to dislodge congealed material not removed by suctioning.

Second and Third Weeks

Suctioning is also used at subsequent office visits to remove loose crusts and clots, but aggressive debridement is avoided because it encourages bleeding. An effective method to debride crusts is irrigation, as described previously.

By the end of the third week after surgery, mucosa usually has formed over most of the operative area and the OMC and maxillary sinus ostium can be visualized. Remaining crusts may cover granulation tissue, which should be cauterized with silver nitrate on a wooden applicator.

Evaluation of Results

By the end of the sixth week after surgery, nasal mucosa and mucociliary flow have been reestablished in most patients, and the patient is ready to evaluate the results of surgery.

SUMMARY

Different approaches have been developed and various techniques reported for safe and effective management of sinus disorders by endoscopic endonasal sinus surgery. The two-handed video endoscopic technique permits the surgeon to use two hands to manipulate instruments and, by displaying the view through the endoscope on a video monitor, allows the surgeon to maintain a broader perspective during the procedure than with traditional endoscopic surgery techniques. By careful evaluation of the patient and the suspected sinus disorder, and with a knowledge of a variety of approaches to surgery for the wide range of sinus problems, the surgeon can manage sinus disease effectively by the least invasive technique.

REFERENCES

1. Kennedy DW, Zinreich SJ, Rosenbaum AE, et al: Functional endoscopic sinus surgery: Theory and diagnostic evaluation. Arch Otolaryngol 111:576–582, 1985.
2. Kennedy DW: Functional endoscopic sinus surgery, technique. Arch Otolaryngol 111:643–649, 1985.
3. Stammberger H: Endoscopic endonasal surgery—new concepts and treatment of recurring rhinosinusitis. I. Anatomic and pathophysiological considerations. II. Surgical technique. Otolaryngol Head Neck Surg 94:143–156, 1986.
4. Messerklinger W: Endoscopy of the Nose. Baltimore: Urban and Schwartzenberg, 1978.
5. May M, Mester SJ, O'Daniel TG, Curtin HD: Decreasing the risks of endonasal endoscopic sinus surgery by imaging techniques. Op Tech Otolaryngol Head Neck Surg 1:89–91, 1990.

6. Huerter JV Jr, Lydiatt WM, Gupta SK, et al: The effect of intranasal oxymetazoline on serum levels of cocaine after intranasal cocaine application. Am J Rhinol 5:235–239, 1991.
7. May M, Hoffmann DF, Sobol SM: Video endoscopic sinus surgery: A two-handed technique. Laryngoscope 100:430–432, 1990.
8. May M, Sobol SM, Korzec K: The location of the maxillary os and its importance to the endoscopic sinus surgeon. Laryngoscope 100:1037–1042, 1990.
9. Draf W: Operating microscope for endonasal sinus surgery. First International Symposium: Contemporary Sinus Surgery. November 4–6, 1990, Pittsburgh.
10. Amedee RG, Mann WJ, Gilsbach JM: Microscopic endonasal surgery of the paranasal sinuses and the parasellar region. Arch Otolaryngol Head Neck Surg 115:1103–1106, 1989.
11. Dixon H: Microscopic sinus surgery, transnasal ethmoid and sphenoidectomy. Laryngoscope 93:440–444, 1983.
12. May M, Sobol SM, Korzec K: Nasopharyngeal balloon catheter enhances endoscopic sinus surgery in the awake patient. Op Tech Otolaryngol Head Neck Surg 1:142–143, 1990.
13. Wigand ME: Transnasal ethmoidectomy under endoscopic control. Rhinology 19:7–15, 1981.
14. Goldman J: Complications of intranasal ethmoidectomy: A review of 1000 consecutive operations. Laryngoscope 89:433, 1979.
15. May M, Har-EL G: Endoscopic sinus surgery: Green, yellow, red color-coded measurements for safety. Op Tech Otolaryngol Head Neck Surg 1:126–127, 1990.
16. Stankiewicz J: Blindness and intranasal endoscopic ethmoidectomy: Prevention and management. Otolaryngol Head Neck Surg 101:320–329, 1989.
17. Schaefer SD, Close LG: Endoscopic management of frontal sinus disease. Laryngoscope 100:155–160, 1990.
18. Hoffman DF, May M. Endoscopic frontal sinus surgery: Frontal trephine permits a "two-sided" approach. Op Tech Otolaryngol Head Neck Surg 2:257–261, 1991.
19. Hayes DM, Hoshaw TC. A simple method for identifying the nasofrontal duct ostium during ethmoidectomy. Presented at the First International Symposium on Contemporary Sinus Surgery, Pittsburgh, November 1990.
20. May M: Frontal sinus surgery: Endonasal endoscopic ostioplasty rather than external osteoplasty. Op Tech Otolaryngol Head Neck Surg 2:247–256, 1991.
21. Draf W: Endonasal micro-endoscopic frontal sinus surgery, the Fulda concept. Op Tech Otolaryngol Head Neck Surg 2:234–240, 1991.
22. Wigand ME, Hosemann WG: Endoscopic sinus surgery for frontal sinusitis and its complications. Am J Rhinol 5:85–89, 1991.
23. DeFreitas J, Lucente FE: The Caldwell Luc procedure: Institutional review of 670 cases 1975–1985. Laryngoscope 98:1297–1300, 1988.
24. Paugh DR, Sullivan MJ: Myospherulosis of the paranasal sinuses. Otolaryngol Head Neck Surg 103:117–119, 1990.
25. Martin SC, May M: Endoscopic sinus surgery: Is hospitalization justified? Op Tech Otolaryngol Head Neck Surg 2:241–243, 1991.

6
Results of Surgery

MARK MAY, M.D., F.A.C.S.
HOWARD L. LEVINE, M.D., F.A.C.S.
BARRY SCHAITKIN, M.D.
SARA J. MESTER, R.T.(R)

The reported success rates in larger series of patients for either traditional sinus surgery or endoscopic sinus surgery (ESS) are generally high (Table 6–1).[1-17] In addition, the reported overall success rates are within a similar range for the two types of sinus surgery.

An investigation of the bases for the reports of sinus surgery results shown in Table 6–1, however, revealed a lack of consistency in the methods used to evaluate and report results, both among surgeons performing traditional sinus surgery procedures and those performing ESS. In this chapter we discuss these reports of sinus surgery results, and the reporting systems used, to help identify factors to be taken into consideration in reporting the outcome of sinus surgery. Then, we describe the system devised by May and Levine to report results of sinus surgery, and we report the results, classified according to this system, of the 1709 ESS procedures performed by Levine (1100 procedures) and May (609 procedures) over the past 5 years.

CONSIDERATIONS FOR SYSTEMS TO REPORT RESULTS OF SINUS SURGERY

We reviewed five reports of 75 or more patients who underwent one or more traditional sinus surgery procedures,[1-5] and 10 reports of 75 or more patients who underwent ESS.[6-15] From this review, our experience,[16,17] and a review of other literature,[18-30] we identified several factors important to accurate reporting of sinus surgery results.

Traditional Sinus Surgery

Preoperative Factors

A review of the results of traditional sinus surgery shows that the outcome of surgery can be affected by conditions or historical factors present preoperatively. Sogg,[1] for example,

Table 6–1 Results After One or More Traditional Versus Endoscopic Sinus Surgery Procedures Reported for Groups of 75 or More Patients Followed for 6 Months or Longer

SURGERY TYPE	PT. REPORTED/ TOTAL PT.	FOLLOW-UP PERIOD	SYMPTOM-FREE (%)	IMPROVED (%)	OVERALL SUCCESS (%)
Traditional Surgery					
Sogg[1]	146/185	6–13 yr			69
Lawson[2]	90/600	2–14 (av. 3.5) yr			73
Friedman/Katsantonis[3]	1178 procedures				85
Stevens/Blair[4]	75/87	6 mo–11 yr			90
Malotte et al.[5]	81/98	av. 23–40 mo	27	48	93
Endoscopic Surgery					
Wigand/Hosemann[6]	220/500 (?)		24	58	79–93
Kennedy et al.[7]	75/75	4–32 mo	33	59	92
Schaefer et al.[8]	100/100	1–20 mo	10	83	93
Toffel et al.[9]	113/170	6 mo	90	10	100
Rice[10]	100/100	2 yr	83	16	99
Vleming/DeVries[11]	146/165	2–24 mo			73
Stammberger/Posawetz[12]	500/4500	8–12 mo			95
Matthews[13]	132/155	median 10–13 mo			91
Lazar et al.[14]	103/210	3–36 mo			84
Gaskins[15]	303/303	median 12 mo			92
Levine[16]	221/250	12–42 mo	79	19	79–88
Hoffman, May et al.[17]	91/100	4–21 mo			98

grouped patients with sinus disease into: (1) those with polyps and allergy, (2) those with polyps but no allergy, (3) those with allergy and no polyps, and (4) those with neither polyps nor allergy. In that study, traditional sinus surgery was successful in removing signs of disease in 72% of patients with infection alone, 76% of those with infection and allergy, and 83% of those with polypoid disease but not allergy. The success rate was only 51% for patients with *both polypoid disease and allergy*, however. Fifteen *revision procedures* were required among the patients in this series, 11 in 10 of 76 patients with polyps and 4 in 70 patients without polyps.

In Lawson's[2] study patients were grouped according to whether they had allergy, asthma, aspirin sensitivity, or history of previous surgery; disease was characterized from radiologic findings as *focal or diffuse* and according to whether polyposis was present. Forty percent of Lawson's patients had previously undergone surgery involving the sinuses, but the effect of this variable on results was not reported. Lawson found that the overall success of the *index procedure* (the procedure, whether initial or revision, considered as the first procedure for this report) in relieving signs of disease was 73%, and the difference for those with polyps versus those without polyps was not significant. There was, however, a statistically significant difference in success of the procedure in those *with asthma* (50%) versus those without asthma (88%).

Asthma and the extent of disease as factors in the success of sinus surgery were also investigated by Friedman and colleagues.[3,19] Friedman and Katsantonis[3] noted that for 1037 sphenoethmoidectomies performed over an 8-year period, the *polyp recurrence* rate was 19% for the approximately half of procedures in patients with asthma and 11% for procedures in patients without *asthma*. The authors also noted reduction in steroid requirements among most asthmatic patients in this study after the procedure. The report of these results did not, however, indicate how many patients underwent multiple procedures or how many revision procedures were performed. The follow-up period also was not specified.

Stevens and Blair[4] studied the recurrence of *polyps* among 75 patients followed for 6 months to 11 years after initial surgery. The initial overall recurrence rate was 25%, with time to *first revision* ranging from 3 months to 10 years (mean, 4 years). They considered surgery to have failed in the eight patients whose polyps recurred after the second or third procedure.

Malotte et al[5] were able to obtain follow-up data on 81 of 98 patients who underwent transantral sphenoethmoidectomy for chronic hyperplastic rhinosinusitis; 29 of these patients had previously undergone sinus surgery. All patients underwent *radiographic* examination and most underwent CT, and the results in all patients showed evidence of pansinusitis. Only eight patients who returned for follow-up evaluation required revision surgery. The overall success rate was 75% after an average *follow-up period* of 23 to 40 months.

In the foregoing review, several factors important to consider in reporting the success of sinus surgery were italicized. First, preoperative conditions such as asthma, allergy, and aspirin sensitivity can affect the outcome of sinus surgery. Second, the type of sinus condition present, especially the presence of polyps, can affect outcome. Third, imaging modalities and other objective measures may be used to estimate the extent of disease preoperatively.

A fourth factor that must be considered when evaluating these reports of sinus surgery outcome is the number of revision procedures represented by the results. Some reports count results as successful or unsuccessful after only one procedure; others evaluate results after an index procedure (whether or not numbers and types of previous sinus operations are provided) or after a specified number of revision procedures.

Timing for Evaluation Results

A fifth consideration in evaluating the results of sinus surgery is the length of follow-up before results are evaluated. Because it is almost always possible for sinus problems to recur, each report can only represent the success of surgery for a certain time frame: the follow-up period. Lawson,[2] for example, pointed out that polyps did not recur in his patients until 15 to 48 months (mean, 30 months) after surgery. Thus, timing of evaluation, based on the natural history of the sinus disorder present, can have a large effect on whether the results reported accurately reflect the long-term rate of success of the procedure.

A sixth factor is whether rates of success are reported for the total number of patients treated or procedures performed, or for the number of patients and procedures evaluated during the specified follow-up period.

Outcome Measures

A seventh factor and a critical consideration in developing a system to classify and grade the results of a surgical treatment is the measure of outcome. That is, what determines success or failure? Because in most cases sinus surgery is performed as an elective procedure to relieve symptoms, how well the operation achieves this goal should be a major factor in determining the success of the procedure. In Sogg's study,[1] patients were questioned about their symptoms and feelings regarding the long-term outcome of sinus surgery. However, the basis for reporting results was *relief of signs of disease*, not improvement in symptoms. Lawson[2] also considered symptoms in evaluating return of sinus disease but not as a measure of outcome of surgery.

Kimmelman et al[18] classified results of transantral ethmoidectomy versus external ethmoidectomy according to whether patients: (1) were symptom-free, (2) had improvement in symptoms, (3) had improved symptoms with antibiotic therapy, (4) required additional surgery, (5) required surgical treatment of a complication, (6) were lost to follow-up care, or (7) had conditions other than sinusitis. Kimmelman et al's system, or a modified version of this system, has been widely used to judge the success of sinus surgery. Malotte et al,[5] for example, used a modified Kimmelman system to classify their results of transantral sphenoethmoidectomy.

In another study, Friedman et al[19] staged chronic hyperplastic rhinosinusitis in 100 patients by computed tomography (CT). Their categorization of disease as focal, multifocal, or diffuse was not, however, predictive of success of surgical outcome: 81 to 92% of patients in all categories had improvement in disease on CT. In addition, Friedman et al did not correlate objective findings with symptoms. Levine,[16] Hoffman et al,[17] and Matthews et al[13] have also failed to find a correlation, either between preoperative CT findings and symptoms or between postoperative CT findings and relief of symptoms. Thus, objective measures of sinus surgery outcome may be included as the eighth factor to be taken into consideration in devising a classification system for surgical results, although the validity of such measures are in dispute.

Endoscopic Sinus Surgery

The preoperative factors and considerations for timing the evaluation of results of ESS are similar to those reported for nonendoscopic sinus surgery. Methods to report outcome measures are more varied, however. Relief of symptoms of sinus dysfunction is the key variable in whether ESS is successful, but authors have used a number of systems to classify symptomatology. In addition, other objective means to evaluate success of ESS have been investigated.

In reviewing their results of performing more than 1000 endoscopic sinus operations, Wigand and Hosemann[6] noted the importance of choice of surgical procedure and of long-term follow-up care to the success of ESS (although more than half of the patients on whom they performed surgery did not return for such care). They evaluated the results of surgery on the basis of relief of symptoms and tried to correlate this indicator with results of endoscopy. Of the 220 patients who did return for follow-up between 3 and 5 years after surgery, Wigand and Hosemann[6] found relief or improvement in symptoms (headache/facial pain, obstructed nasal breathing, nasal discharge, disturbance of smell or taste, or sore throat) in 79 to 93%. On endoscopy, however, they found a normal ethmoid sinus in only 52% and a normal maxillary sinus in only 72% of patients.

Poor correlation between endoscopic findings and symptomatology was also demonstrated in a study by Kennedy et al.[7] They reported results of endoscopic middle meatal antrostomy in 75 patients (117 procedures), 62 of whom returned for endoscopic evaluation of the patency of the maxillary sinus ostium. One third (25) of the patients were asymptomatic and 44 of the 75 had improved symptoms; in only six patients were symptoms unchanged from preoperative severity, and none had worse symptoms after surgery. Despite residual symptoms in two thirds of patients, endoscopy showed that the ostium was patent in 98% of patients. Were an open sinus drainage system the only requirement for normal sinus function, one would expect freedom from symptoms in all patients with no endoscopic evidence of obstruction.

Schaefer et al[8] also used endoscopy and patient reports of symptom relief to evaluate the results of ESS in patients with sinusitis only, polyps only, or both. They reported a success rate of 93% overall, but their follow-up period of 1 to 20 months was too short to provide long-term results in patients with polyps. Toffel et al[9] also reported excellent results in terms of symptom relief or improvement in patients with sinusitis, with or without polyps, but their follow-up period of 1 year was also too short to evaluate results of surgery for polyps.

The 2-year follow-up reported by Rice[10] was too short to evaluate the long-term results of ESS in the 25% of his patients who had polyps. Nevertheless, it is impressive that 83% of the patients in this series remained symptom-free 2 years after surgery and 16 other patients (10 with medical therapy and six with revision surgery) sustained improvement in symptoms.

Vleming and deVries[11] judged the results of ESS to treat sinusitis or polyps on the basis of endoscopic findings (63% good and 37% poor) and patient reports of symptom status as symptom-free or much improved (51%), improved (22%), or poor (no change or worse than before surgery, 27%). They took their subjective and objective results together to obtain a 76% success rate in patients without polyposis, a 90% rate in patients with polyposis, and a 56% rate in those with headache. In another report of 263 procedures in 105 patients with polyposis, subjective results were good in 86% with a median follow-up of 2 years after one or more operations, but only 61% of patients were free of polyp recurrence.[22] The system for reporting results of sinus surgery that Vleming and DeVries[11] described is widely used. It does not, however, take into account whether additional treatment, either medical or surgical, was provided.

Stammberger and Posawetz[12] rated results of surgery according to type of previous surgery, and symptoms such as headache. Interestingly, in their series of 500 patients, when headache was the only symptom of sinus disease it was relieved completely in 88% of cases. This is in contrast to the 56% rate reported by Vleming et al.[22] Stammberger and Posawetz[12] found that ESS is least likely to be successful when polyps and multiple allergies resistant to allergic therapy are present. They also found a poor correlation between abnormal mucosa seen endoscopically and recurrence of symptoms.

Matthews et al[13] also noted a lack of correlation between endoscopic findings and patients' evaluations of success of surgery. Ninety-one percent of patients, when surveyed a median of 12 months after the procedure, stated that they believed the surgery was beneficial. They found statistically significant correlations between opacification of the sphenoid sinus and poor outcome (but no relationship between opacification of other sinuses and outcome) and significantly better improvement in symptoms when a concomitant septoplasty was performed for deviated septum than when no deviated septum was present. Patients in this study with pain as one of their symptoms also had superior results compared with those without pain; this last result is similar to the finding of Stammberger and Posawetz[12] that ESS was associated with a high rate of success in relieving headache.

In a report on ESS in children, Lazar et al[14] found that nasal drainage and persistent cough were the most common complaints of sinus disorder, but objective measures such as the character of drainage or cough were not correlated with the type of disease. Results of allergy testing were positive in 46% of these children. The outcome of surgery in this series was categorized on the basis of endoscopic findings (20% adhesions, 10% granulation tissue, 11% significant crusting, and 7% polyposis), and judged on parents' answers to a questionnaire regarding symptoms. Responses, obtained from nearly half of the children's parents, showed marked or moderate improvement in 83 to 85% of children who had complained preoperatively of chronic headache (128 children), chronic nasal discharge (132 children), chronic nasal obstruction (168 children), or chronic cough (153 children). The researchers noted, however, that most of the parents responding to the questionnaire were those whose children had experienced marked improvement or cure of symptoms. Factors they identified in failure of sinus surgery in children included long chronicity of sinus disease, allergies, immune deficiencies, cystic fibrosis, or presence of immotile cilia syndrome.

Other factors were considered by Lund et al,[23] who studied 12 men and 12 women with chronic rhinosinusitis, some with polyps and asthma and half with allergies. Three quarters had previous nasal or sinus surgery. In addition to CT imaging and rigid endoscopy of the nasal cavity, all patients underwent mucociliary function testing before the operation. All symptoms were significantly improved after the operation, and ciliary beat frequency was also significantly increased for the group as a whole. Olfaction did not improve overall, however, and anterior rhinomanometry failed to demonstrate any significant change in total nasal airway resistance after surgery.

Gaskins[15] proposed a comprehensive system for staging chronic sinusitis before sinus surgery and for reporting results. His system takes into account the anatomic extent of disease, as determined by endoscopic and radiographic examination ("site"); sinus surgery history ("surgery"); presence and extent of polyps ("polyps"); presence and control of infection ("infection"); and immunologic status ("immune"). In each of these five categories a score between 0 and 4 may be assigned, depending on the extent of disease present. Thus, if inflammation is limited to the ostiomeatal complex (OMC), a score of 1 would be assigned in the "site" category, for example. The patient's scores in each category are then averaged to provide a "staging score" between 0 and 4 that corresponds to stage 0–IV sinus disease.

Gaskins scored patients' responses to surgery as 2 (asymptomatic), 1 (symptoms present but improved), 0 (symptoms unchanged), −1 (symptoms somewhat worse), or −2 (symptoms much worse). Finally, he calculated the percent of patients in each stage as a function of response to surgery, both with relation to severity of each of five symptoms (congestion, obstruction, sinusitis, headache, and polyps) and overall.

Using this system, Gaskins was able to make very specific and quantitative observations about the relationship of preoperative disease and the quality of surgical results among the 303 patients in his study. For example, he determined quantitatively that his patients with stage I disease had a 90% chance of experiencing excellent results of surgery; furthermore, he showed that the failure rate essentially doubled for stages II and III, although the overall response rate remained good for patients with disease in any of the first three stages (I–III). Gaskins also associated stages of disease with choice of surgical procedure: he found ESS suitable for treating stage I–III disease, and an external technique more appropriate for stage IV disease.

Despite the refinement of Gaskins's system for staging sinus disease and reporting results, it does not address the need to time follow-up evaluations so as to identify late failures of surgery. Another issue that appears from our review of reporting systems is that in many cases a subsample of the patient population is selected for reporting but the selection process is not fully described. We have also found disparities in presentation of information, such as numbers of patients versus procedures. Such differences in reporting statistical information make comparison of results among studies very difficult if not impossible. Thus, any reporting system is only useful if this type of information is supplied in a standardized way.

SINUS SURGERY RESULTS REPORTING SYSTEM OF MAY AND LEVINE

To improve case selection for and the success of ESS, we have developed a sinus surgery results reporting system that takes preoperative factors into account, qualifies and quantifies the outcome of surgery, and addresses the time frame for follow-up evaluations and care. Our goal in developing this system was to help ourselves and other clinicians: (1) identify the patients for whom sinus surgery is appropriate, (2) choose the surgical approach that will provide the best results for each patient, (3) predict the success of ESS in relieving sinus disease symptoms, and (4) evaluate success or failure in a systematic and reproducible way.

The reporting system we propose draws on the systems devised by others.[11,15,18,19] As did the majority of reporters whose systems we reviewed, we classify disease and identify factors preoperatively that have been shown to affect the outcome of sinus surgery (Table 6–2),[24]

Table 6–2 Classification System for Reporting Results of Sinus Surgery—Severity of Disease State Preoperatively

I. Anatomic variations, including one or more of the following
  A. Turbinoseptal deformity (TS) (determined endoscopically after decongestion):
    1. TS-1: Medial and lateral aspect of middle turbinate visible
    2. TS-2: Anterior attachment of middle turbinate partially obscured by lateralized septum
    3. TS-3: Anterior attachment of middle turbinate completely obscured
    4. TS-4: Septum impacted into lateral nasal wall anterior to attachment of middle turbinate
  B. Narrowed infundibulum or mucosal contact after decongestion associated with one or more of following (determined by endoscopic examination or CT scan):
    1. Paradoxical turbinate
    2. Concha bullosa
    3. Lateralized uncinate
    4. Bulla ethmoidalis
    5. Haller cell
    6. Agger nasi cells (narrow nasofrontal recess)
    7. Other or combination of above
II. Inflammatory disease, acute or chronic (determined by history, endoscopy, and CT scan)
  A. Types of disease:
    1. Mucosal thickening (hyperplastic sinusitis)
    2. Mucosal contact
    3. Retained secretions (mucoid to purulent)
    4. Fungal or bacterial
    5. Barosinusitis
    6. Mucopyocele
    7. Traumatic
    8. Other
  B. Severity (graded by CT and reported as right side, left side, or both):
    1. 1+: limited to ostiomeatal complex (structures between middle turbinate and lateral nasal wall)
    2. 2+: incomplete opacification of one or more major sinuses (frontal, maxillary, sphenoid)
    3. 3+: total opacification of one or more major sinuses but not all
    4. 4+: total opacification of all sinuses
III. Allergic rhinitis (determined by history, endoscopic examination, and allergy tests)
IV. Polyps (reported as right side, left side, or both) severity (graded by endoscopic examination):
    1. 1+: anterior attachment of middle turbinate visible
    2. 2+: anterior attachment of middle turbinate obscured
    3. 3+: nasal cavity filled to vestibule
    4. 4+: nasal cavity filled to nares
    5. 5+: nasal cavity filled to lip
V. Presence of unfavorable prognostic factors
  A. Previous sinus surgery
  B. Reactive airway disease (asthma, chronic bronchitis)
  C. ASA triad (Samter's syndrome: asthma, polyps, aspirin sensitivity)
  D. Allergic sinobronchial aspergillosis
  E. Kartagener's syndrome
  F. Dysmotility syndrome
  G. Cystic fibrosis
  H. Immune disorder

and we base the success of our results on the patient's evaluation of symptom relief at follow-up visits (Table 6–3).[24]

Proposed Management of Nasosinus Disease by Endoscopic Sinus Surgery

We recommended and performed surgery for patients: (1) who had chronic symptoms related to nasosinus disease, (2) whose symptoms persisted in spite of adequate medical management, (3) with abnormalities on endoscopy or CT, and (4) after they had been completely informed of the potential risks of surgery and decided that the potential for relief of symptoms was greater than the potential adverse effects of the procedure (see Appendix, Endoscopic Sinus Surgery Protocol).

We used the endonasal endoscopic approach in all cases, and our overall goal was to relieve obstruction in the OMC. The planned extent of surgery was based on whether disease was focal or diffuse. For example, patients with narrowing of the infundibulum due to an anatomic condition, such as a lateralized uncinate process draping a prominent bulla ethmoidalis, were treated by removing the obstruction, in this case the uncinate process and bulla ethmoidalis. When the preoperative CT showed opacification of anterior and posterior ethmoid cells, interpreted as thickened mucous membrane due to hyperplastic sinusitis, the anterior and posterior ethmoid cells were opened.

A total sphenoethmoidectomy with marsupialization of the sphenoid, ethmoid, and maxillary sinuses was performed for patients with massive polyposis or hyperplastic mucosa associated with asthma, Samter's syndrome (asthma, polyposis, and aspirin sensitivity), dysmotility problems, cystic fibrosis, or a granulomatous disorder. In patients with symptoms referable to the frontal sinus region and with CT evidence of disease in this area, we opened the nasofrontal recess.

Evaluation of the results of treatment included patient chart review, follow-up visits, and telephone surveys (for those who had not returned in the past 4 months). As shown in Table 6–3, results in groups I–IV were considered successful, and results in group V were considered failures.

Table 6–3 Classification System for Reporting Results of Sinus Surgery—Patient's Assessment of Relief of Symptoms Postoperatively*

I.	Symptom-free	
II.	Symptom-free after one additional therapy	
	A. Medical treatment	
	B. Revision surgery	
III.	Improved (3 most prominent symptoms)	
IV.	Improved with maintenance	
	A. Medical therapy	
	B. Revision surgery	
V.	Same or worse (surgical failure)	
VI.	Lost for follow-up	

*Minimum reporting period for each patient is 6 months; list symptoms as of last evaluation, i.e., 1 year, 10 years, and state this duration of follow-up (a minimum of 36 months is suggested for polyps).

Results of Endoscopic Sinus Surgery in Levine and May Patient Series

The results for 1100 of the first 1165 patients operated on by Levine using ESS are tabulated in Table 6–4; Table 6–5 shows results by symptom. The results for 609 of the first 692 patients operated on by May using ESS are shown in Table 6–6, and Table 6–7 shows results by symptom for 400 of May's group of patients.

In comparing Tables 6–5 and 6–7 it may be noted that similar numbers of patients complained of similar symptoms in each series, even though Levine's report covers 1100 patients and May's only 400 patients. We attribute the lower proportion of all patients with complaints in Levine's series to different techniques for gathering information about symptoms: Levine recorded preoperative symptoms volunteered by patients and evaluated relief of these symptoms postoperatively; May questions patients about each symptom pre- and postoperatively. Thus, May's series averages more symptoms per patient than Levine's series. Nevertheless, as a comparison of Tables 6–5 and 6–7 shows, ESS had about the same success in relieving symptoms in the two series.

Improvement in symptoms after one ESS procedure was calculated by adding patients for the two surgeons in groups I, IIA, III, and IVA. In Levine's series 888 patients (81%) had successful results after one operation and in May's series 462 (76%) had successful results after one operation. The proportion of successful results improved after two or more procedures to 95% for Levine's patients and 87% for May's patients.

Effects of Disease on Results in May's Series

May's results were analyzed further to identify any differences in patients who underwent surgery to treat anatomic, hyperplastic, infectious, or polypoid disease. Influences on

Table 6–4 Results of Endoscopic Sinus Surgery in 1100 Patients Operated on by Levine and Followed for 6–52 Months

RESULTS CATEGORY	PATIENTS: NO.	(%)
I. Symptom-free	294	(27)
II. Symptom-free after one additional therapy		
A. Medical treatment	248	(22)
B. Revision surgery	71	(6)
III. Improved	175	(16)
IV. Improved with maintenance		
A. Medical treatment	171	(16)
B. Revision surgery	89	(8)
V. Same or worse	52	(5)
Total	**1100**	**(100)**
VI. Lost to follow-up	65	(6)

Overall Results:
81% improved after initial surgery
<u>14% improved after revision surgery</u>
95% overall success

Group I = 27%
Groups I–III = 71%
Group IV = 24%
Group V = 5%

Table 6–5 Symptom Profile of 1100 of Levine's Patients Preoperatively and at Last Evaluation (6–52 months postoperatively)*

SYMPTOM	NO. PTS. WITH SYMPTOM PREOPERATIVELY	NO. (%) PTS. IMPROVED POSTOPERATIVELY
Nasal stuffiness	243	223 (91.8)
Nasal airway obstruction	317	267 (84.2)
Postnasal discharge	330	208 (63.0)
Eye pressure/pain	189	153 (81.0)
Headache	126	94 (74.6)
Facial pressure	367	307 (83.7)
Taste/smell changes	191	155 (81.2)
Chronic cough	114	84 (73.7)

*Preoperative symptom profile is based on information volunteered by patients. Postoperative profile is based on patients' responses to questions about the symptoms they complained of preoperatively.

Table 6–6 Results of Endoscopic Sinus Surgery in 609 Patients Operated on by May and Followed for 6–48 Months

RESULTS CATEGORY	PATIENTS: NO.	(%)
I. Symptom-free	168	(28)
II. Symptom-free after one additional therapy		
A. Medical treatment	37	(6)
B. Revision surgery	22	(4)
III. Improved	151	(25)
IV. Improved with maintenance		
A. Medical treatment	106	(17)
B. Revision surgery	43	(7)
V. Same or worse	82	(13)
Total	**609**	**(100)**
VI. Lost to follow-up	83	(14)

Overall Success:
76% improved after initial surgery
11% improved after revision surgery
87% overall success

Group I = 28%
Groups I–III = 63%
Group IV = 24%
Group V = 13%

Table 6–7 Symptom Profile of the First Consecutive 400 of May's Patients Preoperatively and at Last Evaluation (6–48 months postoperatively)*

SYMPTOM	NO. PTS. WITH SYMPTOM PREOPERATIVELY	NO. (%) PTS. IMPROVED POSTOPERATIVELY
Nasal stuffiness	368	317 (86)
Postnasal discharge	316	277 (88)
Headache	260	221 (85)
Facial pressure	229	212 (93)
Rhinorrhea	203	186 (92)
Taste/smell changes	179	170 (95)
Eye pressure	169	167 (99)

*Each patient was surveyed pre- and postoperatively regarding presence of each symptom listed on the Endoscopic Sinus Surgery Protocol (Appendix).

Table 6–8 Results of Sinus Surgery Grouped According to Disease for 609* of May's Patients Followed for 6–48 Months

DISEASE[†]	TOTAL PATIENTS	GRADE I–III No. (%)	GRADE IVA, IVB No. (%)	GRADE V No. (%)
Anatomy	208	146 (70)	37 (18)	25 (12)
Hyperplasia	196	121 (62)	37 (19)	38 (19)
Infection	28	19 (68)	8 (29)	1 (4)
Polyposis	117	71 (61)	34 (29)	12 (10)
Triad	60	21 (35)	33 (55)	6 (10)
Total	**609**	**378 (62)**	**149 (25)**	**82 (13)**

*Total 692 patients, 83 lost to follow-up.
[†]Disease status preoperatively: Anatomy = anatomic variations; Hyperplasia = hyperplastic disease; Infection = suppurative infection; Triad = ASA triad (Samter's syndrome).

results of asthma, nasal allergy, previous surgery, or Samter's syndrome (ASA triad) were also sought. The results are summarized in Table 6–8. A review of the data indicates that disease correlated best with results for patients with results in grades I–III.

As shown in Table 6–8, ESS achieved grade I–III results less often in patients with ASA triad (35% of 60 patients) than in those with other conditions (61 to 70%). However, the failure rate in those with ASA triad compares favorably with that for patients with polyposis (10%) or suppurative infection (4%). Furthermore, in 33 (55%) of the 60 patients with ASA triad symptoms were improved only with additional treatment (grade IVA or IVB). Thus, the best results (grade I–III) were obtained in only about half the proportion of patients with ASA triad as for any of the other conditions.

Probst et al[25] noted that even in patients without ASA triad but with polyps, 35% have been found sensitive to aspirin, 40 to 70% had bronchial asthma, and 29% had rhinitis. The likelihood is thus high that another component of ASA triad will be present even if the full triad is not, and the additional factor could be expected to have an effect on the success of ESS. In May's series of patients this was verified by the finding of 39% grade I–III results in patients with asthma and polyps versus 55% in patients with asthma but without polyps (Table 6–9). Additionally, the 39% success rate in those with asthma and polyps is close to the 35% success rate in those known to have the full triad. Regarding effects on treatment, Probst et al[25] note that surgical treatment of polyposis has been thought by some to lead to worse symptoms of asthma in those with both factors; however, there is evidence that polypectomy actually improves symptoms of asthma, or at least makes asthma less difficult to manage.[3]

Effects of Preoperative Factors on May's Results

May's results were next analyzed for the influence on surgical success of asthma, allergy, previous surgery, or ASA triad, with polyposis versus without polyposis. It was found, not surprisingly, that ESS gave the best results in patients with anatomic variations or infection and in the absence of polyposis, asthma, allergy, previous surgery, or ASA triad (Tables 6–8 and 6–9). Grade I–III results were achieved in 70% of patients operated on for anatomic

Table 6–9 Results of Sinus Surgery Grouped According to Preoperative Factors for 609* of May's Patients Followed for 6–48 Months

FACTOR[†]	TOTAL PATIENTS	GRADE I–III No. (%)	GRADE IVA, IVB No. (%)	GRADE V No. (%)
NO POLYPOSIS				
Normal	296	204 (69)	49 (17)	43 (14)
Asthma	44	24 (55)	12 (27)	8 (18)
Allergy	68	43 (63)	18 (26)	7 (10)
Surgery	24	15 (62)	3 (12)	6 (25)
Subtotal	432	286	82	64
POLYPOSIS				
Normal	69	45 (65)	16 (23)	8 (12)
Asthma	18	**7 (39)**	9 (50)	2 (11)
Allergy	15	10 (67)	5 (33)	0
Surgery	15	9 (60)	4 (27)	2 (13)
Subtotal	117	71	34	12
ASA triad	60	**21 (35)**	33 (55)	6 (10)
Total	609	378	149	82

*Total 692 patients, 83 lost to follow-up.
[†]Factor present preoperatively: Surgery = previous sinus surgery; ASA triad = asthma, aspirin sensitivity, and polyps (Samter's syndrome).

problems and in 68% of those with infection (Table 6–8). The rates of success (grade I–III results) were somewhat worse in patients with polyposis (61%) or hyperplasia (62%) (Table 6–8). The success rates were notably worse, however, for patients without polyposis but with asthma (55%) (Table 6–9). The poorest results were noted in those with asthma *and polyposis* (39%) and ASA triad (35%).

Based on these observations, a poorer prognosis for a grade I–III result can be expected for patients with a combination of polyposis and asthma. Furthermore, it is clear from these data that of all factors ASA triad carries the worst prognosis for success of ESS in relieving symptoms (Tables 6–8 and 6–9). The prognosis is almost as poor for those with asthma and polyps, probably because many of these patients actually may have ASA triad. Of any single factor alone, asthma carries a somewhat worse prognosis than polyps, allergy, or previous surgery.

REVISION ENDOSCOPIC SINUS SURGERY

Sixty-five (those with grade IIB or IVB results, Table 6–6) or 11% of the 609 patients in May's series underwent revision ESS. The proportion in Levine's series (160 of 1100 patients, or 15%) was similar. These rates may be compared to a revision rate of 9.4% in another study[26] in which 63 patients (16 children less than 16 years old and 47 adults) of 673 required a revision procedure after ESS for chronic recurrent sinusitis.

Reasons for Revision Surgery

Reasons for revision surgery include polyposis, adhesions, and persistent disease.

Polyposis

The most common reason (in 16 of 65 of May's patients) for performing revision surgery was to treat recurrent polyposis. For these 16 patients, the time from index ESS until recurrence of symptoms of polyposis was 2 to 3 years.

Polyps were also a common reason for revision surgery in many other series we reviewed.[1,4,15,21,23]

Adhesions

Another reason for failure of the index ESS procedure was symptoms due to adhesions or synechiae between the middle turbinate and the lateral wall of the nose (in 15 of 65 of May's patients). In one report by Schaefer et al[8] adhesions occurred in 6 of 100 patients and were a factor in revision surgery performed in four patients. In another report, nearly half of patients who required revision surgery had fibrosis between the lateral nasal wall and the middle turbinate.[26] Symptoms of adhesions occur within the first 6 months after surgery. This problem is directly related to the extent of surgery. Adhesions between the middle turbinate and lateral nasal wall do not occur after nonendoscopic endonasal sinus surgery because the middle turbinate is removed as part of the procedure.[27]

Avoiding Adhesions

Recommendations have been made to decrease adhesions complicating ESS. Schaefer et al.[8] listed four maneuvers to prevent scarring between the middle turbinate and lateral nasal wall: (1) remove the agger nasi cells and mucous membrane at the angle formed by the anterior attachment of the middle turbinate and lateral nasal wall, (2) excise loose fragments of bone and mucous membrane from the ethmoid sinus and lateral aspect of the middle turbinate, (3) preserve the mucous membrane on the lateral surface of the middle turbinate, and (4) clean the ethmoid cavity frequently in the postoperative period. Stankiewicz[29] suggests placing a spacer between the middle turbinate and lateral nasal wall, as well as frequent postoperative debridement of the nose until healing has occurred.

Another way to prevent adhesions involving the middle turbinate is to remove the bulky portion of this structure, a course recommended by Toffel[30] in all cases. Toffel recommends this course because the middle turbinate may be a source of pathologic obstruction of drainage from the OMC as well as a locus for formation of adhesions. After resecting the middle turbinate, Toffel places a spacer between the middle turbinate and lateral nasal wall for 5 days postoperatively. He reported adhesions in only 1 of 170 patients with this technique.[30]

These observations have been borne out for endoscopic procedures as well. We found that in our patients middle turbinate adhesions and maxillary sinus ostial stenosis did not occur when more extensive surgery was performed for advanced disease. This lower incidence of adhesions was the result of removing the middle turbinate and enlarging the maxillary sinus ostium.

Persistent Disease

Failure and the need for revision ESS may be due to persistent or recurrent disease, confirmed by postoperative endoscopic examination or CT scan, involving the agger nasi-nasofrontal region or the sphenoid sinus. Another cause of failure is persistent obstruction of the maxillary sinus ostium. In these cases the surgeon finds, on postoperative endoscopy, that a large patent maxillary antrostomy created in the posterior fontanelle does not connect with the natural ostium. In these cases, the natural ostium is often obstructed.

Friedman and Katsantonis[27] reported that revision surgery was needed after transantral sphenoethmoidectomy in 6.3% of cases in which an inferior meatal antrostomy was performed but only 2.8% of cases when the middle meatus was marsupialized with antrostomy. This observation supports the importance of a patent middle meatus antrostomy to increase the success rate of sinus surgery for inflammatory disease.

Polyps and Frontal Sinus: Delayed Failure

Except for polyps, which tend to recur in 3 or 4 years after surgery, the only condition that does not become apparent within 6 months of surgery is frontal sinus obstruction due to recurrent disease or postoperative scarring of the nasofrontal recess. In May's experience with traditional surgery, the need for frontal sinus revision surgery may not become apparent until 5 to 15 years after the index procedure.

Treatment-Resistant Disease

A small proportion of patients failed to respond to ESS, even after a revision procedure. Typically, postoperative endoscopy in these patients shows a normally mucosalized ethmoid cavity and a clear view into the frontal, maxillary, and sphenoid sinuses, and CT scans show apparently normal anatomy, but symptoms persist. The reason for failure in these cases could not be determined. The three most common symptoms to persist in such patients with treatment-resistant disease are postnasal drainage, combined loss of taste and smell, and nasal stuffiness.

Symptoms present preoperatively that appear to be associated with a lower rate of surgical success are isolated complaints of postnasal discharge, headache, or cough. Postnasal discharge as an isolated symptom may be due to mucositis, and surgery is not effective in relieving this problem. Headache and cough as isolated symptoms are not usually related to nasosinus disease. Typically, headache due to nasosinus disease is felt as pressure, fullness, or dull aching around the eyes, forehead, and face, and this symptom occurs in conjunction with other symptoms and signs of sinus involvement. When headache is the only presenting symptom, the differential diagnosis includes, among other conditions, temporomandibular, myofascial, or cervico-craniofacial neuralgic syndromes. Patients with isolated cough should undergo a thorough evaluation for pulmonary involvement before sinus surgery is considered.

SUMMARY

The results of ESS reported in this chapter show that the procedure can alleviate chronic symptoms and improve the quality of life for a very high proportion of patients with disease in the area of the OMC. The endoscopic approach allows precise visualization and surgical treatment of disease in the narrow cleft between the middle turbinate and the lateral nasal wall, leaving uninvolved structures untouched. This focal management minimizes morbidity and is associated with an 80 to 90% or better success rate, even in patients with predisposing factors such as asthma, allergy, or ASA triad. Consideration of results in grades I–III versus those in grade IV, however, shows that patients with ASA triad are more likely than those with other factors to require additional medical and/or surgical therapy for relief of symptoms.

In patients in the authors' series who required revision surgery, symptoms were due in the majority of cases to recurrent polyposis or adhesions. When the space between the middle turbinate and lateral nasal wall has been carefully cleared of obstructions, relief from symptoms can be lasting. The results of ESS reported to date indicate that this procedure is effective in relieving symptoms in selected patients when meticulous postoperative and follow-up care are provided.

REFERENCES

1. Sogg A: Long-term results of ethmoid surgery. Ann Otol Rhinol Laryngol 98:699–701, 1989.
2. Lawson W: The intranasal ethmoidectomy: An experience with 1,077 procedures. Laryngoscope 101:367–371, 1991.
3. Friedman WH, Katsantonis GP: The role of standard technique in modern sinus surgery. Otolaryngol Clin North Am 22:759–775, 1989.
4. Stevens HE, Blair NJ: Intranasal sphenoethmoidectomy: 10-year experience and literature review. J Otolaryngol 17:254–258, 1988.
5. Malotte MJ, Petti GH, Chonkich GD, Rowe RP: Transantral sphenoethmoidectomy: A procedure for the 1990s? Otolaryngol Head Neck Surg 104:358–361, 1991.
6. Wigand ME, Hosemann WG: Results of endoscopic surgery of the paranasal sinuses and anterior skull base. J Otolaryngol 20:385–390, 1991.
7. Kennedy DW, Zinreich SJ, Kuhn F, et al: Endoscopic middle meatal antrostomy: Theory, technique, and patency. Laryngoscope 97(8, pt. 3) Suppl 43, 1987.
8. Schaefer SD, Manning S, Close LG: Endoscopic paranasal sinus surgery: Indications and considerations. Laryngoscope 99:1–5, 1989.
9. Toffel PH, Aroesty DJ, Weinmann RH: Secure endoscopic sinus surgery as an adjunct to functional nasal surgery. Arch Otolaryngol Head Neck Surg 115:822–825, 1989.
10. Rice DH: Endoscopic sinus surgery: Results at 2-year followup. Otolaryngol Head Neck Surg 101:476–479, 1989.
11. Vleming M, deVries N: Endoscopic paranasal sinus surgery: Results. Am J Rhinol 4:13–17, 1990.
12. Stammberger H, Posawetz W: Functional endoscopic sinus surgery. Eur Arch Otorhinolaryngol 247:63–76, 1990.
13. Matthews BL, Smith LE, Jones R, et al: Endoscopic sinus surgery: Outcome in 155 cases. Otolaryngol Head Neck Surg 104:244–246, 1991.
14. Lazar RH, Younis RT, Gross CW: Pediatric functional endonasal sinus surgery: Review of 210 cases. Head Neck 14:92–98, 1992.
15. Gaskins RE: A surgical staging system for chronic sinusitis. Am J Rhinol 6:5–12, 1992.
16. Levine HL: Functional endoscopic sinus surgery: Evaluation, surgery, and follow-up of 250 patients. Laryngoscope 100:79–84, 1990.
17. Hoffman DF, May M, Mester SJ: Functional endoscopic sinus surgery-experience with the initial 100 patients. Am J Rhinol 4:129–132, 1990.
18. Kimmelman CP, Weisman RA, Osguthorpe JD, Kay SL: The efficacy and safety of transantral ethmoidectomy. Laryngoscope 98:1178–1182, 1988.

19. Friedman WH, Katsantonis GP, Sivore M, Kay S: Computed tomography staging of the paranasal sinuses in chronic hyperplastic rhinosinusitis. Laryngoscope 100:1161–1165, 1990.
20. Eichel B: The intranasal ethmoidectomy: A 12-year perspective. Otolaryngol Head Neck Surg 90:540–543, 1982.
21. Freedman HM, Kern EB: Complications of intranasal ethmoidectomy: A review of 1,000 consecutive operations. Laryngoscope 89:421–432, 1979.
22. Vleming M, Stoop AE, Middelweerd RJ, deVries N: Results of endoscopic sinus surgery for nasal polyps. Am J Rhinol 5:173–176, 1991.
23. Lund VJ, Holmstrom M, Scadding GK: Functional endoscopic sinus surgery in the management of chronic rhinosinusitis. An objective assessment. J Laryngol Otol 105:832–835, 1991.
24. May M: Reporting results of sinus surgery: A classification system. Op Tech Otolaryngol Head Neck Surg 2:244–246, 1991.
25. Probst L, Stoney P, Jeney E, Hawke M: Nasal polyps, bronchial asthma and aspirin sensitivity. J Otolaryngol 21:60–65, 1992.
26. Lazar RH, Younis RT, Long TE, Gross CW: Revision functional endonasal sinus surgery. Ear Nose Throat J 71:131–133, 1992.
27. Friedman WH, Katsantonis GP: Transantral revision of recurrent maxillary and ethmoid disease following functional intranasal surgery. Otolaryngol Head Neck Surg 106:367–371, 1992.
28. Kennedy DW: Functional endoscopic sinus surgery: Technique. Arch Otolaryngol 111:643–649, 1985.
29. Stankiewicz JA: Complications in endoscopic intranasal ethmoidectomy: An update. Laryngoscope 99:686–690, 1989.
30. Toffel PH: Chronic nasal obstruction. Curr Ther Otolaryngol Head Neck Surg 4:283–287, 1990.

7
Complications of Endoscopic Sinus Surgery

MARK MAY, M.D., F.A.C.S.
HOWARD L. LEVINE, M.D., F.A.C.S.
BARRY SCHAITKIN, M.D.
SARA J. MESTER, R.T.(R)

Even when performed by the most experienced surgeons, using a traditional or an endoscopic approach, sinus surgery may be associated with complications. In this chapter on complications of sinus surgery we describe how we report complications, review complications reported by surgeons performing traditional sinus surgery versus endoscopic sinus surgery (ESS), review the complications experienced by patients of the senior authors (H.L. and M.M.), and discuss complication recognition, management, and prevention.

SYSTEM FOR REPORTING SINUS SURGERY COMPLICATIONS

Classification

Complications are usually classified broadly as major or minor, but how these categories are defined varies. We believe that a review of sinus surgery complications should point to ways surgeons might improve results and decrease complications of future procedures. Thus, for our review of reports by other surgeons[1-17] and of our own experiences, we classified complications according to whether they resolved spontaneously, were corrected with treatment, or were permanent (lasted beyond 1 year). Major complications were those that usually required treatment to prevent permanent serious sequelae or that caused permanent serious sequelae despite treatment; other complications were considered minor.

We further classified major complications as resulting from violation of orbital, intracranial, vascular, or lacrimal structures. We considered all intracranial violations to be major complications, even if repaired at the time of occurrence and there were no postoperative sequelae. Permanent lacrimal duct obstruction is also considered a major complication, whether or not it requires treatment. Classification of other complications as major or minor is shown in Table 7–1.

Incidence

The incidence of complications has been reported by some authors as number of complications per total procedures performed. For example, Vleming et al[12] recently published the most complete and thorough analysis to date of complications of sinus surgery, focusing on the number of complications per procedure they performed. We believe it is the patient's experience of the complication that is significant for an elective procedure, however, and so we report the incidence of complications with the denominator as the number of patients who underwent surgery, not the number of procedures performed.

Table 7–1 Classifying Reported Complications of Sinus Surgery*

CATEGORY	TREATMENT CATEGORY	COMPLICATION
Major	Correctable with treatment	Orbital hematoma (postseptal) Loss of vision Diplopia Cerebrospinal fluid leak Meningitis Brain abscess Focal brain hemorrhage Hemorrhage requiring transfusion Carotid artery injury Epiphora (dacryocystorhinostomy)
	Permanent	Blindness Diplopia Central nervous system deficit(s) Death
Minor	Temporary, requires no treatment	Periorbital emphysema Periorbital ecchymosis Dental or lip pain or numbness
	Temporary, correctable with treatment	Adhesions requiring treatment Epistaxis requiring packing Bronchospasm Infection (sinus)
	Permanent if persists beyond 1 Year	Dental or lip pain or numbness Anosmia

*Incidences should be reported as (1) numbers of patients with major or minor complications and (2) total numbers of major and minor complications in the series.
Example: For a series of 100 patients:

    Patient A   **Patient B**
    cerebrospinal fluid leak   periorbital emphysema
    meningitis   periorbital ecchymosis
    periorbital ecchymosis

Major complications: 1 patient/100 patients = 1%
                                2 complications/100 patients = 2%
Minor complications: 2 patients/100 patients = 2%
                                3 complications/100 patients = 3%

We also believe it is most helpful to report the incidences of major and minor complications separately. For example, if, in a series of 50 patients, one patient experiences a cerebrospinal fluid (CSF) leak (major complication) and periorbital ecchymosis (minor complication) after bilateral ESS and another patient who underwent only unilateral ESS experiences periorbital emphysema and periorbital ecchymosis (minor complications), the incidence of major complications for this series is 1 of 50 patients or 2%, and the incidence of minor complications is 3 of 50 patients or 6%.

REPORTED COMPLICATIONS OF TRADITIONAL AND ENDOSCOPIC SINUS SURGERY

The results of our review of complications of sinus surgery for large series of patients[1-17] are shown in Table 7–2 and summarized in Table 7–3. A number of factors must be taken into consideration when evaluating the incidences reported here.

Differences in Enumeration

Reported Incidence per Patient

First, in some reports[3,7] the incidence of complications was reported per procedure rather than per patient; because most patients undergo bilateral procedures, we divided the number of procedures listed by 2 to obtain an estimate of the number of patients reported on in these cases. For these surgeons, the incidences cited in Table 7–2 are higher than the incidences cited in the original report.

Full Disclosure of Complications Reported

A second factor in reporting incidences of complications is whether authors report all of the complications that occurred, especially minor complications. In one report,[6] for example, minor complications were not enumerated although they were mentioned, and in another report minor complications were not discussed at all.[7] In a third report,[13] major and minor complications were noted for a subset of 500 patients of a total of 4500, and only major complications were mentioned for the larger group.

Because the overall results of reporting indicate a higher incidence of minor complications than major complications, we may suppose that all series have some minor complications and that there are likely to be more minor complications than major complications for a given series. However, accurate reporting of complication incidences is the only way to determine the true risk-to-benefit ratio for a procedure. For this reason, we have been meticulous in detailing the complications of our patients undergoing ESS.

Types of Complications Reported

A third discrepancy arises in the assortment of "other" minor complications reported (Table 7–2). The relationship of some of these complications to the sinus surgery is not clear, and in one case (cerebrovascular accident occurring 4 days after the operation)[4] the authors stated that they believed the complication was not, in fact, attributable to the surgery.

Table 7–2 Complications of Traditional Endonasal Versus Endoscopic Sinus Surgery Procedures Reported for Groups of 75 or More Patients, 1987–1990

SURGERY TYPE	TOTAL PTS.	MAJOR NO. PATIENTS WITH COMPLICATIONS					MINOR NO. PATIENTS WITH COMPLICATIONS				
		ORBIT.	INTRACRAN.	HEMORRH.	LACRIMAL	ORBIT.	ADHES.	EPISTAX.	ASTHMA	OTHER*
Traditional										
Sogg[1]	146	—	—	—	—	3	—	1	—	—
Lawson[2]	600	2	3	—	2	3	—	2	—	—
Friedman/Katsantonis[3]	589‡‡	—	2[s]	—	—	1	—	7	17	2
Stevens/Blair[4]	87	3	—	3	—	6	—	2	—	—
Freedman/Kern[5]	565‡	4	2[ǁ]	2	1	—	—	10	4	2
Eichel[6]	123	1	2	1	—	("several," all temporary)			
Total	2110	10	9	6	3	13	—	22	21	4
Incidences:		0.47%	0.43%	0.28%	0.14%	0.62%	—	1.0%	1.0%	0.19%

Overall incidence major complications: 28/2110 = 1.3%
Overall incidence minor complications: 60/2110 = 2.8%

Endoscopic Sinus Surgery										
Wigand/Hosemann[7]	500†	—	10	1	—	1	(not reported)		
Kennedy et al[8]	75	—	—	—	2	—	—	—	—	—
Schaefer et al[9]	100	—	—	—	—	2	6	2	2	2
Toffel et al[10]	170	—	—	1	—	—	1	5	—	—
Rice[11]	100	—	—	—	—	3	7	—	—	—
Vleming et al[12]	593	2	2	2	1	16	11	7	1	3
Stammberger[13]/Posawetz	500 (4500)	(2)	1 (3)	1	—	9	6	10	—	6
Matthews et al[14]	155	—	—	—	—	—	(not reported)		
Lazar et al[15]	210	—	—	—	3	5	—	3	—	3
Stankiewicz[16]	90‡	1¶	1	—	—	8	6	8	—	1
Stankiewicz[17]	90	—	1	—	—	1	—	5	—	—
Total	2583	3	14	5	6	45	37	40	3	15
Incidences:		0.12%	0.54%	0.19%	0.23%	1.7%	1.4%	1.6%	0.12%	0.58%

Overall incidence of major complications: 28/2583 = 1.1%
Overall incidence of minor complications: 140/2583 = 5.4%

Study	N									
Levine and May										
Levine (1986–91)	1165	—	4	3	—	16	20	7	35	16
Incidences:			0.34%	0.26%		1.4%	1.7%	0.6%	3%	1.4%
		Incidence of major complications: 7/1165 = 0.6%								
		Incidence of minor complications: 94/1165 = 8.0%								
May (1987–91)	943	1	6	1	3	20	15	6	3	7
Incidences:		0.1%	0.6%	0.1%	0.3%	2.1%	1.6%	0.6%	0.3%	0.7%
		Incidence of major complications: 11/943 = 1.2%								
		Incidence of minor complications: 51/943 = 5.4%								
Total	2108	1	10	4	3	36	35	13	38	23
Incidences:		0.05%	0.47%	0.19%	0.14%	1.7%	1.7%	0.6%	1.8%	1.0%
		Overall incidence of major complications: 18/2108 = 0.85%								
		Overall incidence of minor complications: 145/2108 = 6.9%								

*Other complications are discussed in the text; numbers represent only those related to sinus surgery.
†Number of patients was estimated to be half the number of procedures reported.
‡More than one complication listed per patient.
§Pneumocephalus and frontal mucocele also reported.
‖Patient with meningitis also had partial cranial nerve III palsy and sensorineural hearing loss among 28 complications in 26 patients.
¶Temporary blindness reported as one of 26 complications in 19 patients.

For nonendoscopic endonasal surgery the "other" complications reported included atrophic rhinitis[3]; cerebrovascular accident, hypotension, vomiting[4]; anxiety reaction, pneumonitis secondary to aspiration of blood, dental pain, fever of unknown origin, and anosmia.[5] For ESS reported on by other authors, "other" minor complications included frontal sinusitis,[9] mucocele or wound infection,[12] inflammation or granulomatous reactions of soft tissues due to retention of a surgical sponge or infiltration of antimycotic ointment,[13] severe otalgia in a pediatric series,[15] and tooth pain or closure of a natural ostium.[16]

Only the other complications that relate to sinus surgery (atrophic rhinitis, dental pain, anosmia, and infection) have been included in this report. The other complications experienced by Levine's and May's patients included dental or lip pain or numbness (9 Levine, 3 May), anosmia (7 Levine, 1 May), and infection (3 May).

Reporting Numbers of Patients Versus Complications

A fourth factor to consider in reporting incidence of complications is whether any patients experienced more than one complication (as shown in our example in the previous section). For all but four of the series reviewed,[3,5,12,16] it appeared that each patient experienced only one complication. We determined this from the fact that authors used the words "patients," "complications," and "cases" interchangeably and only one number was reported for each complication.

For this reason, and because we believe that patients contemplating undergoing ESS would like to know their chances of experiencing any complication (not whether the procedure is bilateral or unilateral), we tabulated complication rates for all of the series together using patients as the numerator (Table 7–2).

Surgeon's Learning Curve

The fifth factor we identified as affecting rates of complications of sinus surgery is the surgeon's learning curve for a new procedure. Stankiewicz reported on the first series of 90 patients on whom he performed ESS[16] and later reviewed this experience in light of his second 90 patients.[17] There were 26 complications in 19 of the first 90 patients, and one complication in each of two patients in the second series.[17] The complication rate of 29% (26 complications in 90 patients) in this surgeon's first 90 patients is the highest in reports we reviewed, whereas the complication rate for the next 90 patients (1% major, 1% minor) is comparable to the overall rate for the other series we reviewed.

Wigand and Hosemann[7] did not detail the types of surgery performed or the number of patients who underwent the 1000 procedures they report (as noted in Table 7–2, the number of patients was estimated at 500). However, the high incidence of CSF leakage they report occurred early in their experience and was due to an aggressive approach for removing polyps from the ethmoid roof (Wigand ME. Personal communication, 1992).

These results follow the trend we would expect; that is, that the early part of the "learning curve" for any surgical procedure is associated with a higher complication rate than the later part of the curve. Other surgeons in the series we are reporting on also have higher complication rates associated with smaller numbers of patients operated on to the date of the report. This was true for those performing traditional sinus surgery[4] and those performing ESS.[8]

Table 7–3 Summary of Major and Minor Complications of Traditional Versus Endoscopic Sinus Surgery for Large Series of Patients

SERIES	TOTAL PATIENTS NO.	INCIDENCE OF COMPLICATIONS MAJOR	MINOR
Levine and May	2108	0.85%	6.9%
Endoscopic sinus surgeons	2583	1.1%	5.4%
Nonendoscopic surgeons	2110	1.3%	2.8%

The overall complication rate may not drop over time in teaching programs because in these circumstances ESS is being performed partially by residents under supervision of a staff member.[12]

None of the surgeons whose results we reviewed, however, was immune to complications of surgery, even though they are experienced and well-known in the field. Our belief is that, by calculating rates based on a large number of reports of sizable patient series, we have diluted the effects of individually low or high rates and determined overall rates for complications that a typical surgeon might expect to achieve after a moderate amount of experience.

Type of Procedure

A sixth factor that might have affected the reported incidence of sinus surgery complications is the type of surgery performed. Friedman and Katsantonis[3] predicted, for example, that the complication rates of endonasal endoscopic approaches to treat massive disease are likely to be high, especially if such approaches are used by less experienced surgeons. In addition, the complications reported by Wigand and Hosemann[7] occurred early in their experience when they were using an aggressive approach to remove polyps from the ethmoid roof (Wigand ME. Personal communication, 1992).

The senior authors (H. L. and M. M.) noted a correlation between use of the canine fossa approach and dental or lip pain or numbness.

Vleming et al[12] noted significantly higher incidences of all complications except adhesions when the middle turbinate, an important surgical landmark, was absent. In contrast, we found that previous surgery, even when the middle turbinate had been removed, did not affect the incidence of complications.

Categorization of Complication

A seventh factor that was taken into account for our calculations of complications of sinus surgery was variations in reporting adverse events as major or minor complications.

Orbital Hematoma

Orbital hematoma (retrobulbar hemorrhage), for example, is usually considered a major complication. In four patients in one report it resolved without treatment and the authors considered this complication to be in the "less severe" category.[5] However, we consider all postseptal bleeding into the orbit to be a major complication.

Bleeding

These same authors[5] listed 12 hemorrhages as major complications, but only two patients required transfusion. Because in our classification system only bleeding treated by transfusion was considered a major complication, we classified these complications as two major complications and 10 minor complications. In another series[10] one of six patients with epistaxis 48 hours or more after surgery required transfusion, and we categorized this event as a major complication.

Adhesions

Adhesions have also been difficult to evaluate as complications. We considered adhesions to be complications of ESS if they were symptomatic, as indicated by the need for treatment (revision surgery or office lysis).

Position of the Surgeon During Operation

Lawson[2] and Freedman and Kern[5] made the interesting observation that the majority of complications in their series of patients occurred on the patient's right side. This might be attributed to creating an awkward angle of approach to the sinus cavity for a right-handed surgeon who would be standing on the right side of the patient. This problem has not been noted, however, by the senior authors (M.M. and H.L.) or others[12] using the endoscopic technique.

Complications for Traditional Versus Endoscopic Sinus Surgery

There were some notable differences between complications following traditional surgery and those following ESS. One surgeon reporting on traditional sinus surgery[1] and three reporting on ESS[9,11,14] indicated that no major complications occurred in their series. We believe the relatively small numbers of patients in these series might explain the very low incidence of major complications reported. As more patients are added to these series, a major complication is likely to occur with either traditional or endoscopic surgery.

Orbital Complications

One difference that is notable between the two types of surgery is the incidence of major versus minor orbital complications. In the series of traditional sinus surgery reports the incidence of major orbital complications (retrobulbar hematoma) was 0.47%, versus 0.05% (Levine and May) to 0.12% for ESS. The incidence of minor orbital complications (preseptal ecchymosis), however, was higher in the ESS series (1.7%) than in the traditional sinus surgery series (0.62%). Of note is that the incidence of minor orbital complications in a series of patients 16 years or younger (5 of 210, 2.4%)[15] was comparable to the incidence in adults (40 of 2373, 1.7%).

The higher incidence of major orbital complications with traditional sinus surgery is likely related to the greater extent of surgery via a traditional endonasal approach. The higher incidence of minor orbital complications with ESS is likely related to the frequency with which the uncinate process is removed during this procedure, with the risk of violation of the lamina papyracea. This higher incidence of minor orbital complications with ESS contributed significantly to the higher overall incidence of minor complications with endoscopic techniques.

Vascular Complications

Wigand and Hosemann[7] are the only surgeons to report penetration of the carotid artery, which occurred when the sphenoid sinus septum was removed.

Adhesions

The second minor complication that occurred noticeably more often with ESS versus traditional endonasal approaches was adhesions. This complication was peculiar to ESS in this series of reports, which is not surprising because the occurrence of adhesions is related to removal of the middle turbinate. If the middle turbinate is removed, as with traditional sinus surgery, adhesions do not occur. During ESS, in contrast, the middle turbinate is usually preserved[2] and adhesions may occur.

AUTHORS' INCIDENCES OF ENDOSCOPIC SINUS SURGERY COMPLICATIONS

The incidences of complications reported by the senior authors (H.L. and M.M.) are shown at the end of Table 7–2. The senior surgeons share a similar philosophy regarding surgical management of patients with sinus disease. Both of us believe, as set forth by Stammberger and Kennedy, that the goal of sinus surgery should be to restore function while limiting surgery to the treatment of disease evident endoscopically and by computed tomography (CT). Furthermore, the senior surgeons have collaborated in organizing ESS workshops and resident teaching programs.

Nevertheless, there are minor variations in our techniques and thus one would expect differences in our complication rates. Major complications occurred somewhat more frequently in May's series (11 of 943, 1.2%) than in Levine's series (7 of 1165, 0.6%), for example. However, minor complications occurred slightly more often in Levine's series (94 of 1165, 8.0%) than in May's series (51 of 943, 5.4%). An explanation for these differences was sought by looking for differences in our techniques for ESS.

Major Complications

Orbital Complications

No patients in Levine's series and only one patient in May's series experienced a major orbital complication of ESS. In this patient retrobulbar hemorrhage developed secondary to transection and subsequent retraction of the anterior ethmoid artery. As previously reported,[18] formation of the hematoma was evidenced by proptosis, pupil dilation, decreasing vision, and increasing intraorbital pressure as measured by tonometry (to 45 mmHg). Pressure decreased after lateral canthotomy and inferior cantholysis,[19] but bleeding did not stop until ligation of the anterior ethmoid artery through an external ethmoid approach. The patient required transfusion, and, although vision returned to preoperative level over the next 10 days, the patient was left with a permanent small temporal scotoma.

A modification in technique, use of the double-ended maxillary sinus ostium seeker (see Chapter 5 and later in this chapter), is credited with absence of any subsequent instances of orbital penetration in May's series.

Dural Complications

CSF leakage was the major complication most often reported by either Levine (four patients) or May (six patients). One of Levine's patients had a massive maxillary-ethmoid-sphenoid sinus mucocele; the CSF leak occurred when the lining of the mucocele was peeled away because the lining was found to be attached to the dura. From this experience, Levine recommends not disturbing mucosa lying against the roof of the ethmoid sinus, even when a mucocele is present.

A similar problem occurred on stripping hyperplastic mucosa attached to the roof of the ethmoid sinus; this led to small CSF leaks in three of May's patients. In the fourth case the CSF leak occurred with an attempt to enter the sphenoid sinus (see Chapter 5; the posterior nasal choana, nasal septum, and posterior attachment of the middle turbinate should be used as guides, supplemented by C-arm lateral fluoroscopy in cases of uncertainty as to the location of the sphenoid or posterior ethmoid sinus). The fifth patient in whom CSF leak occurred in May's series had an extremely thin vertical plate of the olfactory groove, where the middle turbinate attaches to the roof of the ethmoid sinus. The vulnerability of this anatomic area is detailed in a report of a histologic study by Kainz and Stammberger.[20]

In the sixth patient the dura was penetrated by a suction cannula at the completion of the procedure. This occurred because the cannula was placed in the nose without direct visualization and it penetrated the roof of the ethmoid sinus through an area of bony dehiscence. Dural violation was suspected by the depth of penetration of the cannula, and the CSF leak was found by inspection of the roof of the ethmoid sinus. The leak was repaired and the patient recovered from general anesthesia with no signs or symptoms of central nervous system deficit, despite postoperative CT scan evidence of a focal area of hemorrhage in the frontal lobe. The patient was hospitalized and the dural violation managed with neurosurgical consultation, intravenous antibiotic drugs, and observation; after discharge the patient was prescribed oral antibiotics for 10 days and phenytoin (Dilantin) prophylactically for 6 months. Three years have passed with no evidence of sequelae.

In addition to a conservative approach to managing mucosa over the roof of the ethmoid sinus, May uses landmarks to enter the basal lamella posteriorly rather than anteriorly (see Chapter 5). These modifications in technique have resulted in no CSF leaks in the last 210 patients operated on by May.

Minor Complications

The incidences of minor complications are related in some cases to elements of operative technique or patient care.

Orbital Ecchymosis or Edema

Orbital complications of ESS usually occurred in May's series during removal of a thinned, lateralized uncinate process that hugged the lamina papyracea. Orbital fat was noted in 33 patients, but only 21 patients developed signs or symptoms of orbital penetration. The patient who developed retrobulbar hematoma has already been discussed; of the 20 patients with minor orbital complications, 17 had periorbital ecchymosis and three had subcutaneous emphysema. Preseptal signs of orbital penetration cleared over 10 days for all patients with minor complications.

Adhesions

Symptomatic adhesions occurred in both Levine's and May's patients. These adhesions were primarily due to lateralization of the middle turbinate, and less often to stenosis of a surgically enlarged maxillary antrostomy.

Bleeding

A difference between Levine's and May's series of patients in the incidence of postoperative bleeding led to a change in routine care of Levine's patients. Postoperative bleeding was found to be more often a problem in Levine's patients, in whom a postoperative dressing was rarely used, than in May's patients, in whom an intranasal dressing and an external "moustache" dressing (see Chapter 5) were used routinely.

Both surgeons now agree that patients who have significant oozing of blood during surgery should have an intranasal and moustache dressing put in place in the operating room. If, by 2 hours after surgery, the moustache dressing has remained dry, the intranasal dressing may be removed. Otherwise, the moustache dressing is changed and rechecked in 2 more hours. If dry, then the intranasal dressing can be removed; otherwise, it is left in place until the next morning.

Asthma

Because the proportions of asthmatic patients in Levine's and May's series are similar, we looked for differences in technique to explain the much higher incidence of perioperative bronchospasm in Levine's patients with asthma. We identified Levine's preference for using local anesthesia versus May's preference for general anesthesia as a possible source of the variation. This seems a reasonable explanation because with local anesthesia, patients' airways are exposed to more secretions during and after surgery, and this exposure might trigger laryngobronchospasm in patients with reactive airway disease. Our suspicion was strengthened by the relatively high incidence of bronchospasm in patients operated on (routinely under local anesthesia) by Friedman and Katsantonis[3] (Table 7–2).

As a result of these observations, Levine now prefers to use general anesthesia, particularly for patients with reactive airway disease (asthma or ASA triad).

Dental or Lip Pain or Numbness

The different incidences of dental or lip pain or numbness in Levine's and May's series relate directly to the numbers of patients who underwent canine fossa puncture. Early in their experiences with ESS, both surgeons used the canine fossa approach often to visualize and remove cysts and polyps from the maxillary sinus. As they have gained confidence with more experience approaching the maxillary sinus endonasally through an enlarged maxillary antrostomy, Levine and May rarely use the canine fossa approach and, the incidences of changes in dental or lip sensation have decreased.

Anosmia

The occurrence of anosmia has been related directly to scarring in the olfactory area (between the septum and middle turbinate). Such scarring usually occurs in patients undergoing ESS for recurrent nasal polyposis.

PREVENTION AND MANAGEMENT OF COMPLICATIONS

This section describes the appearance of major and minor complications and their prevention and management.

Orbital Penetration

Orbital penetration may lead to one of three major or two minor complications, depending on which zone of the orbit is penetrated (Fig. 7–1).

Zone A

No complications may result if the lamina papyracea is violated but the periorbita is not. If the periorbita is also violated, *periorbital ecchymosis* (Fig. 7–2) or *subcutaneous emphysema* (Fig. 7–3) may result.

One way to prevent orbital penetration in zone A during ESS is to take care when removing the uncinate process, especially when the uncinate process is lateralized or the lamina papyracea is dehiscent. Frequently, the uncinate process is lateralized when the septum is deviated, with or without a concha bullosa or a lateralized paradoxical turbinate (Fig. 7–4). May now uses a double-ended maxillary sinus ostium seeker to move the uncinate process away from the lamina papyracea before sectioning the uncinate process (Fig. 7–5).

Stankiewicz[21] reported maneuvers to prevent or limit orbital penetration. To prevent violation of the lamina papyracea, he recommends keeping two fingers on the globe to

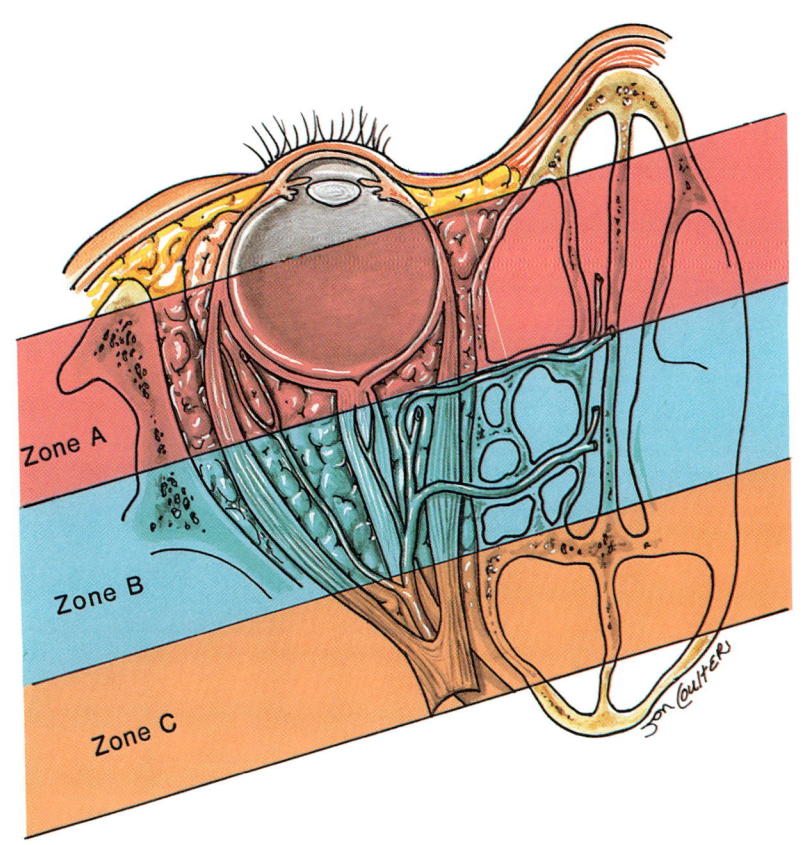

Figure 7–1. The lines used to divide the ethmoid box into surgical-anatomic compartments have been extended laterally through the orbit to delineate zones of orbital vulnerability.

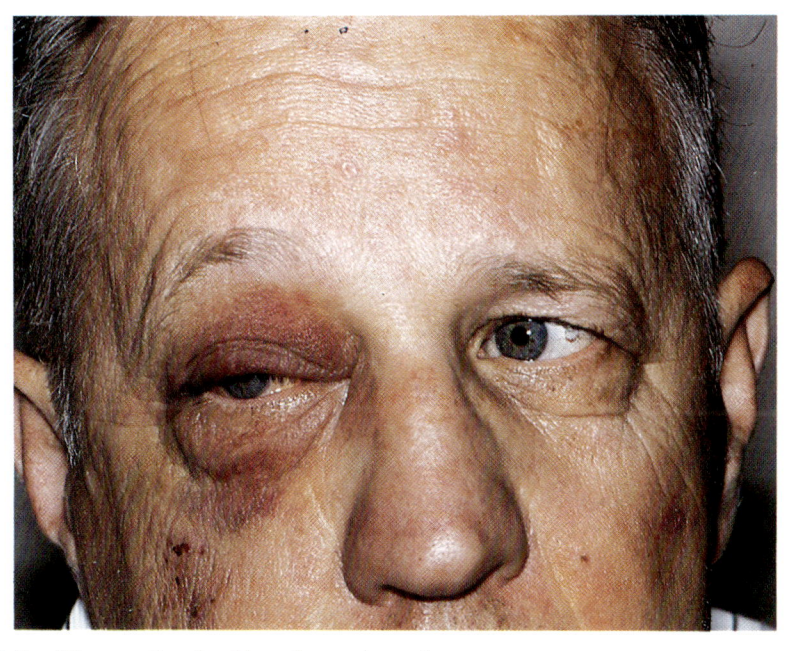

Figure 7–2. (Figure continued and legend on next page.)

205

206 *Endoscopic Sinus Surgery*

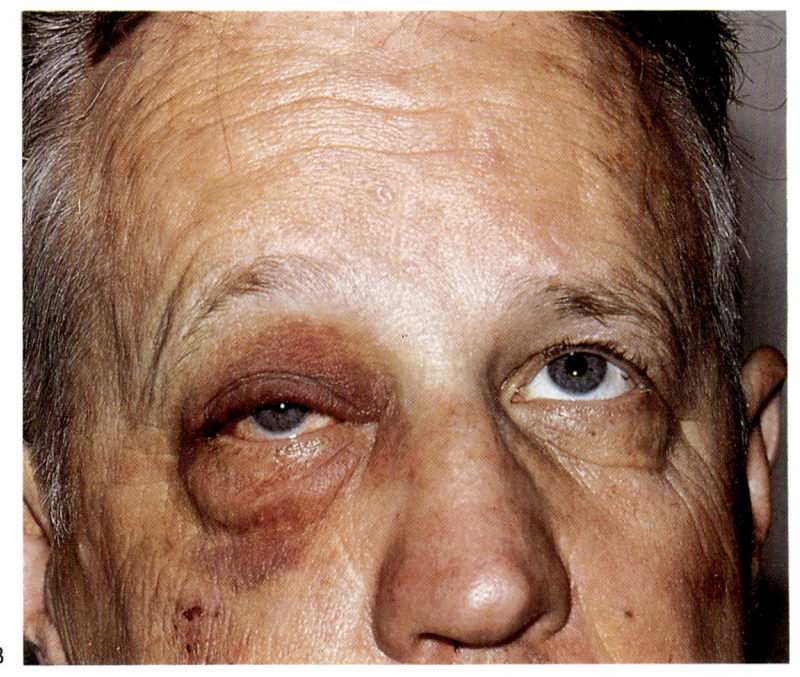

Figure 7–2. (*Continued*). **A**, **B**: Periorbital ecchymosis, due to orbital penetration on the right side, 1 day after endoscopic sinus surgery. Limitation in extraocular muscle movement is apparent rather than real; preseptal rather than orbital soft tissues have been affected.

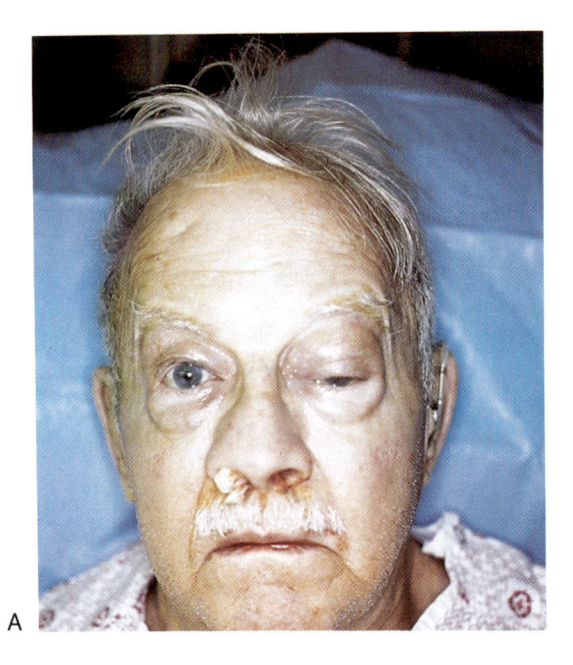

Figure 7–3. (Figure continued and legend on next page.)

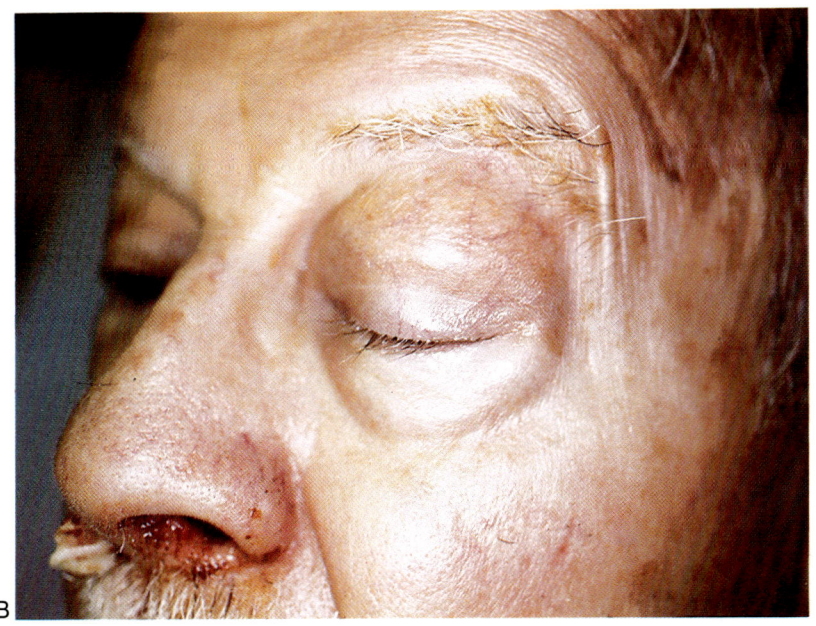

Figure 7–3. **A**, **B**: Subcutaneous emphysema immediately after orbital penetration during endonasal sinus surgery. This complication can occur suddenly and frighten staff as well as the patient, although vision is not altered and pupils retain equal tone and responsivity to light. Positive-pressure ventilation during emergence from general anesthesia was thought to be the cause of this patient's complication.

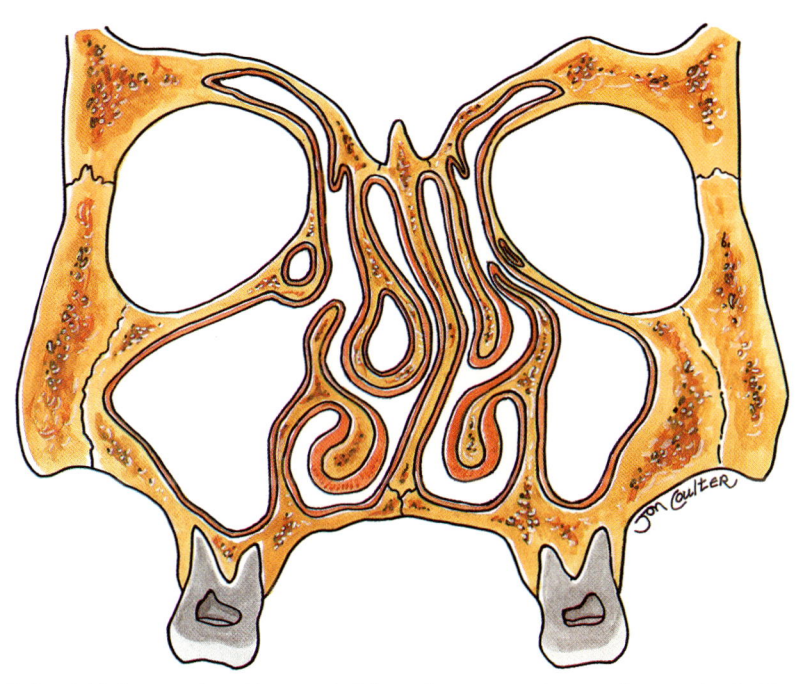

Figure 7–4. Orbital penetration with removal of the uncinate process is most often associated with a deviated nasal septum and lateralized turbinate and uncinate process.

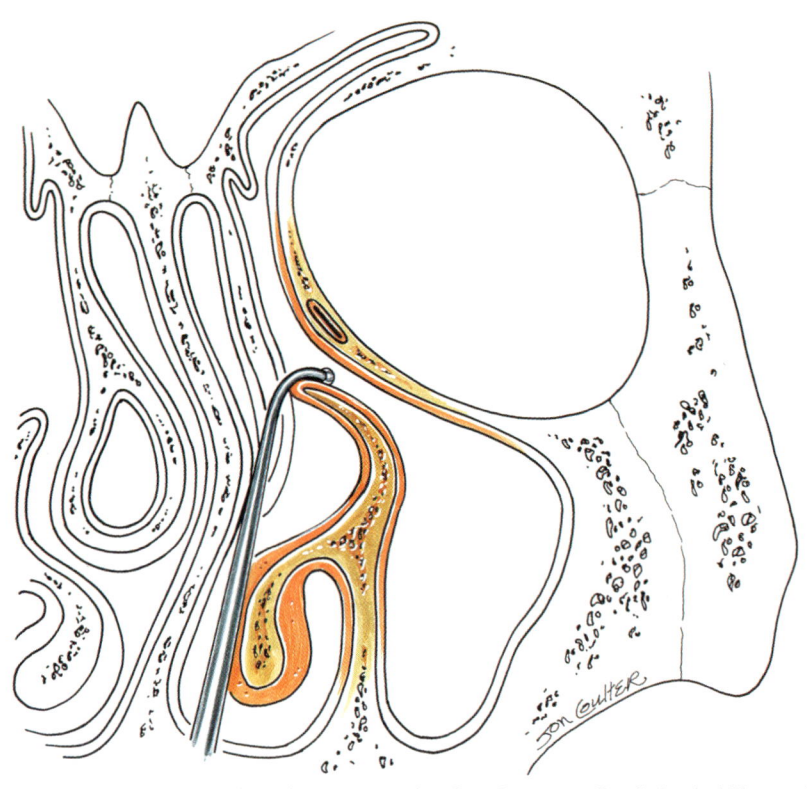

Figure 7–5. A double-ended maxillary sinus ostium seeker (Storz Instrument Co., St. Louis, MO, item 629820) is used to displace the uncinate away from the orbit to avoid orbital penetration.

palpate for vibrations transmitted from the nasal cavity. If the surgeon suspects violation of the orbit, the fingers may also be used to apply gentle pressure on the globe while watching intranasally for movement of the lamina or bulging of intraorbital fat through the lamina (Fig. 7–6). Fat should be distinguishable by its yellow, globular, greasy appearance, and removing material bulging from the area of the lamina papyracea to check whether it is fat (placed in water, fat floats but mucosa does not) is discouraged.

To prevent subcutaneous emphysema (Fig. 7–3) when the lamina papyracea has been violated in zone A, positive pressure insufflation by mask is discouraged during emergence from general anesthesia, and the patient should be told not to blow the nose for a week after surgery.

Preseptal ecchymosis resulting from penetration of the orbit in zone A usually resolves spontaneously over 5 to 10 days. Nurses in the patient care unit are instructed to notify the surgeon if periorbital fullness or bleeding occurs so that the nature and location (preseptal versus retrobulbar) of the collection can be determined. Although there are signs and symptoms that distinguish one from the other, as will be discussed, CT findings are definitive (Fig. 7–7).

Complications 209

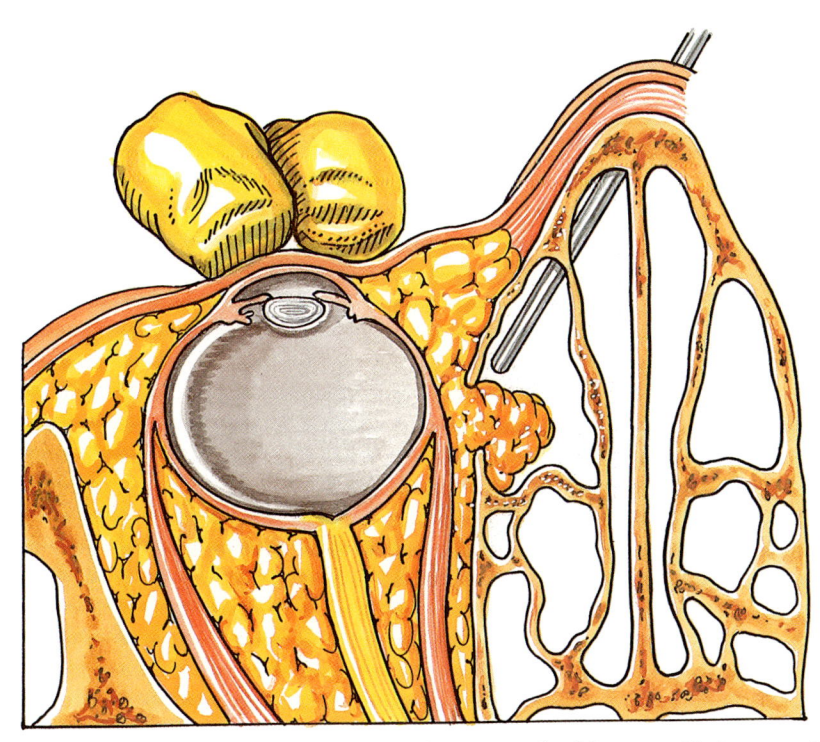

Figure 7–6. If the orbit has been entered, applying gentle pressure to the globe may enable the surgeon looking through the endoscope to see orbital fat pouching into the nose.

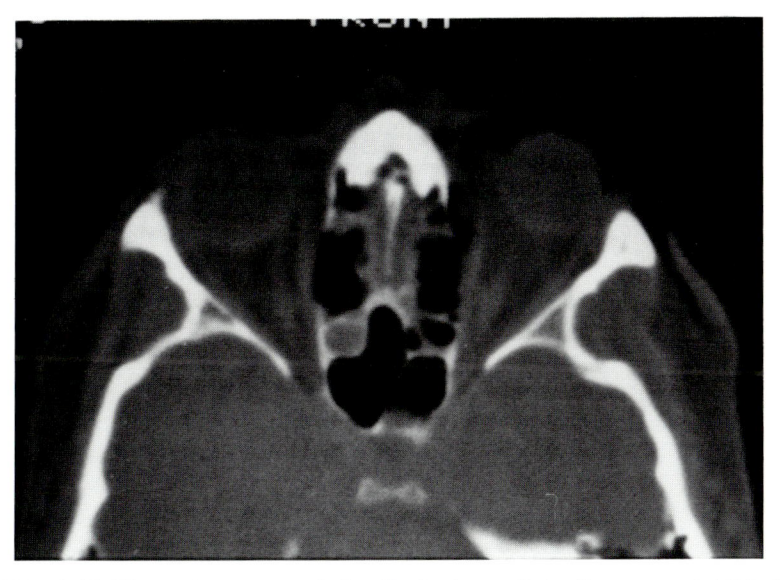

Figure 7–7. Axial CT scan shows preseptal air collection in a patient with severe periorbital edema and ecchymosis. This finding rules out retrobulbar involvement.

Zones B and C

Penetration of the orbit in zone B may result in *retrobulbar hematoma*, a major complication with threat of vision loss or diplopia resulting from damage to the medial rectus muscle.

To avoid violating zone B, an axial CT scan should be examined preoperatively and at the time of surgery so that the surgeon can appreciate the shape of the ethmoid complex. A wedge-shaped versus oblong ethmoid complex puts the orbit at greater risk because the ethmoid cells lie closer to the optic nerve and orbital cone. On occasion, a lateralized posterior ethmoid cell may actually envelop the optic nerve (Onodi cell) (Fig. 7–8).

Signs of retrobulbar hemorrhage are dramatic and usually occur during surgery:[21,22] (1) the eyelids become ecchymotic, (2) the globe becomes proptotic, (3) intraorbital tone increases, (4) extraocular muscle movement becomes limited, (5) the pupil on the affected side dilates and becomes less responsive to light, and (6) vision may diminish with progression of pressure. Figure 7–9 shows steps to be taken to evaluate orbital penetration.[21]

Retrobulbar hemorrhage may occur when biting forceps used in zone B to grasp polyps or infected tissue are inadvertently used to grasp and remove orbital material (Fig. 7–10). Alternatively, this complication may result from tearing the anterior ethmoid artery (Fig. 7–11).

Usually, retrobulbar hemorrhage is self-limiting and will respond to conservative measures,[16,20,22] including: (1) removing packing; (2) administering diuretic medications, such as mannitol or acetazolamide, and steroid drugs, intravenously; and (3) consultation with an ophthalmologist.

If the hematoma progresses, especially if intraorbital pressure increases and visual acuity decreases, the orbit should be decompressed and hemorrhage controlled without delay: once vision is impaired, pressure must be relieved within 60 to 90 minutes to prevent permanent deficit.[16,20,22] If retrobulbar hemorrhage is due to a lacerated anterior ethmoid artery that has retracted into the orbit, an external procedure is usually necessary to manage the tear (Fig. 7–12). Lateral canthotomy and inferior cantholysis (Fig. 7–13) should be performed to reduce temporarily intraorbital pressure until the bleeding can be managed definitively. The surgeon more experienced in ESS may decompress the orbit intranasally using the endoscope[23]; an external ethmoidectomy may be necessary if endonasal structures cannot be visualized because of disease or the effects of surgery.

Steps in evaluation and management of retrobulbar hematoma are listed in Table 7–4.

Optic nerve damage may occur as a result of violation of the lamina papyracea during ethmoid or sphenoid sinus surgery in zones B and C. The nerve may be prominent in the lateral wall of the posterior ethmoid sinus (Onodi cell) or the sphenoid sinus, and in 4% of cases the nerve is dehiscent, separated from the sinus cavity only by its sheath and sinus mucosa.[24] Blindness that occurs intraoperatively or postoperatively is evaluated as for retrobulbar hemorrhage (Table 7–4).

Optic nerve decompression may be indicated, particularly in cases of delayed blindness, because decompression has been shown effective to treat traumatic optic nerve injury.[25,26] Although delayed blindness would imply that the optic nerve has not been transected, before considering optic nerve decompression to relieve blindness magnetic resonance imaging (MRI) should be performed to evaluate the possibility of surgical disruption of the nerve.

Complications 211

Onodi cell

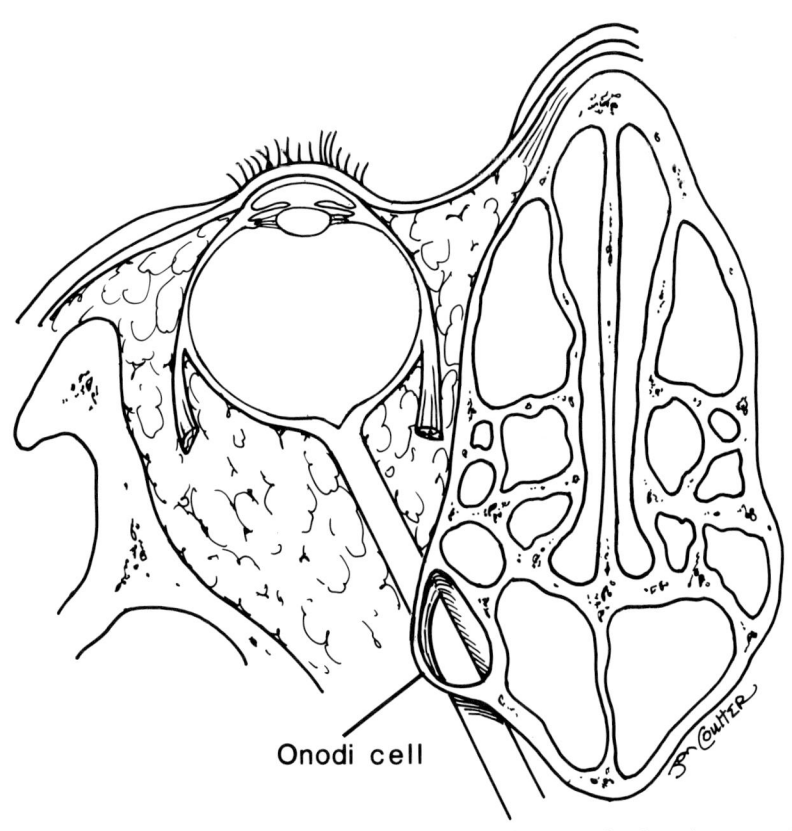

Figure 7–8. A laterally pneumatized posterior ethmoid cell (Onodi cell) may envelop the optic nerve, making it vulnerable to injury during sinus surgery. This situation may be identified on an axial CT scan.

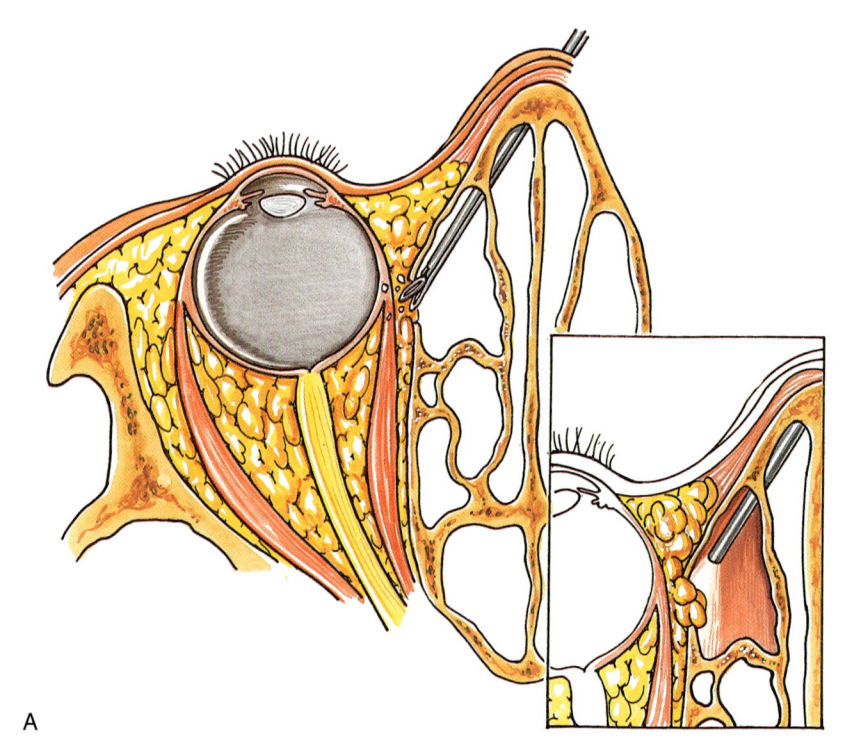

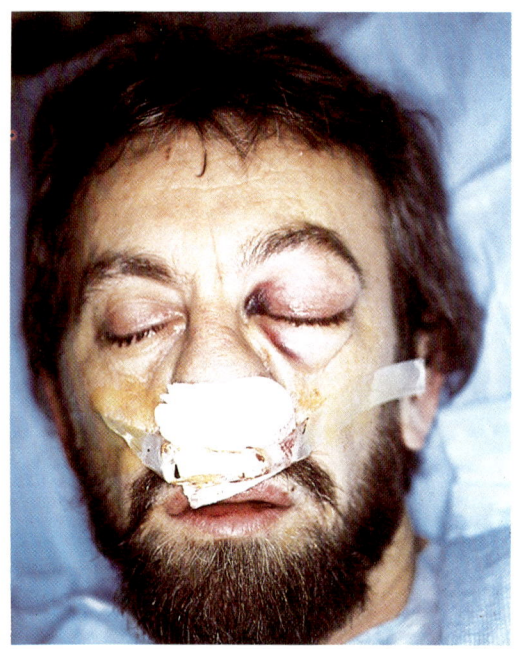

Figure 7–9. Mechanism of orbital penetration and steps to evaluate this complication. **A**: Entry into the orbit in zone A reveals fat. **B**: Fullness and ecchymosis of the left eyelids are evident immediately postoperatively. (Figure continued on next page.)

Complications 213

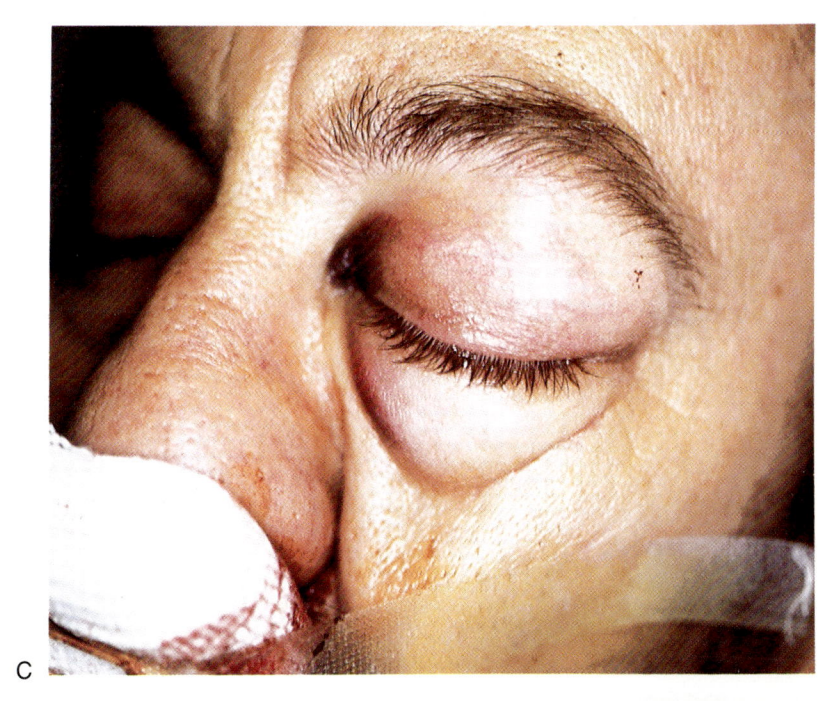

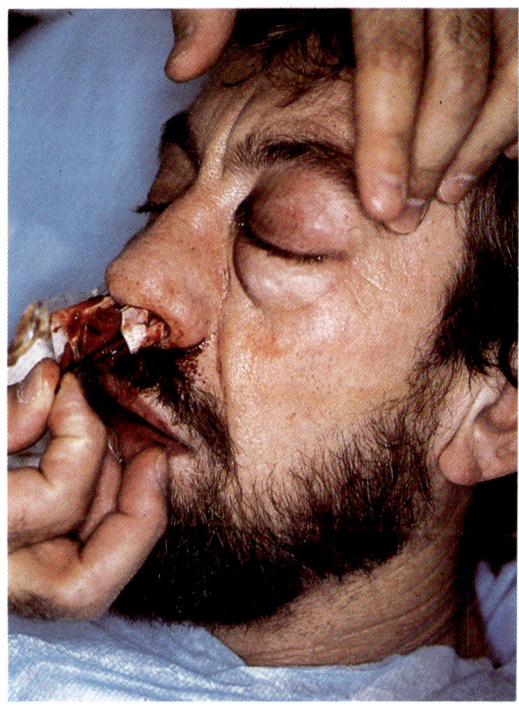

Figure 7–9. (*Continued*). **C**: Fullness and echymosis of left eyelids. **D**: First step in management is to remove packing. (Figure continued on next page.)

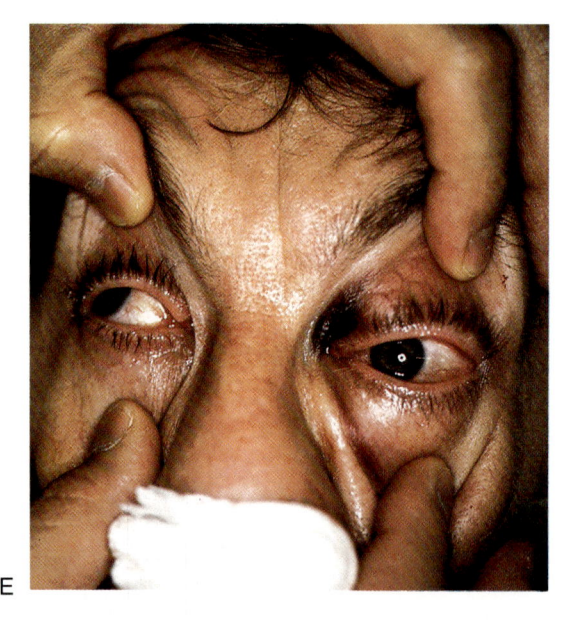

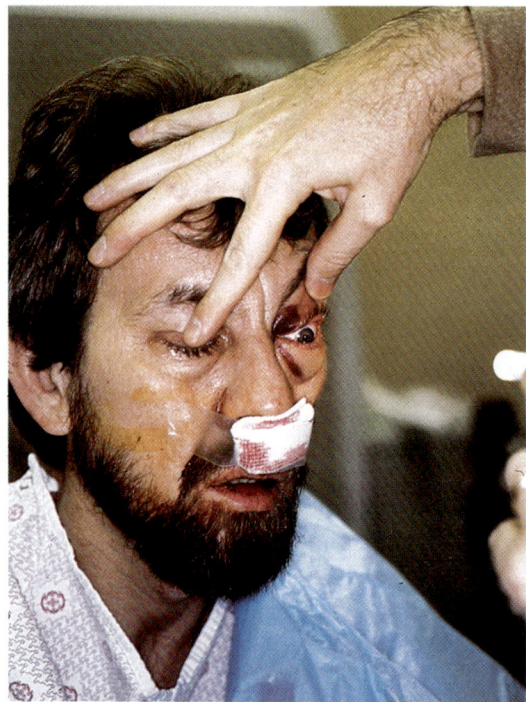

Figure 7–9. (*Continued*). **E:** A check of the eyes for extraocular muscle movement shows apparent limitation of medial gaze on involved left side. **F:** Pupils are checked for size and reactivity to light. (Figure continued on next page.)

Complications 215

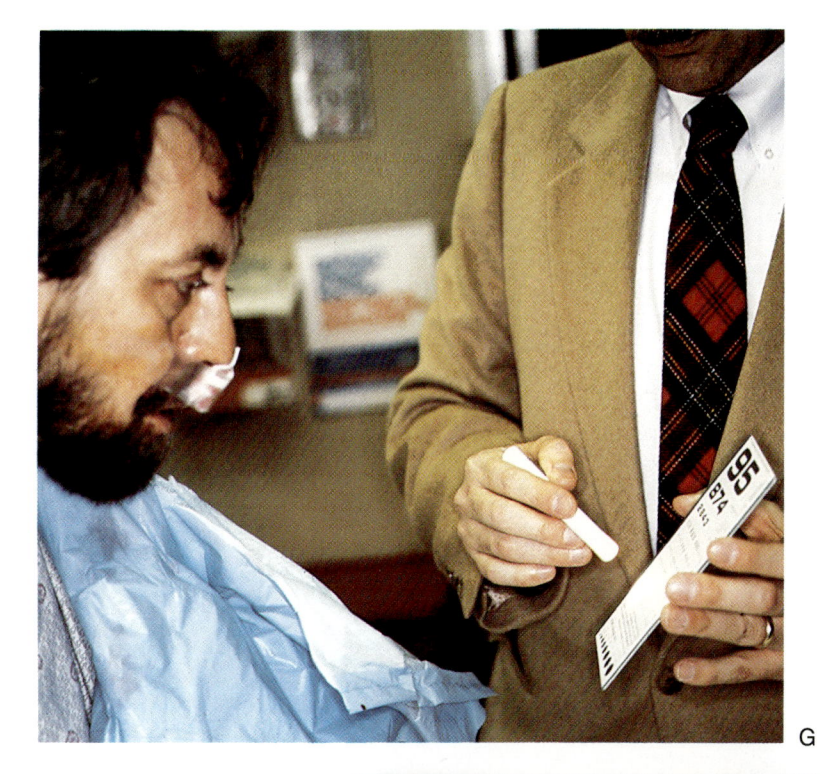

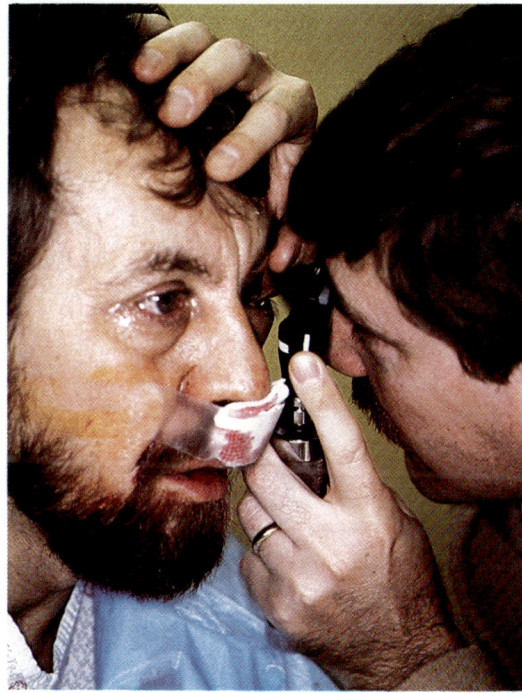

Figure 7–9. (*Continued*). **G**: Visual acuity is checked in both eyes. **H**: Ophthalmologist performs fundoscopic examination. (Figure continued on next page.)

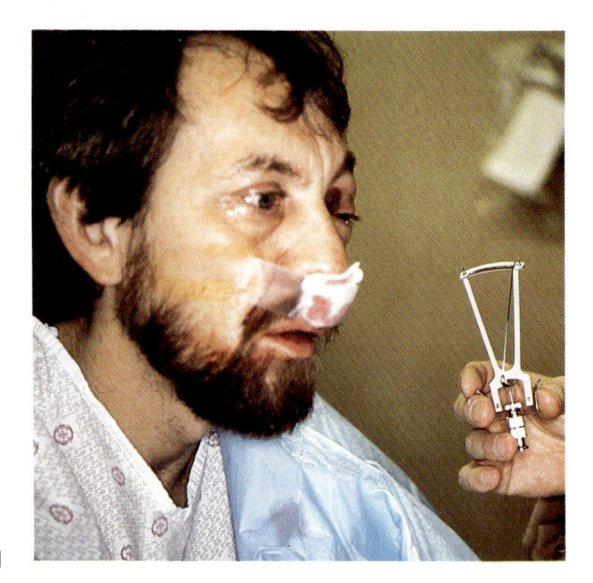

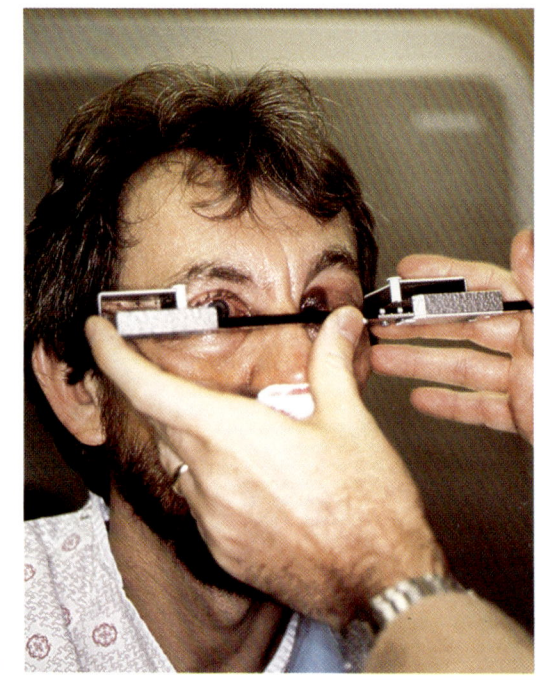

Figure 7–9. (*Continued*). **I**: Orbital tone is measured. **J**: Presence of true exophthalmos is checked with Hertl exophthalmometer. (Figure continued on next page.)

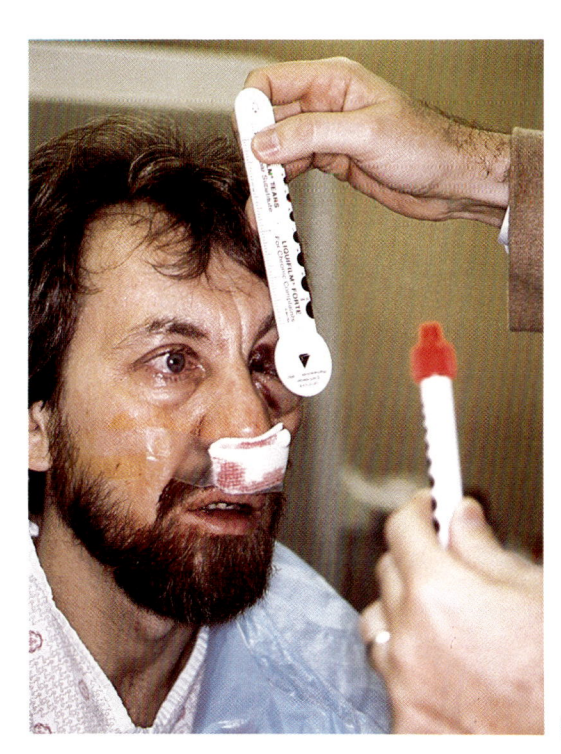

Figure 7–9. (*Continued*). **K**: Vision for red is checked because this is last function to be lost with optic nerve ischemia.

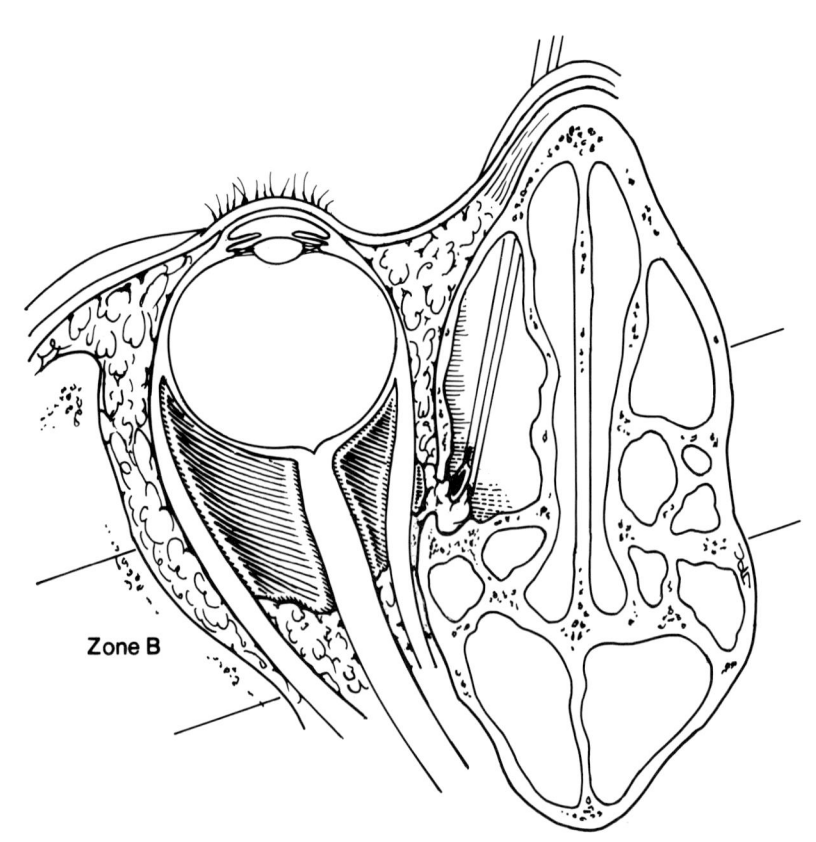

Figure 7–10. Retrobulbar hemorrhage may be associated with violation of the orbit in zone B if orbital fat is grasped and pulled out of the retrobulbar region. The other mechanism for retrobulbar hemorrhage is violation of the anterior ethmoid artery with retraction of the artery into the orbit.

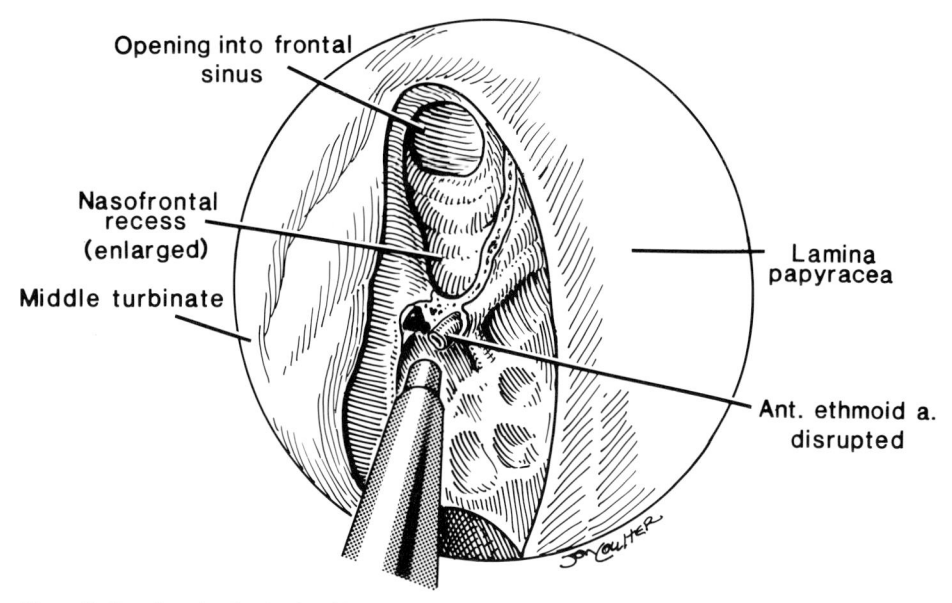

Figure 7-11. Anterior (Ant.) ethmoid artery (a.) has been torn at the junction of the nasofrontal recess with the roof of the ethmoid sinus. Artery is shown end-on and bleeding is being controlled with suction cautery.

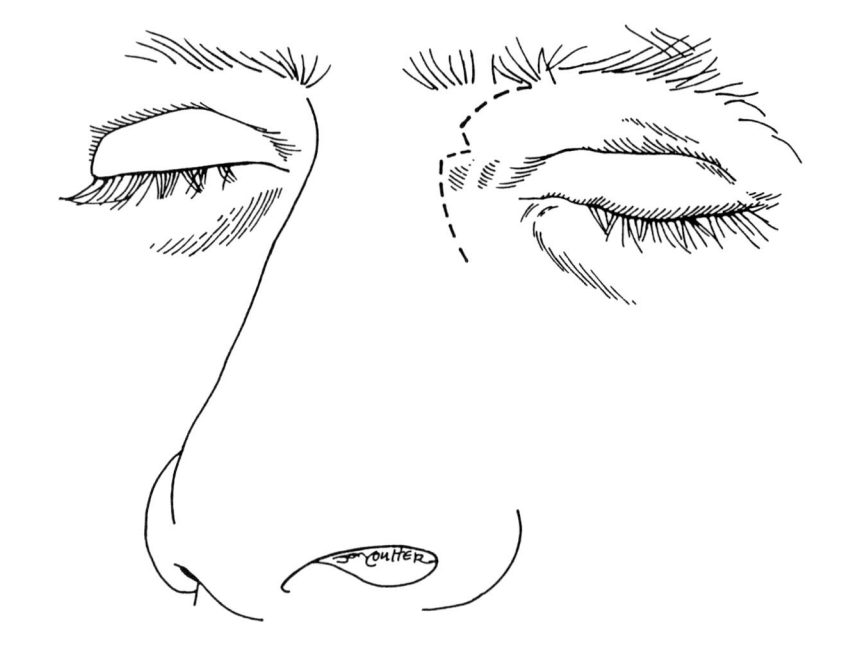

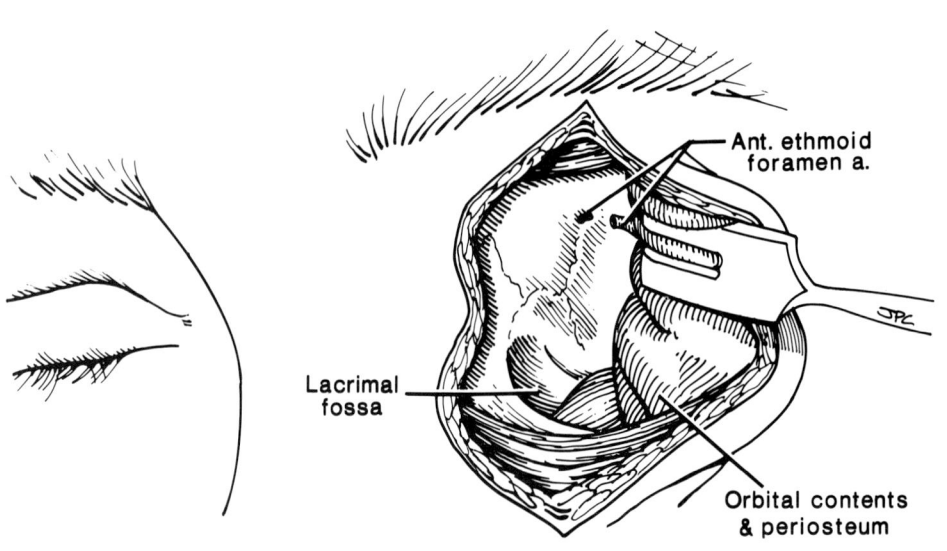

Figure 7–12. If an injured anterior (Ant.) ethmoid artery (a.) retracts intraorbitally and retrobulbar hemorrhage occurs, bleeding can be controlled via an external ethmoid approach. **A**: A "seagull" or "flying bird" incision is made and extended through skin to the periosteum over the ethmoid bone. **B**: Periosteum is elevated off the ethmoid bone to reveal the anterior ethmoid foramen and the artery coursing from the periosteum into the orbit. (Figure continued on next page.)

Complications 221

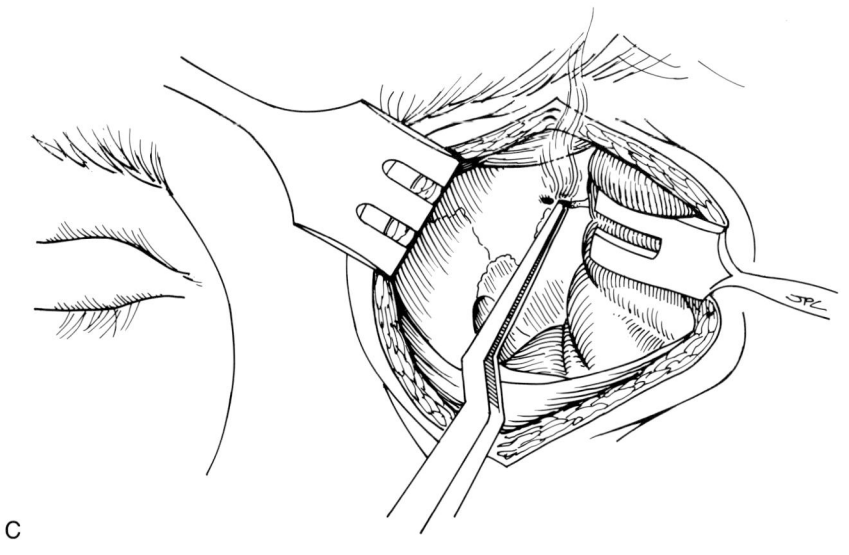

Figure 7–12. (*Continued*). **C**: Wet-field bipolar cautery is used to stop bleeding.

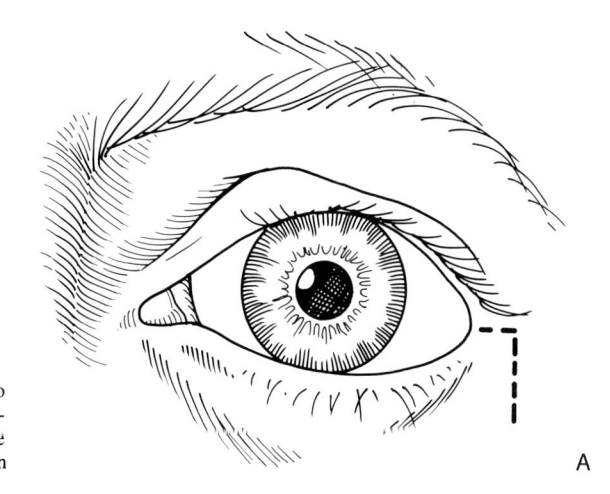

Figure 7–13. Decompression of the orbit to manage retrobulbar hemorrhage with increased ocular tension. **A**. Incision in the lateral canthal region. (Figure continued on next page)

222 Endoscopic Sinus Surgery

Lateral canthotomy

Inferior cantholysis

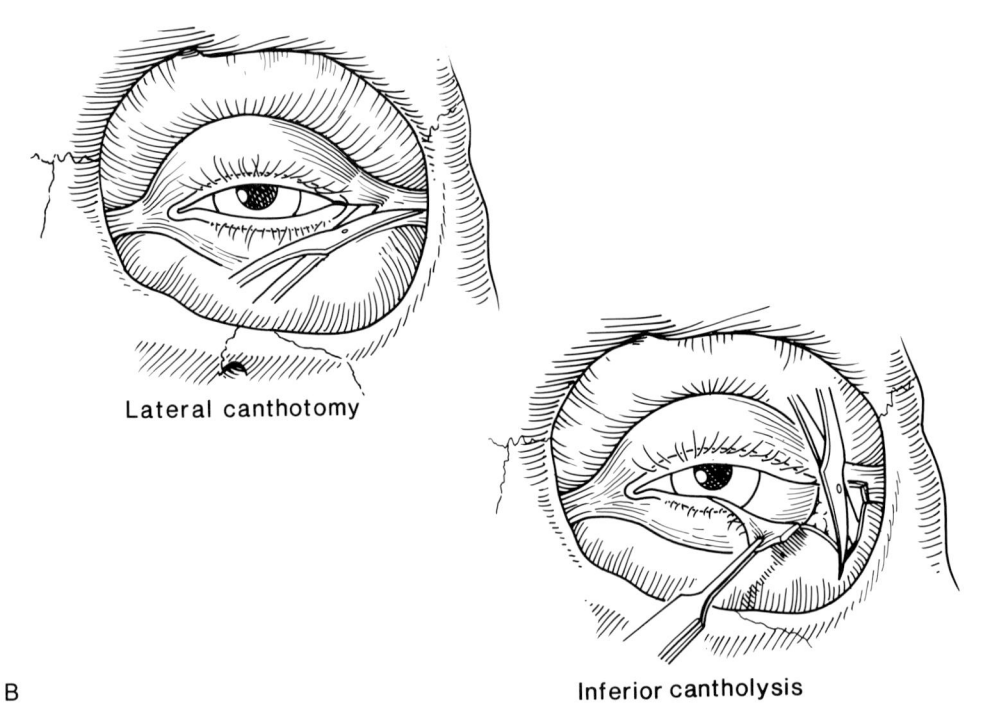

B

Figure 7–13. (*Continued*). **B**: Procedures for lateral canthotomy and inferior cantholysis. (Modified with permission from Thompson et al.[20])

Table 7–4 Steps in Evaluation and Management of Retrobulbar Hemorrhage*

Evaluation
Remove nasal packing
Obtain objective measures of:
- Extraocular muscle movement
- Pupillary size and reaction to light
- Visual acuity and visual fields of both eyes

Perform fundoscopic examination
Determine orbital tone
Assess for true exophthalmos
Check vision for red

Management

Medical (normal vision)	Surgical (vision impaired) 60-90 minute window
Remove packing	Lateral canthotomy
Consult ophthalmologist	Inferior cantholysis
Administer diuretics (mannitol, acetazolamide) and steroids IV	Orbital decompression Anterior ethmoid artery ligation

*Modified from Stankiewicz.[21]

Diplopia

Diplopia may occur with retrobulbar hemorrhage or with minor ocular complications (preseptal hemorrhage or emphysema). When caused by pressure alone this sign usually resolves as the primary condition improves. If the medial rectus or superior oblique muscle is damaged directly,[27] however, the prognosis is very poor for recovery of function, even with surgical intervention.[21] Fortunately this complication is quite rare.

Dural Complications of ESS

Leakage of Cerebrospinal Fluid

Pathognomonic of CSF leak is the "washout" sign: clear fluid leaking through a defect in the dura washes away blood from the ethmoid roof (Fig. 7–14). As with penetration of the orbit, when a dural tear occurs the anesthesiologist should be informed and should avoid assisted ventilation by bag and mask when the patient is emerging from general anesthesia, because of the danger of inducing pneumocephalus. Patients are instructed not to blow the nose for 3 weeks postoperatively for the same reason.

Many endonasal techniques have been reported effective in closing dural tears;[28-31] the technique we use involves removing disease from the area of the dural tear and rotating the middle turbinate over the defect (Fig. 7–15). If the middle turbinate is not available, then fascia, fat, or muscle is taken from the patient's scalp or abdomen. The tissue graft is held in place with a nasal dressing for 48 hours, during which time antibiotic medications are administered.

After repair of a CSF leak, if minimal CSF drainage is noted and continues beyond 3 to 5 days, an intrathecal drain may be placed. Although such a drain may be beneficial, it increases the risk of intracranial infection and pneumocephalus. It may be prudent, especially if drainage is more than minimal, to return the patient to the operating room and explore the site of the dural tear. Most cases of CSF leakage occur when mucosa is removed from the roof of the ethmoid, without associated instrument penetration of the dura. If an instrument did penetrate the dura, however, a CT scan should be obtained to evaluate for intracranial damage.

Brain Injury

Penetration of the brain is a potentially fatal complication of paranasal sinus surgery[32] that must be treated aggressively. The defect in the dura should be closed as described for management of CSF leakage, and an evaluation for central nervous system deficits should be carried out. Neurosurgical consultation should be obtained—immediately if a sudden change in vital signs, especially bradycardia and hypotension, occurs while the patient is under general anesthesia. Such a change may indicate intracranial hemorrhage.

A CT scan should be obtained and reviewed in consultation with the neurosurgeon to determine the extent of brain damage (Fig. 7–16); elective neurosurgery may be decided on if there is evidence of continued bleeding (Fig. 7–17).

224 *Endoscopic Sinus Surgery*

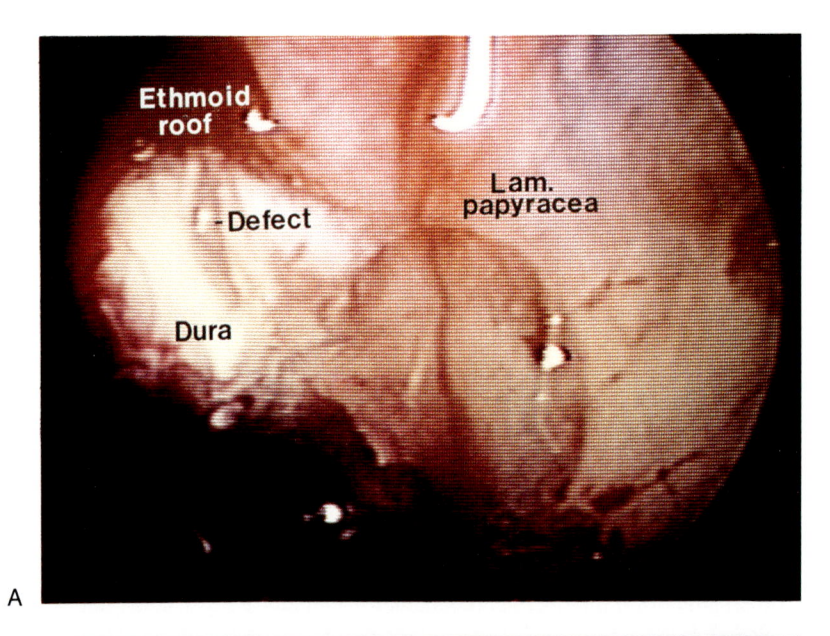

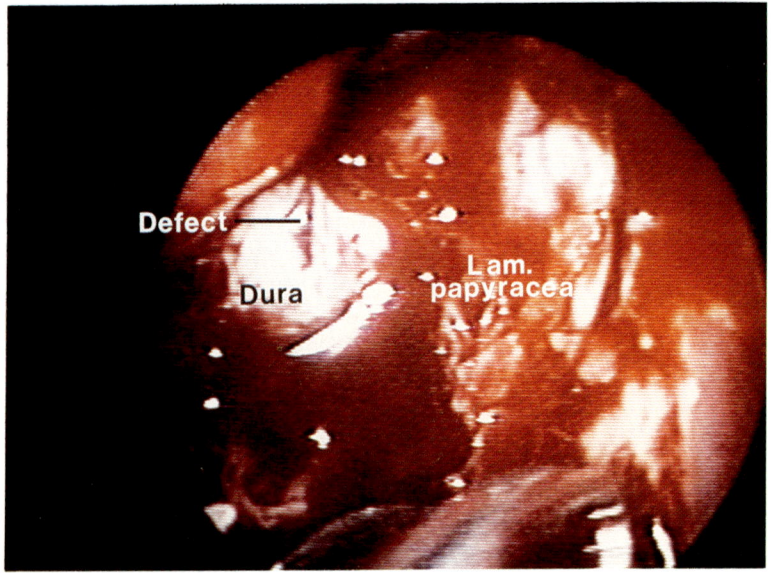

Figure 7–14. A, **B**: The "washout" sign is pathognomonic for CSF leak. As clear CSF exits through the dural tear, it washes out blood in the area of the leak. Lam.: lamina.

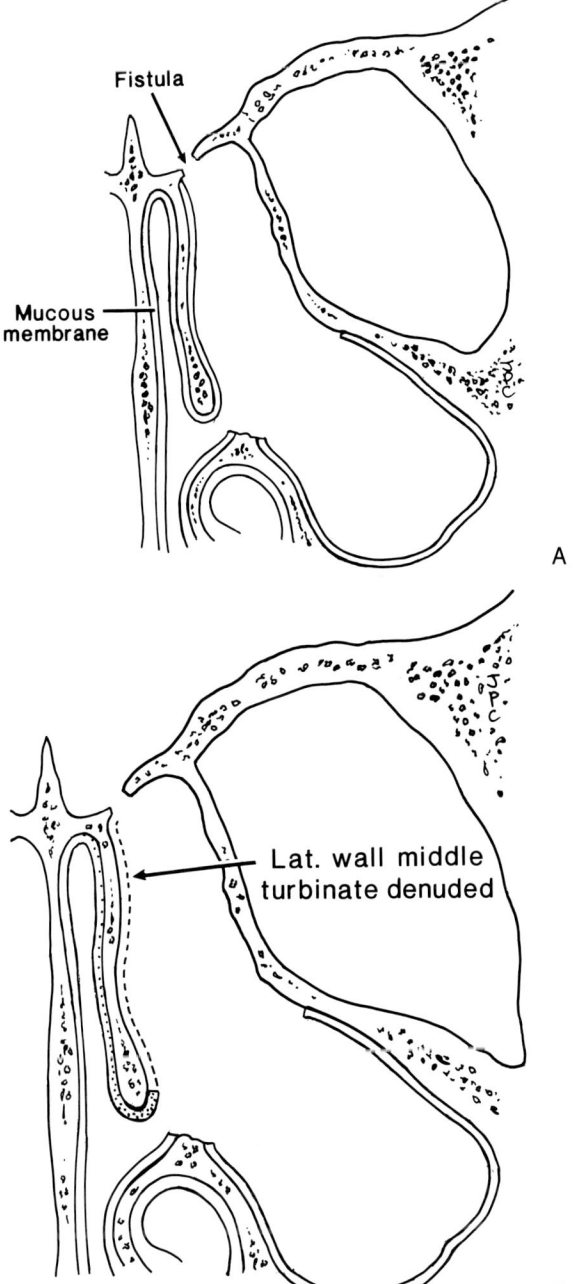

Figure 7–15. A CSF leak occurring during endoscopic sinus surgery should be closed. Ideally a vascularized tissue flap made from the middle turbinate is used to cover the defect. **A**: Note proximity of middle turbinate to dural tear. **B**: Lateral (Lat.) wall of middle turbinate is denuded. (Figure continued on next page.)

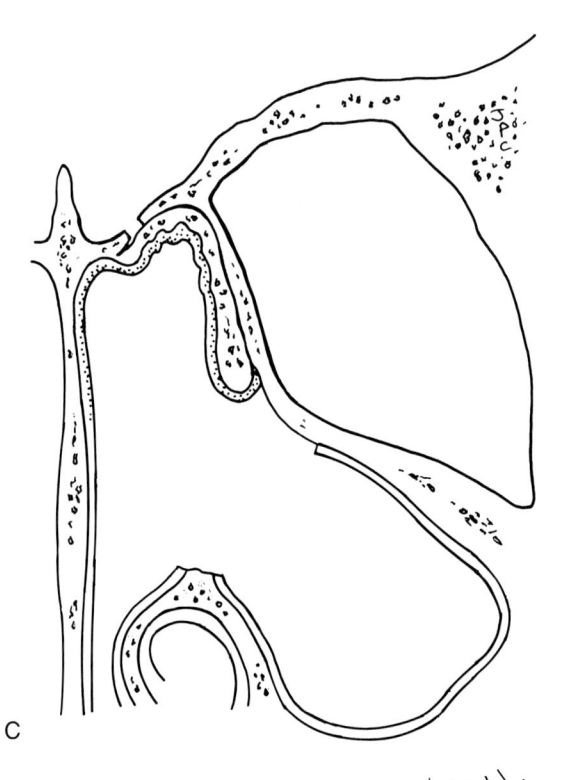

Figure 7–15. (*Continued*). **C**: Middle turbinate is rotated over dural defect. **D**: Lateral view shows cut across superior attachment of middle turbinate, made so as to preserve the blood supply via the sphenopalatine artery (a.). Ant.: anterior; eth.: ethmoid. (Figure continued on next page.)

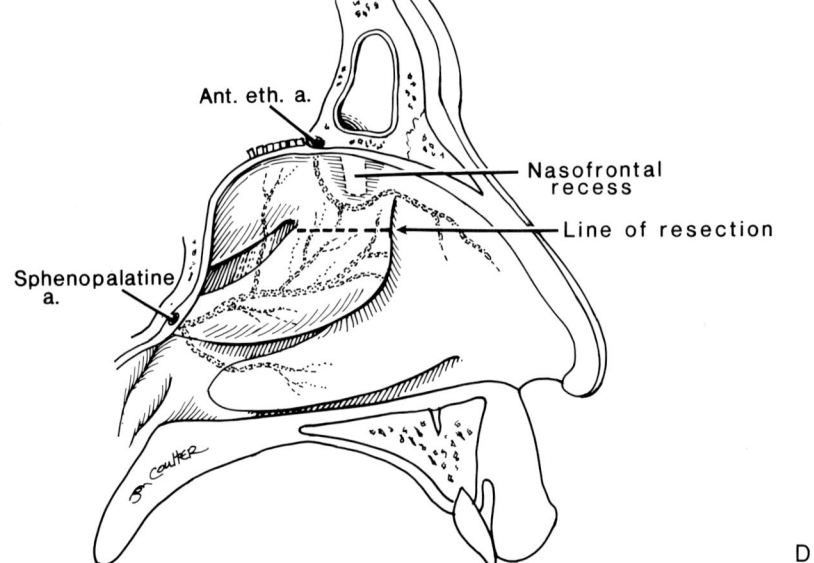

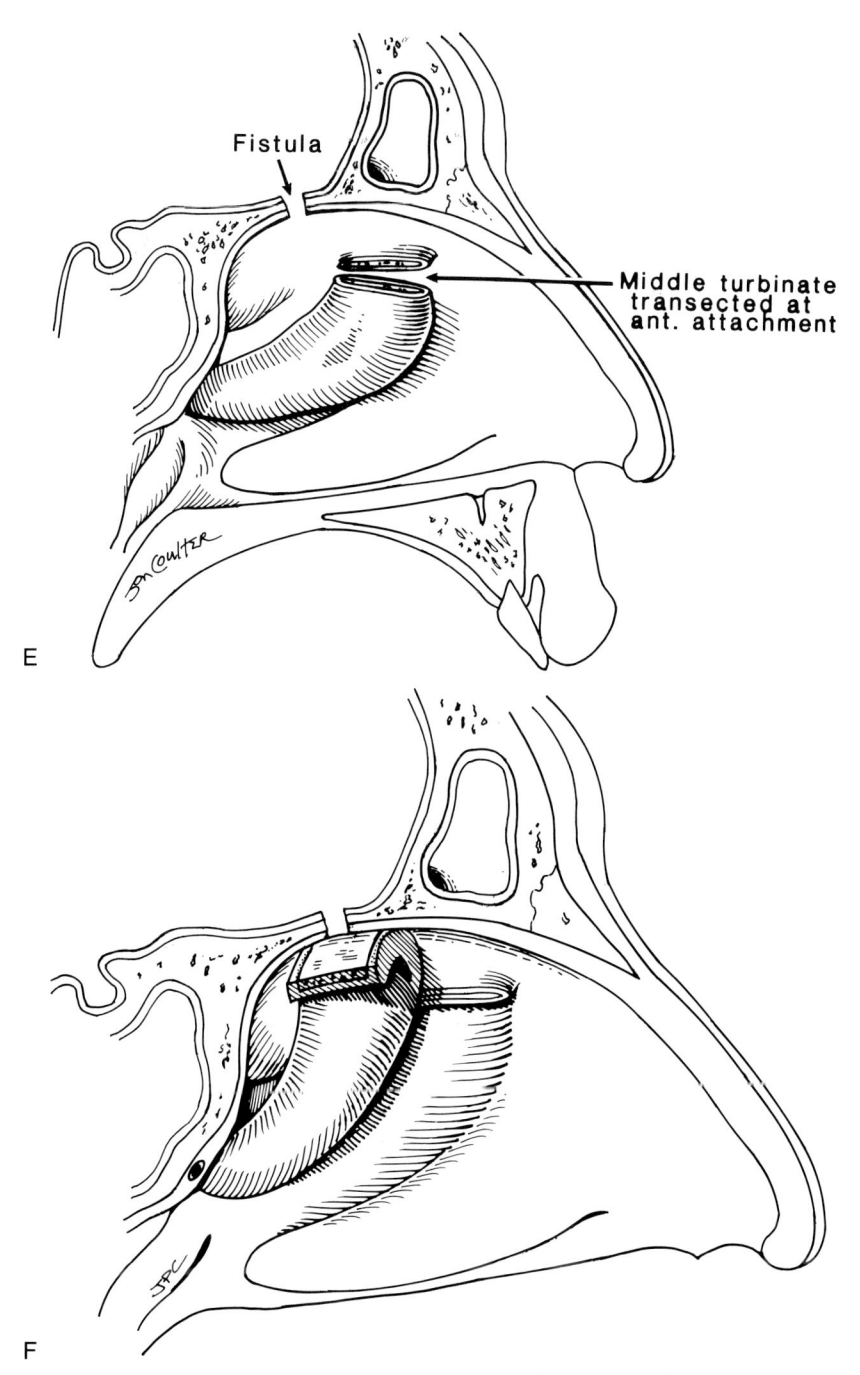

Figure 7–15. (*Continued*). **E**: Transection of the middle turbinate. **F**: Separation of the middle turbinate from its superior attachment and displacing it posteriorly provides coverage of the dural defect without obstruction of the nasofrontal recess and area of the maxillary sinus ostium. ant.: anterior.

228 *Endoscopic Sinus Surgery*

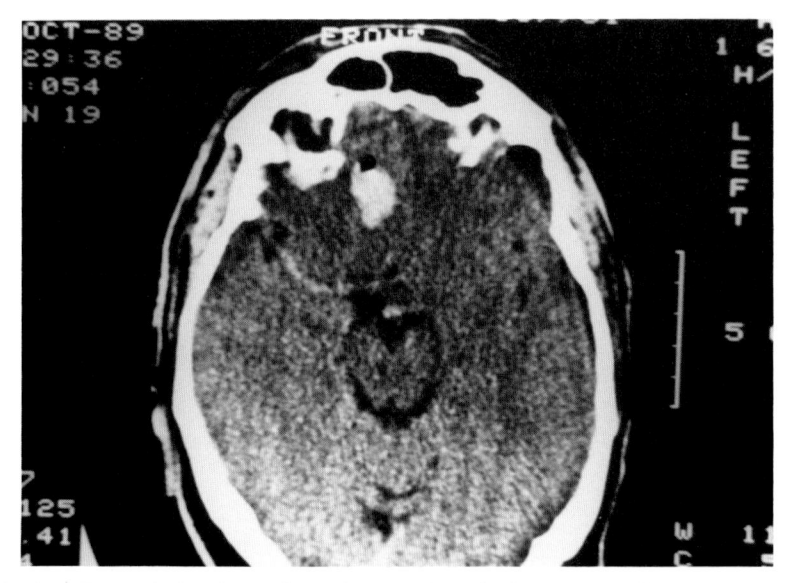

Figure 7–16. CT scan obtained hours after endonasal endoscopic sinus surgery with penetration of the brain parenchyma by suction. Focal hemorrhage is evident, but the patient suffered no sequelae, either immediately postoperatively or during a 3-year follow-up.

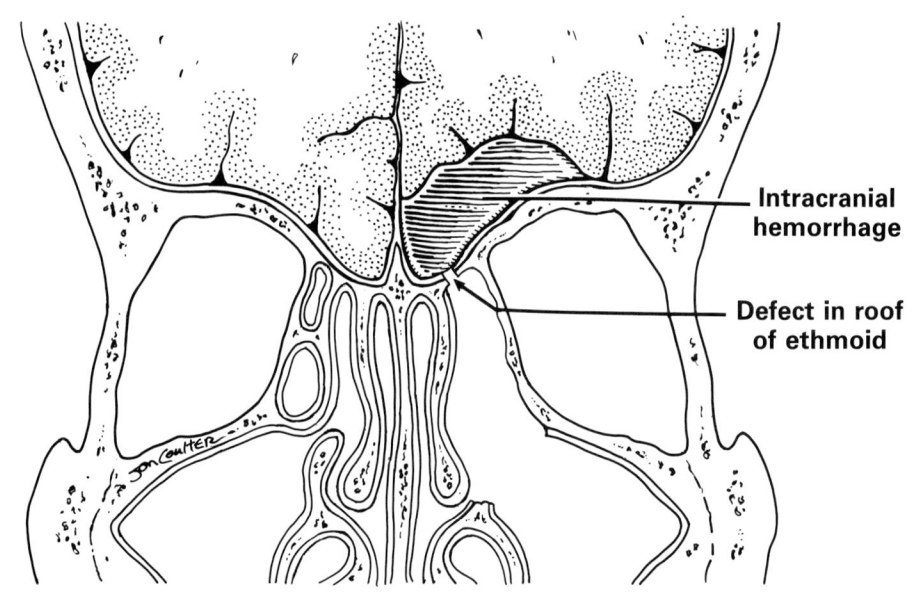

Figure 7–17. A CT scan or magnetic resonance image can show penetration of the roof of the ethmoid sinus or dura. Such penetration may lead to subdural or epidural hemorrhage, requiring immediate neurosurgical intervention to prevent permanent neurologic sequelae.

Bleeding

Bleeding associated with surgery may occur intraoperatively, immediately postoperatively (within 24 hours), or later in the postoperative period (delayed bleeding). Bleeding from the anterior ethmoid or sphenopalatine arteries during surgery was discussed in Chapter 5, and management of anterior ethmoid artery bleeding was discussed in this chapter under "Orbital Penetration" (Figs. 7–11 and 7–12). In this section we will discuss management of carotid artery hemorrhage and postoperative bleeding.

Carotid Artery Injury

The carotid artery is rarely injured during sinus surgery, but any procedure that involves zone C carries the risk of this serious complication. In one case in which this occurred, the sphenoid sinus septum was apparently abnormally thin and attached to a thin-walled carotid canal.[7]

Violation of the carotid artery is immediately evidenced by profuse hemorrhage that must be controlled the instant it is recognized. To control the hemorrhage, the patient's nose and oropharynx must be packed with whatever materials are available. Blood volume is replaced by crystalloid solutions until blood is available for transfusion.

The patient is assessed for neurologic deficits, which may involve allowing the patient under general anesthesia to awaken. Management of carotid artery injuries will vary, depending on the experience of those available for consultation. Ideally, angiography will delineate the defect and the defect can be occluded by balloon.

The risk of violating the carotid artery is decreased by: (1) studying preoperative axial CT scans of the sphenoid sinus to identify this structure in the superolateral wall of the sphenoid sinus, noting its special relationship to the optic nerve, (2) recognizing that carotid canal dehiscences have been identified in 8 to 25% of specimens,[24,33] (3) remembering that an intersphenoid sinus septum may actually be attached to a thin carotid artery canal (manipulation of such a septum was, in fact, the cause of the carotid artery hemorrhage reported by Wigand and Hosemann[7]), and (4) avoiding reaching into the sphenoid sinus with forceps; rather, material should be drawn out of this sinus with suction.

Postoperative Bleeding

Bleeding during the first 24 hours after surgery usually arises from raw edges of mucosa left after removal of the middle turbinate, or after surgery in a patient with massive polyposis or history of previous surgery. When postoperative bleeding occurs, we make a dressing of a non-Latex finger cot stuffed with cottonoids and lubricated with mupirocin (Bactroban) (see Chapter 5) and place it in the nose. It is unusual for a patient to have further bleeding after this dressing is removed 24 hours later.

If blood oozes out after the dressing is removed, spraying the operative area with oxymetazoline (Afrin Nasal Spray) often stops the oozing. If frank bleeding restarts, however, the nose may need to be repacked. Should this procedure fail to stop bleeding, the patient is taken to the operating room for endoscopic localization and cautery of the source of bleeding. Most often, such postoperative bleeding arises from the territory of the sphenopalatine artery, either along the face of the sphenoid sinus or from the posterior aspect of the residual middle turbinate.

Three patients in May's series had delayed hemorrhage due to premature separation of crusts within the nasal or sinus cavity. This problem can be minimized by: (1) keeping the cavity moist through provision of humidified air and topical application of saline spray to the nose and (2) allowing crusts to separate on their own. Postoperatively, these crusts, formed of blood clots, serve as a biologic dressing and are only disturbed if the patient experiences nasal stuffiness, pressure, or pain. In these cases gentle suction is used to dislodge loose crusts.

Lacrimal Complications

Epiphora, caused by lacrimal duct damage, is an annoying complication of ESS[34] that often can only be corrected by a secondary surgical procedure.[35] The lacrimal duct is most often damaged when remnants of the uncinate process are removed or the maxillary sinus ostium is enlarged using side-biting forceps (Fig. 7–18). This is because the uncinate process diverges as a wing of the lacrimal bone.

In fact, this close relationship between the uncinate process and the lacrimal bone probably results in lacrimal duct damage occurring more often than surgeons believe. A clue to such damage is a patient's comment that when he or she blows the nose, air comes into the eye. These patients have, in effect, undergone inadvertent dacryocystorhinostomy (DCR). When the duct is crushed and lacrimal outflow is blocked, however, symptoms will occur (Fig. 7–19). Symptomatic lacrimal duct injury can be evaluated (Fig. 7–20) and managed (Fig. 7–21) quite well endoscopically.

The best way to prevent damage to the lacrimal duct is to use care when removing bone with the side-biting forceps. When the forceps are used to enlarge the maxillary sinus ostium, for example, the blade of the forceps should be kept within the infundibulum and not placed in the maxillary sinus.

Adhesions and Stenoses

Adhesions are more likely to develop in patients with massive disease, a very tight ostiomeatal complex, or a history of previous sinus surgery. Attempts to preserve the middle turbinate during ESS also seem to be more often followed by this complication, because adhesions can be anticipated anywhere mucosa is denuded or abraded and in close proximity to another structure. These circumstances most often arise between the inferior turbinate and the nasal septum, the middle turbinate and the septum, and the middle turbinate and the lateral nasal wall. Adhesions in the last area are most troublesome if they obstruct drainage from the frontal, anterior ethmoid, and maxillary sinuses into the ostiomeatal complex.

The incidence of adhesions may be lowered by taking care not to abrade or denude mucosa along the lateral surface of the middle turbinate; this often takes great surgical skill, acquired with experience. In addition, when factors predisposing to adhesions are present, a stent may be placed to discourage this complication (see Chapter 5); stents should be left in place for approximately a week postoperatively. Another technique to discourage adhesion of the middle turbinate to the lateral nasal wall is to remove the anterior third of the turbinate.

Stenosis of the maxillary sinus ostium may be discouraged by manipulating the ostium as little as is necessary. A normal ostium should not be disturbed, and when the ostium must be opened, only a portion should be enlarged, preferably the segment toward the posterior

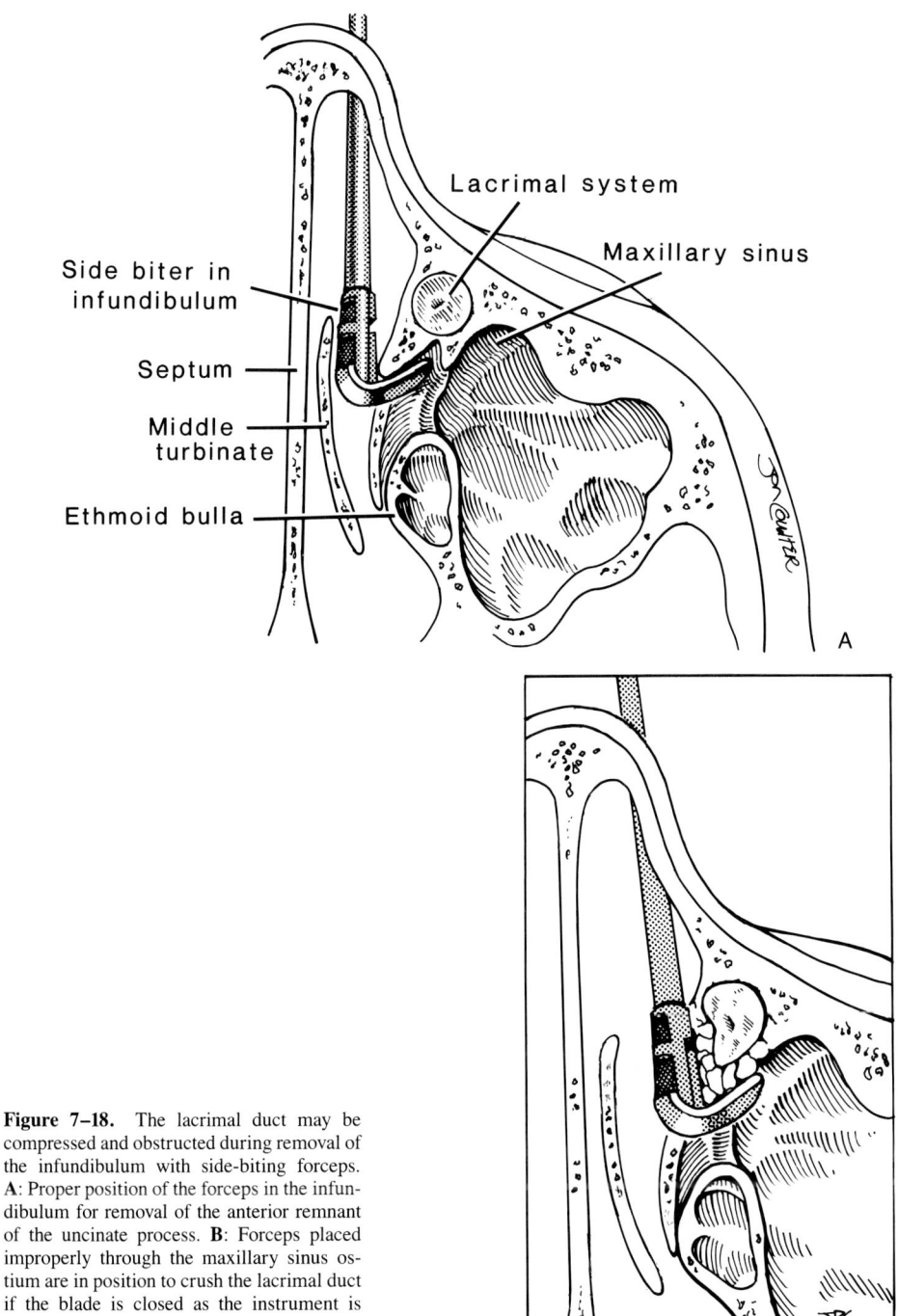

Figure 7–18. The lacrimal duct may be compressed and obstructed during removal of the infundibulum with side-biting forceps. **A**: Proper position of the forceps in the infundibulum for removal of the anterior remnant of the uncinate process. **B**: Forceps placed improperly through the maxillary sinus ostium are in position to crush the lacrimal duct if the blade is closed as the instrument is pulled toward the surgeon.

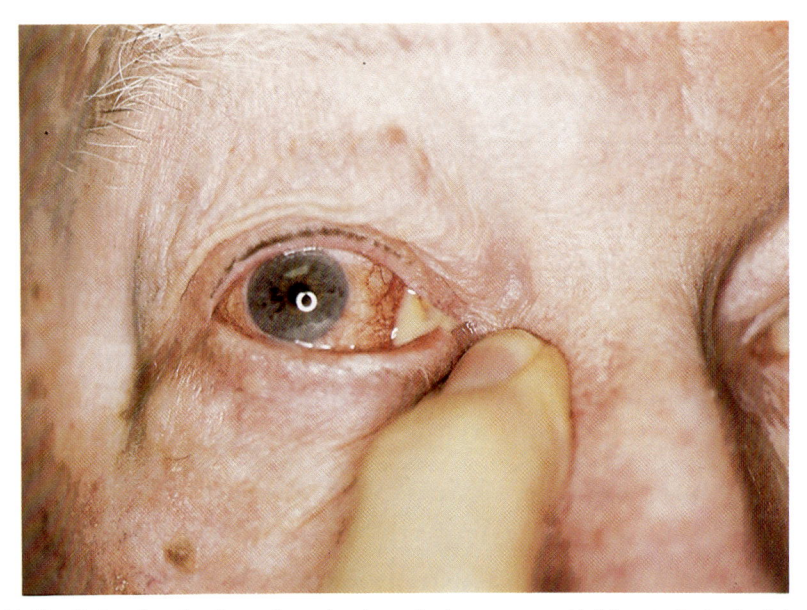

Figure 7–19. Patient 6 weeks after endonasal endoscopic sinus surgery with injury to the lacrimal duct on the right side. Pressing on the lacrimal fossa causes pus collected in the obstructed duct to be expressed through the puncta.

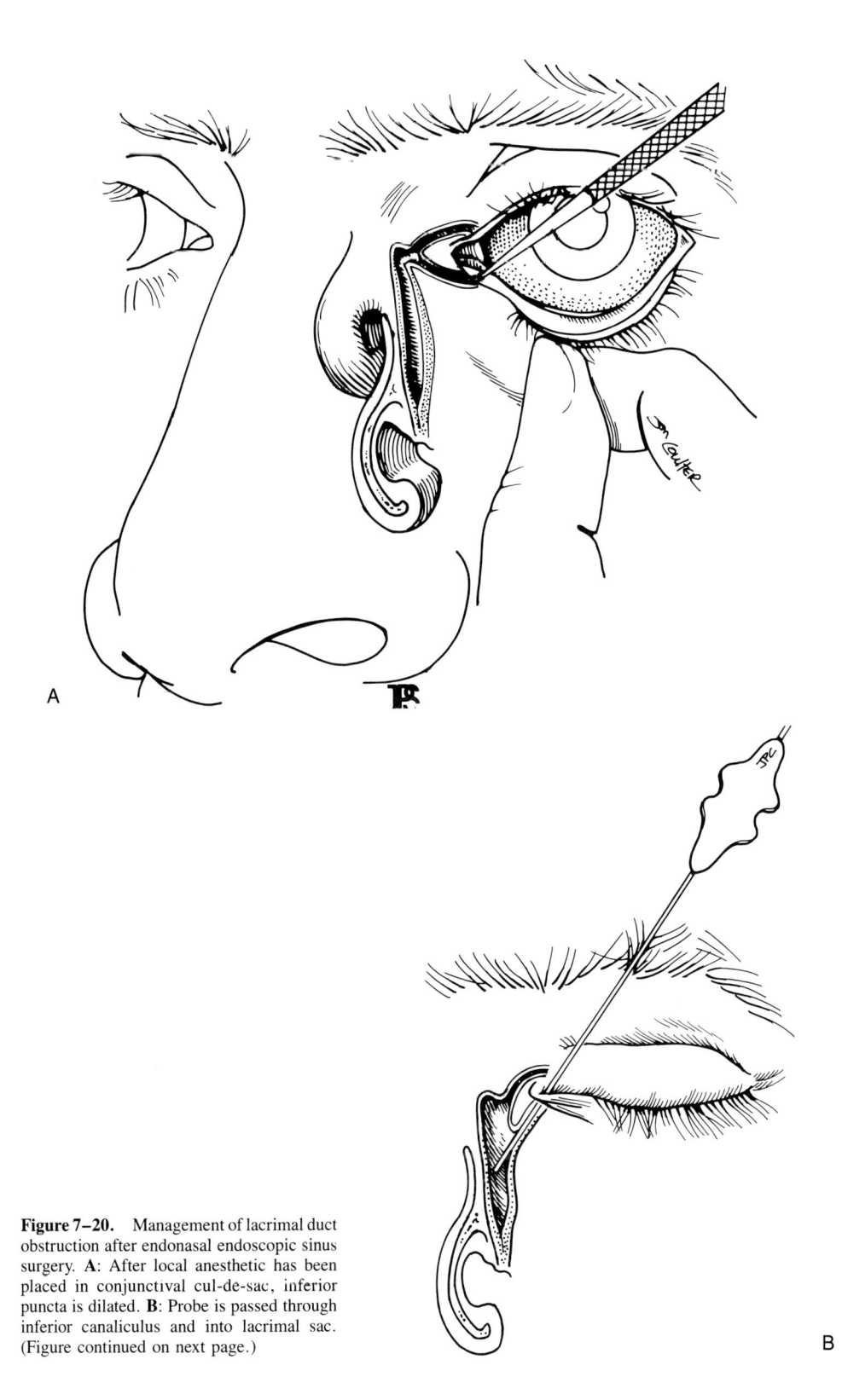

Figure 7–20. Management of lacrimal duct obstruction after endonasal endoscopic sinus surgery. **A**: After local anesthetic has been placed in conjunctival cul-de-sac, inferior puncta is dilated. **B**: Probe is passed through inferior canaliculus and into lacrimal sac. (Figure continued on next page.)

Dye

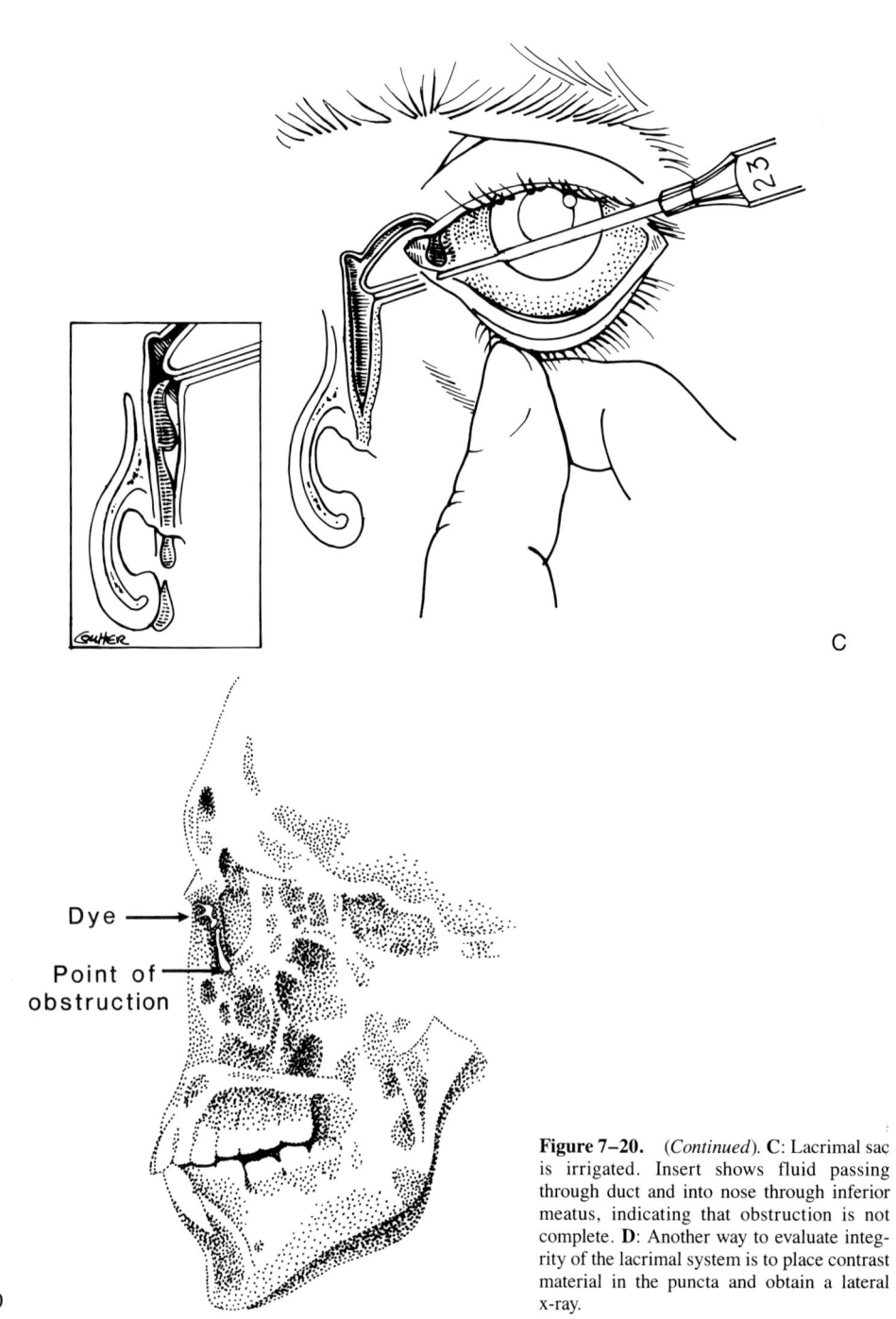

Point of obstruction

Figure 7–20. (*Continued*). **C**: Lacrimal sac is irrigated. Insert shows fluid passing through duct and into nose through inferior meatus, indicating that obstruction is not complete. **D**: Another way to evaluate integrity of the lacrimal system is to place contrast material in the puncta and obtain a lateral x-ray.

Complications 235

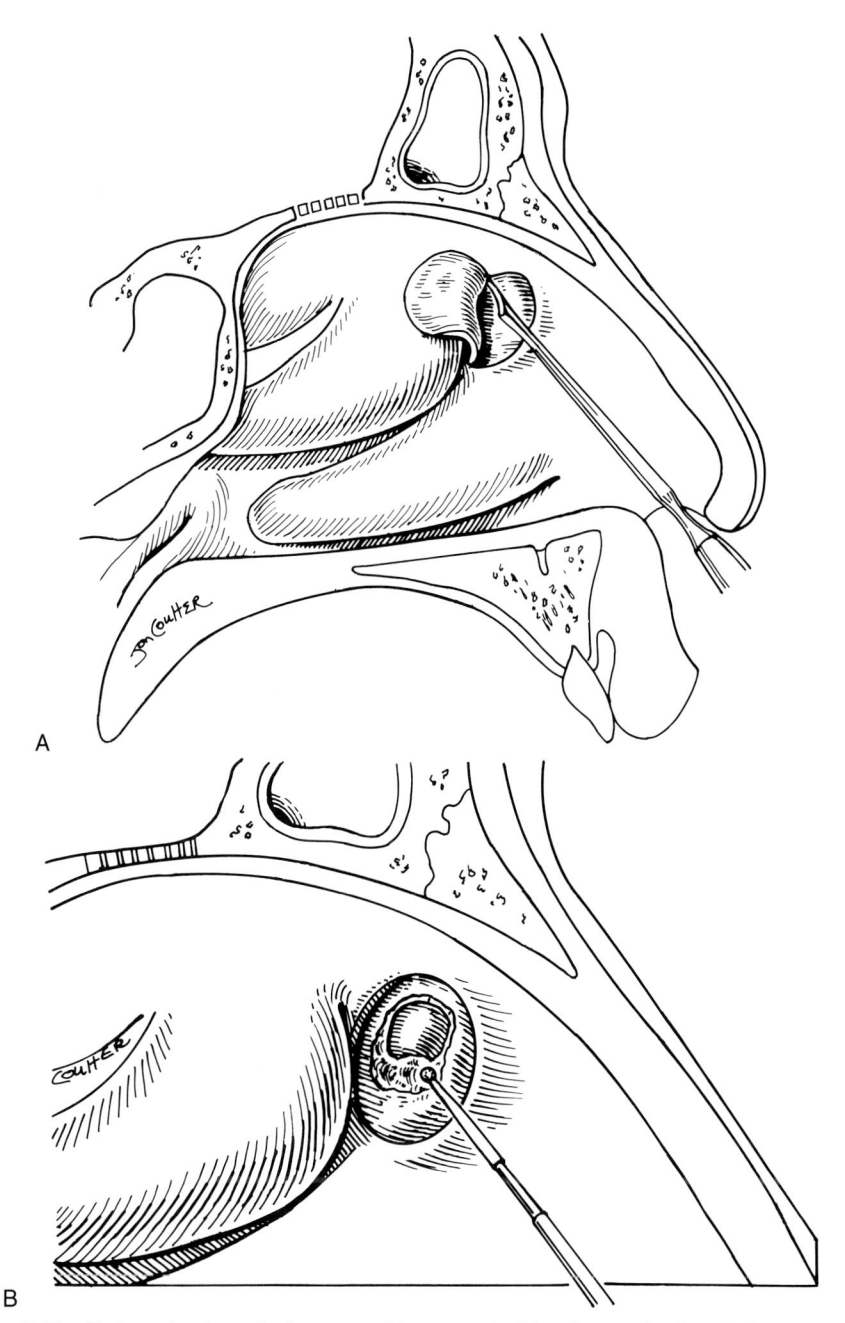

Figure 7–21. Endonasal endoscopic dacryocystorhinostomy. **A**: After the nose has been infiltrated with 1% lidocaine and 1:100,000 epinephrine, a mucosal flap is elevated in front of the anterior attachment of the middle turbinate. **B**: A Xomed Micro-Slim drill (Xomed) is used to thin bone until the lacrimal sac and duct can be identified. (Figure continued on next page.)

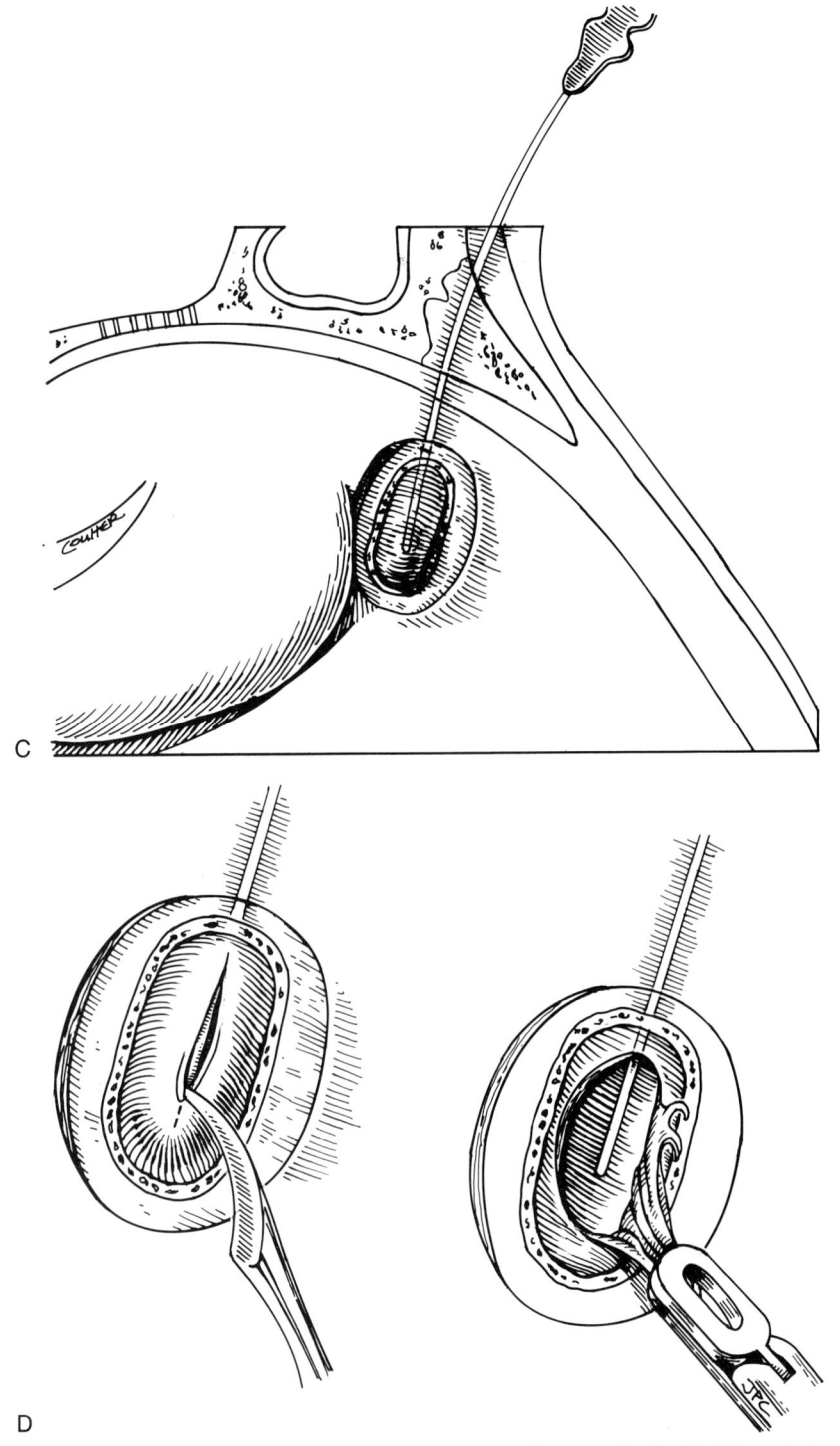

Figure 7–21. (*Continued*). **C**: Sac and duct are probed via the inferior canaliculus. **D**: The probe is used to displace the wall of the lacrimal sac and duct toward the surgeon, so that a sharp beaver knife can be used to open the sac and duct. A large window is removed with grasping forceps. (Figure continued on next page.)

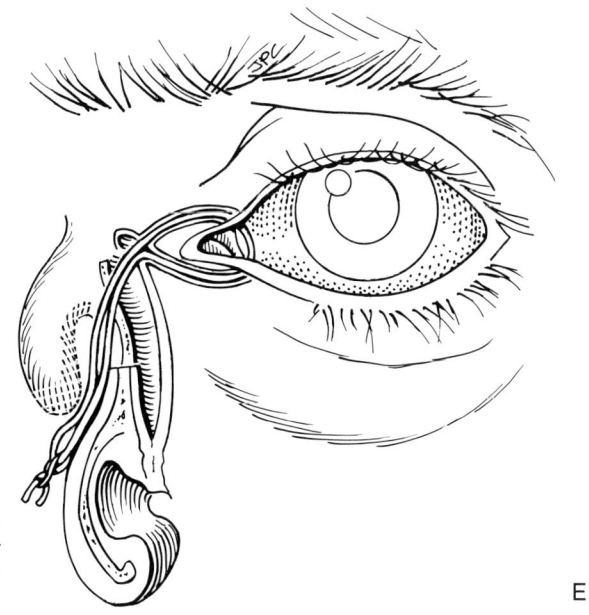

Figure 7–21. (*Continued*). **E**: Silastic tubing is passed through the superior and inferior canaliculi and tied inside the nose. This tubing is left in place for 3 to 6 months.

fontanelle. To enlarge the ostium, a mucosal flap is created by cutting with a sinus scissors from the natural ostium to the posterior extent of the fontanelle in a procedure referred to as a maxillary sinus ostioplasty. The flap created is rotated medially and inferiorly over the inferior turbinate.

When ostium stenosis does occur, it should be treated under direct visualization and monitoring through a canine fossa sinoscopy. The ostium should be opened widely at the expense of the posterior fontanelle and the superior turbinate. Furthermore, a Silastic stent can be left in place up to 3 weeks to keep the ostium patent.

Asthma

Patients should be screened carefully preoperatively to identify those with reactive airway disease or asthma, because in these patients bronchospasm needs to be anticipated and may need to be managed aggressively perioperatively. Consultation with a pulmonary specialist is routine in the care of such patients undergoing sinus surgery, and patients with more severe disease will benefit from hospital admission 24 hours before surgery for administration of steroid medications, inhaled bronchodilators, and chest physiotherapy. General endotracheal anesthesia is preferred for patients with reactive airway disease. Furthermore, one of the special precautions taken for patients with steroid-dependent asthma (patients receiving daily steroid maintenance therapy) includes intravenous administration of a bolus of 100 mg hydrocortisone sodium succinate (Solu-Cortef) at the start of surgery and by continuous intravenous infusion until the patient can resume oral intake of corticosteroid medication. This medication regimen reduces the risk of adrenal insufficiency as well as perioperative bronchospasm. Care of these patients perioperatively was discussed in detail in Chapter 5.

Other Complications

Dental or Lip Pain or Numbness

Changes in sensation in the teeth or lips may result from damage to branches of the infraorbital nerve, which most often occurs with canine fossa puncture. The risk of such injury during this procedure is decreased by keeping lateral on the anterior face of the maxillary sinus, avoiding sliding toward the infraorbital canal, or medially and inferiorly to the roots of the canine and incisor teeth.

The bony wall between the nasal cavity and the maxillary sinus contains branches of the sphenopalatine nerve. If these branches are injured, for example during extensive middle meatal antrostomy or creation of a nasoantral window, neuralgia or dysesthesia may result. Disruption of the nasal branch of the sphenopalatine nerve, such as may occur during septoplasty, may result in incisor dysesthesias.

Infection

Patients who have chronic suppurative sinusitis need intensive antibiotic therapy, perhaps including admission to the hospital for intravenous administration of medications before ESS is performed. If infection is present in the maxillary sinus, a middle meatal maxillary sinus antrostomy is performed and the new opening connected to the natural ostium. Sphenoid sinusitis is treated by removing the entire anterior wall of the sinus to reach and remove disease. Disease obstructing the nasofrontal region is removed to treat frontal sinusitis. All infected sinuses are irrigated and inspected to be sure they are clear of abnormal secretions or fungus deposits (greasy, claylike, yellow or brown material).

Because antibiotic medication is given perioperatively to patients with suppurative disease, material taken for culture is usually sterile unless a fungus infection is present. For this reason, culture specimens are not obtained routinely, unless fungus is suspected.

Anosmia

Disturbance of the olfactory cleft, either by polyps or removal of the special mucous membrane between the middle turbinate and roof of the nose, may lead to disturbances of smell. Patients who experience such disturbance may notice a return of olfaction with a bolus course of steroid medications, which is a good sign in that it indicates that loss of olfaction is probably due to mucosal obstruction rather than damage to the olfactory mucosa. The return of olfaction in these cases is usually temporary, however; when steroids are stopped the sense of smell is again lost.

To prevent disturbances of smell, the olfactory cleft should not be disturbed on the nasal side. Avoidance of this area will also decrease the risk of dural penetration.

Miscellaneous Complications

Toxic Shock Syndrome

Toxic shock syndrome (TSS) is characterized by: (1) body temperature of 38.2°C or greater; (2) exanthem with erythroderma, followed by desquamation; and (3) orthostatic hypotension or shock.[36] TSS is caused by toxins produced by *Staphylococcus aureus* in association with dressings or packing materials left in a closed cavity, and although this syndrome is rare, it has been reported in association with ESS.[37]

Lubricating dressings or packing with antimicrobial agents does not protect against TSS. Therefore, the best way to decrease the risk of this possible complication is not to leave any dressing (Gelfoam, Surgicel, Merocel, gauze, Telfa, or Silastic implants) in the nose.[38] If an intranasal dressing is necessary, the time the material remains in the nose should be kept to a minimum.

Latex Allergy

The incidence of sensitivity to Latex is reported to be as high as 7% among surgical personnel and 40% among spina bifida patients, and anaphylaxis and death have occurred as a result of sensitive persons being exposed to this material.[39,40] For this reason, we specify use of a non-Latex glove to fashion nasal dressings.

Myospherulosis

Placement of petrolatum-containing medications in a surgically created cavity has been reported, although rarely, to cause myospherulosis.[41–44] The mechanism apparently involves a soft tissue reaction to phagocytosis of petrolatum molecules followed by formation of chronic granuloma. The description by Stammberger and Posawetz[13] of a granulomatous complication occurring in five of their patients suggests myospherulosis, and to avoid this complication we coat intranasal dressings with a bactericidal topical medication (mupirocin) that contains propylene glycol instead of petrolatum.

Dilated Pupil During Surgery

Marked dilation of one or both pupils has been noted during ESS. This condition is disconcerting because it suggests serious injury to the optic nerve, but no evidence of such injury has been found and the condition clears spontaneously within an hour after surgery. Singh[45] and Schaefer[46] proposed that dilation is due to injected epinephrine or lidocaine or topically applied phenylephrine, and they recommend that precautions be taken not to introduce these agents into the patient's conjunctiva.

Developing Surgical Skills to Avoid Complications

As was discussed earlier in this chapter, the risk of complications is higher with a new technique. Thus, although the majority of surgeons beginning to perform ESS will have had experience with traditional sinus surgery techniques, engaging in planned learning experiences with ESS is mandatory for the surgeon who wishes to perform ESS effectively, efficiently, and safely.

The surgeon new to endoscopic surgery will notice that depth perception is altered by the monocular lens-rod system of the instrument. Experience with the endoscope can be gained by examining preoperative patients in the office setting, and then using the instrument to remove crusts, old blood, and mucus from sinus cavities of patients who have been operated on by a traditional technique. By using the endoscope to visualize suctioning and manipulating forceps to treat postoperative conditions, the surgeon will acquire the basic skills necessary for intraoperative techniques.

Courses and workshops in endoscopic sinus surgical anatomy, particularly those that include cadaver dissection, will also improve understanding and technique. Finally, the surgeon new to ESS should operate at first on patients with minimal disease who have no history of previous sinus surgery procedures, then progress to more challenging cases.

Some Tips to Avoid Complications of Endoscopic Sinus Surgery

Dicta

1. "Do as little as possible and as much as necessary" (Erik Malte Wigand, First International Symposium on Contemporary Sinus Surgery, November 1990, Pittsburgh, PA).
2. Be conservative: ESS is designed to treat anatomic or inflammatory disease, not cancer.

Generalities

1. Stop if you can't see.
2. Stop if you are not sure where you are.
3. Mark the instruments to make measurements and hang a preoperative lateral x-ray in the operating room for reference.
4. Remember the "learning curve"; do easy cases at first and progress.
5. A 0° endoscope gives the least amount of distortion.
6. The greater the distortion (higher the angle), the higher the risk of getting lost.
7. Keep the field clean and dry.
8. An advantage of local anesthesia: the patient will keep you out of trouble by complaining of pain when surgery approaches the orbit or roof of the ethmoid sinus.
9. Leave the patient's eyes uncovered and watch the pupils.
10. Palpate the globes preoperatively for tone and check during procedure for any change.
11. The "washout" sign means CSF leak—repair it now!

Specific Areas

Ethmoid Sinus:

1. Leave mucosa over the roof of the ethmoid sinus.
2. Remove only enough disease to reestablish drainage, ventilation, and mucociliary transport—and most importantly to relieve symptoms.
3. There is no need to remove every bit of "diseased" tissue; often mucosa that looks "bad" will revert to normal.
4. Beware of the vulnerable area in zone A, between the middle turbinate and the roof of the ethmoid sinus.

Uncinate Process:

1. Palpate the globe while working near the lamina papyracea.
2. Use the double-ended maxillary sinus ostium seeker to palpate the infundibulum and displace the uncinate process away from the orbit.

Maxillary Sinus Ostium:

1. Find the maxillary sinus ostium before penetrating the bulla ethmoidalis and place the ostium seeker into the infundibulum.
2. Always direct the ostium seeker forward and down.
3. To find the maxillary sinus ostium, locate the junction of the vertical and horizontal limbs of the infundibulum at the level of the inferior border of the middle turbinate.
4. Pressure on the posterior fontanelle may force air bubbles or secretions out of the maxillary sinus ostium.

Bulla Ethmoidalis:

- The nasofrontal recess and anterior ethmoid artery are just above and in front of the face of the bulla ethmoidalis.

Sphenoid Sinus:

1. Obtain an axial CT scan (to evaluate optic nerve and carotid artery) in all patients scheduled for sphenoid sinus surgery. Study CT scans preoperatively and have them within view during surgery.
2. Always open an opaque sphenoid sinus: silent areas—infection, mycosis, pyoceles, tumors—may be asymptomatic.
3. Use the C-arm fluoroscope to locate the face of the sphenoid sinus when in doubt.
4. To enter the sphenoid sinus safely, orient to landmarks: junction of the posterior septum, above the posterior attachment of the middle turbinate, the arch of the posterior choana.

Frontal Sinus:

1. Avoid creating frontal sinusitis—don't touch agger nasi cells or nasofrontal recess unless symptomatic.
2. The frontal sinus isthmus is located in the anterior superior aspect of the nasofrontal recess, under the anterior superior attachment of the middle turbinate, close to the lamina papyracea.

Nasal Septum:

1. If a 4 mm endoscope will not fit between the septum and lateral nasal wall or the middle turbinate cannot be medialized enough to enter the ostiomeatal complex, perform septoplasty.
2. Perform ostiomeatal complex surgery on the open side first, then do septal surgery before operating on the closed side.

Middle Turbinate:
- Remove the middle turbinate if lateralized, bulbus, bullous, polypoid, or likely to adhere to the lateral nasal wall.

Basal Lamella:
- Enter the basilar lamella posteriorly.

SUMMARY

Complications will occur with ESS regardless of the training, skill, and experience of the surgeon; therefore, each surgeon needs to learn to recognize complications and treat them appropriately when they occur. Our review has shown that the overall complication rates for nonendoscopic and endoscopic techniques are comparable. What, then, justifies the increased expense for equipment and training for ESS? The answer is that this new technology provides an effective method to teach and learn an endonasal endoscopic approach to diseases of the nose, paranasal sinuses, and contiguous structures in close proximity to the ethmoid sinus—such as the orbit, optic nerve, and pituitary gland. The endonasal route is direct and eliminates the need for external incisions, which significantly reduces patient morbidity. Thus, as the binocular operating microscope revolutionized neuro-otology, the endoscope is revolutionizing rhinology.

REFERENCES

1. Sogg A: Long-term results of ethmoid surgery. Ann Otol Rhinol Laryngol 98:699–701, 1989.
2. Lawson W: The intranasal ethmoidectomy: An experience with 1,077 procedures. Laryngoscope 101:367–371, 1991.
3. Friedman WH, Katsantonis GP: The role of standard technique in modern sinus surgery. Otolaryngol Clin North Am 22:759–775, 1989.
4. Stevens HE, Blair NJ: Intranasal sphenoethmoidectomy: 10-year experience and literature review. J Otolaryngol 17:254–258, 1988.
5. Freedman HM, Kern EB: Complications of intranasal ethmoidectomy: A review of 1,000 consecutive operations. Laryngoscope 89:421–434, 1979.
6. Eichel BS: The intranasal sphenoethmoidectomy: 10-year experience and literature review. J Otolaryngol 17(5):254–259, 1988.
7. Wigand ME, Hosemann WG: Results of endoscopic surgery of the paranasal sinuses and anterior skull base. J Otolaryngol 20:385–390, 1991.
8. Kennedy DW, Zinreich SJ, Kuhn F, et al: Endoscopic middle meatal antrostomy: Theory, technique, and patency. Laryngoscope 97(8, pt. 3) Suppl 43, 1987.
9. Schaefer SD, Manning S, Close LG: Endoscopic paranasal sinus surgery: Indications and considerations. Laryngoscope 99:1–5, 1989.
10. Toffel PH, Aroesty DJ, Weinmann RH: Secure endoscopic sinus surgery as an adjunct to functional nasal surgery. Arch Otolaryngol Head Neck Surg 115:822–825, 1989.
11. Rice DH: Endoscopic sinus surgery: Results at 2-year followup. Otolaryngol Head Neck Surg 101:476–479, 1989.
12. Vleming M, Middelweerd RJ, deVries N: Complications of endoscopic sinus surgery. Arch Otolaryngol Head Neck Surg 118:617–623, 1992.
13. Stammberger H, Posawetz W: Functional endoscopic sinus surgery. Eur Arch Otorhinolaryngol 247:63–76, 1990.
14. Matthews BL, Smith LE, Jones R, et al: Endoscopic sinus surgery: Outcome in 155 cases. Otolaryngol Head Neck Surg 104:244–246, 1991.
15. Lazar RH, Younis RT, Gross CW: Pediatric functional endonasal sinus surgery: Review of 210 cases. Head Neck 14:92–98, 1992.

16. Stankiewicz JA: Complications in endoscopic intranasal ethmoidectomy: An update. Laryngoscope 99:686–690, 1989.
17. Stankiewicz JA: Complications of endoscopic intranasal ethmoidectomy. Laryngoscope 97:1270–1273, 1987.
18. May M, Hillsamer P, Hoffmann DF: Management of orbital hematoma following functional endoscopic sinus surgery. Am J Rhinol 5(2):47–50, 1991.
19. Thompson RF, Glukman JL, Kulwin D, Savoury L: Orbital hemorrhage during sinus surgery. Otolaryngol Head Neck Surg 102:45–50, 1990.
20. Kainz J, Stammberger H: The roof of the anterior ethmoid: A place of least resistance in the skull base. Am J Rhinol 3(4):191–199, 1989.
21. Stankiewicz JA: Blindness and intranasal endoscopic ethmoidectomy: Prevention and management. Otolaryngol Head Neck Surg 101:320–329, 1989.
22. Sacks SH, Lawson W, Edelstein D, Green RP: Surgical treatment of blindness secondary to intraorbital hemorrhage. Arch Otolaryngol Head Neck Surg 114:801–803, 1988.
23. Kennedy DW, Goodstein ML, Miller NR, Zinreich J: Endoscopic transnasal orbital decompression. Arch Otolaryngol Head Neck Surg 116:275–282, 1990.
24. Fujii K, Chambers SM, Rhoton AL: Neurovascular relationships of the sphenoid sinus: A microsurgical study. J Neurosurg 50:31–39, 1979.
25. Takahashi M, Itoh M, Ishii J, Yoshida A: Microscopic intranasal decompression of the optic nerve. Arch Otolaryngol 246:113–116, 1989.
26. Sofferman RA: Transnasal approach to optic nerve decompression. Op Tech Otolaryngol Head Neck Surg 2:150–156, 1991.
27. Mark LE, Kennerdell JS: Medial rectus injury from intranasal surgery. Arch Ophthalmol 97:459–461, 1979.
28. Papay FA, Maggiano H, Dominquez S, et al: Rigid endoscopic repair of paranasal sinus cerebrospinal fluid fistulas. Laryngoscope 99:1195–1201, 1989.
29. Stankiewicz JA: Cerebrospinal fluid fistula and endoscopic sinus surgery. Laryngoscope 101:250–256, 1991.
30. Mattox DE, Kennedy DW: Endoscopic management of cerebrospinal fluid leaks and cephaloceles. Laryngoscope 100:857–862, 1990.
31. Yessenow R, McCabe B: The osteo-mucoperiosteal flap in repair of cerebrospinal fluid rhinorrhea: A 20-year experience. Otolaryngol Head Neck Surg 101:555–558, 1989.
32. Maniglia AJ: Fatal and major complications secondary to nasal and sinus surgery. Laryngoscope 99:267–283, 1989.
33. Kennedy D, Zinreich S, Hassab M: The internal carotid artery as it relates to endonasal sphenoethmoidectomy. Am J Rhinol 4:7–12, 1990.
34. Serdahl CL, Berris CE, Chole RA: Nasolacrimal duct obstruction after endoscopic sinus surgery. Arch Ophthalmol 108:391–392, 1990.
35. Metson R: The endoscopic approach for revision dacryocystorhinostomy. Laryngoscope 100(12):1–4, 1990.
36. Breda SD, Jacobs JB, Lebowitz AS, et al: Toxic shock syndrome in nasal surgery: A physiochemical and microbiologic evaluation of Merocel and Nu Gauze nasal packing. Laryngoscope 97:1388–1391, 1987.
37. Younis RT, Gross CW, Lazar RH: Toxic shock syndrome following functional endonasal sinus surgery. A case report. Head Neck Surg 13:247–248, 1991.
38. deVries N, van der Baan S: Toxic shock syndrome after nasal surgery: Is prevention possible? Rhinology 27:125–128, 1989.
39. Shapiro G: Latex allergy tied to surgical anaphylaxis. Respir News 11(2): 1991.
40. Federal Drug Bulletin. October 1990.
41. McClatchie S, Warambo MW, Bremner AD: Myospherulosis. A previously unreported disease. Am J Pathol 51:699–704, 1969.
42. Paugh D, Sullivan M: Myospherulosis of the paranasal sinuses. Otolaryngol Head Neck Surg 103:117–119, 1990.
43. Kyriakos M: Myospherulosis of the paranasal sinuses, nose, and middle ear: A possible iatrogenic disease. Am J Clin Pathol 67:118–130, 1977.
44. May M: Myospherulosis of the paranasal sinuses. (Letter to the Editor.) Otolaryngol Head Neck Surg 105:136, 1991.
45. Singh J: Pupil dilation during endoscopic surgery. (Letter to the Editor.) Arch Otolaryngol Head Neck Surg 118:105, 1992.
46. Schaefer SD: Response. (Letter to the Editor.) Arch Otolaryngol Head Neck Surg 118:105, 1992.

8
Endoscopic Sinus Surgery in Children

RANDE H. LAZAR, M.D.
RAMZI T. YOUNIS, M.D.
MICHAEL J. GURUCHARRI, M.D.

Sinusitis is one of the most poorly understood disorders that may affect children. Many symptoms of sinusitis may be overlooked or not recognized because the child cannot verbalize them or because the physician believes the sinuses to be too underdeveloped to be the source of a clinical disorder.

Sinusitis is, however, often seen in children, although its incidence in this age group is not known. This inflammatory process in the mucosal lining of the paranasal sinuses may arise from a number of causes, ranging from a simple, localized inflammation to a serious systemic disorder (Table 8–1). Most often, however, this condition is the sequela of an upper respiratory tract infection and/or an allergic condition.[1]

Determining the correct treatment for sinusitis in children can be as difficult as making the diagnosis. Optimally, the condition is managed medically, but after well-established medical regimens have failed, surgery is indicated. In the United States, endoscopic sinus surgery (ESS) is rapidly becoming the technique of choice for adults, and although use of this technique in children has only recently been reported,[2] we believe this procedure is a safe and effective way to manage sinus disease in younger patients as well.

The paranasal sinuses change quite significantly, however, with growth and development of the individual. Therefore, before attempting any surgical intervention for nasosinus disease in a child, the surgeon should have a thorough understanding of normal sinus anatomy for a patient of that age. This chapter reviews developmental anatomy of the paranasal sinuses, sinus pathophysiology with special reference to disease in children, medical treatment of sinus disease in children, and ESS in children.

DEVELOPMENTAL ANATOMY OF THE PARANASAL SINUSES

The four paired paranasal chambers that constitute the paranasal sinuses are filled with air and connected to the nose by small openings, the ostia. These chambers, small in young children, grow at different rates until they reach adult size at various ages. In children, as in

Table 8–1 Etiologic Factors in Pediatric Sinusitis

MECHANISM	FACTOR
Inflammatory	Upper respiratory tract infection
	Allergy
Mechanical	Nasoseptal deformity
	Ostiomeatal complex obstruction
	Turbinate hypertrophy
	Polyps
	Tumor
	Adenoid hypertrophy
	Foreign body
	Cleft palate
	Choanal atresia (unilateral) or posterior nasal stenosis
Systemic	Cystic fibrosis
	Immotile cilia syndrome
	Kartagener's syndrome
	Immunodeficiency
	Cyanotic congenital heart disease
Miscellaneous	Diving, swimming

adults, they are lined with ciliated pseudostratified columnar epithelium interspersed with goblet-type mucous cells.

Ethmoid Sinus

Anterior, middle, and posterior ethmoid sinus cells are usually present bilaterally. The anteromiddle ethmoid cells evaginate from pits in the frontal recess in the third fetal month,[3,4] and the posterior cells evaginate shortly afterward.[5] In children, in contrast to adults, the ethmoid sinus cells are more difficult than the maxillary sinus cells to visualize on plain roentgenographs. The ethmoid sinuses grow by nearly 400% from birth until they reach adult size, at about age 12 years.

Maxillary Sinus

The maxillary sinus, the first to begin development, arises at the third fetal month as an evagination between the inferior and middle turbinates.[3,5] The original maxillary sinus cell is the groove between the uncinate process and the bulla ethmoidalis, which grows rapidly between birth and 3 years, enlarges only slightly between 3 and 7 years, and then grows quickly again from age 7 to 12 years. The maxillary sinus attains its adult size, nearly twice the volume of the neonate sinus, in the late teenage years.[3] With growth and development, the floor of the maxillary sinus, which is 4 mm above the floor of the nose at birth, descends to 4 to 5 mm below the floor of the nose by adulthood.[6]

The ostium of the maxillary sinus is generally located in the superior aspect of the medial wall of the sinus, posterior to the midpoint of the bulla ethmoidalis.[3] Secretions that drain through the maxillary sinus ostium then drain into the infundibulum and through the hiatus semilunaris. The size, shape, and location of the maxillary sinus ostium vary, depending on the degree of pneumatization of the bulla ethmoidalis and the projection of the uncinate process. Accessory ostia may also be found in 15 to 40% of specimens studied.[3,7,8]

Frontal Sinus

Several origins for the frontal sinus have been proposed, but the most often accepted is that the frontal sinus on each side begins as a pit or furrow in the frontal recess.[3] Indistinguishable from the anterior ethmoid cells at birth,[3] the frontal sinus begins to invade the vertical portion of the frontal bone by the age of 4 years,[5] and by the age of 6 years it may be visualized radiographically. Growth of the frontal sinuses is usually complete before the age of 20 years.[3,7]

When fully developed, the frontal sinuses usually are paired pyramid-shaped chambers in the vertical portion of the frontal bone. Substantial variations in the size and shape of the sinus do occur, however, even in the same individual. In some 4% of cases the frontal sinuses are totally absent.[5]

Sphenoid Sinus

The sphenoid sinus on each side evaginates from the respective sphenoethmoid recess. The sinus begins to grow at about age 3 years, and after age 5 it grows rapidly.[3] In adults, the sphenoid sinus may extend superiorly to the sella turcica and posteriorly to the basisphenoid.[3]

Vital structures such as the optic nerve, internal carotid artery, and pituitary gland lie in close proximity to the sphenoid sinus on each side and may appear as indentations in the wall of the sinus.[3,9] The sphenoid sinus ostium is located in the sphenoethmoid recess, 10 to 15 mm superior to the sinus floor.[3]

PATHOPHYSIOLOGY OF SINUSITIS IN CHILDREN

Healthy sinus function requires: (1) patent ostia, (2) a functioning ciliary apparatus, and (3) normal sinus secretions.

Mucus is continuously produced in the sinuses. A healthy ciliary apparatus moves the mucus toward the natural sinus ostia which, when patent, drain mucus into the nose and nasopharynx to be swallowed or expectorated. Conditions that interfere with one or more of these steps can lead to sinusitis (Table 8–1) by mechanisms that will now be discussed.

Ostial Obstruction

The ostiomeatal complex (OMC) (Fig. 8–1) is key in the pathophysiology of sinusitis because this region of the middle meatus contains the ostia of the frontal, maxillary, and ethmoid sinuses. Obstruction of the OMC, and thus the sinus ostia, to which a number of factors may contribute (Fig. 8–2), can cause sinusitis by severely hindering mucociliary flow of secretions.

Endoscopic Sinus Surgery in Children 247

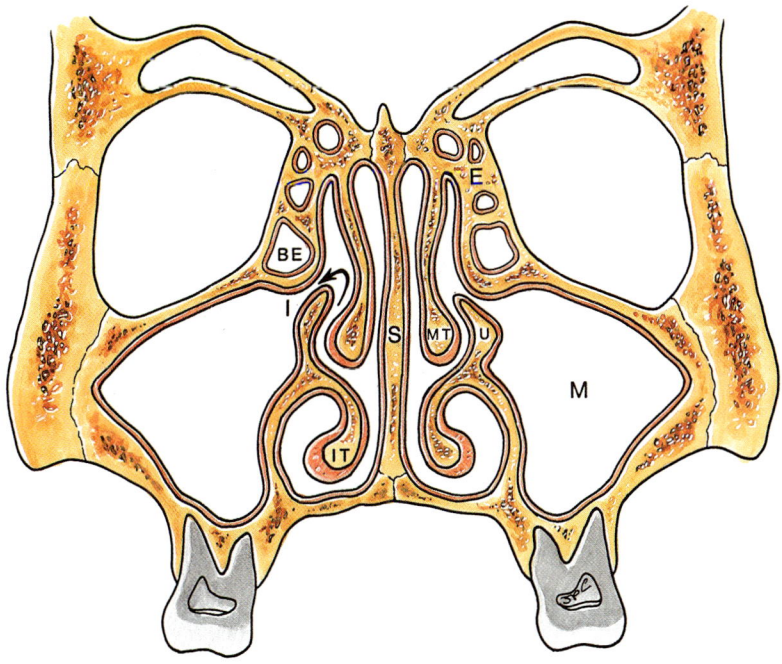

Figure 8–1. Schematic drawing of normal ostiomeatal complex. BE: bulla ethmoidalis; I: maxillary sinus infundibulum; U: uncinate process; IT: inferior turbinate; S: nasal septum; MT: middle turbinate; E: ethmoids; curved arrow: hiatus semilunaris.

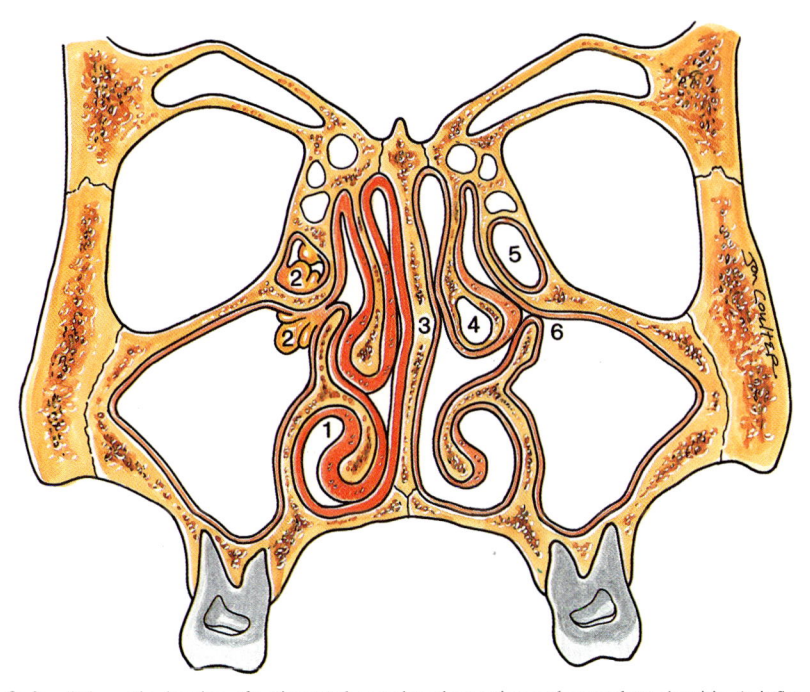

Figure 8–2. Schematic drawing of ostiomeatal complex obstruction and secondary sinusitis. 1: inflammatory (obstructive) changes; 2: polyps (maxillary and ethmoid sinuses); 3: septal deviation; 4: paradoxical middle turbinate and concha bullosa; 5: large bulla ethmoidalis; 6: ostiomeatal complex stenosis.

The most common cause of acute sinusitis in children is obstruction of the sinus ostia by an inflammatory reaction, usually due to an upper respiratory infection or allergic disease, or both (Table 8–1).[1] The inflammatory reaction leads to thickening and engorgement of the sinonasal mucosa that causes ostial obstruction, production of an inflammatory exudate, pooling of secretions, and secondary bacterial infection. Gas exchange is also impaired, leading to hypoxia and promoting the growth of certain bacterial species (anaerobes). In addition to obstructing the ostia, these conditions can result in abnormal mucociliary flow.

By causing mechanical obstruction of mucociliary flow in the OMC, other factors can also cause or contribute to sinusitis in children (Fig. 8–2): polyps; septal deviation; a paradoxical middle turbinate (marked lateral convexity) or concha bullosa (massive enlargement of the middle turbinate, a condition that is more than twice as common in patients with sinusitis versus those without[10]); a large bulla ethmoidalis that narrows the hiatus semilunaris; and OMC stenosis due to marked rotation of the uncinate process. Additional causes of sinusitis due to mechanical obstruction are listed in Table 8–1.

Mucociliary Dysfunction

The mucociliary system is the local sinonasal defense mechanism. When normal levels and activity of lysozymes, secretory immunoglobulin A, and other surface enzymes are present in mucus and when cilia of the sinus mucosa have normal motility, secretions are moved distally by the beating action of the cilia. However, any change in the quality or quantity of mucus or an alteration in ciliary function, number, morphology, or motility may lead to mucociliary dysfunction or ostial obstruction and thus sinusitis.

Change or Abnormality in Mucus

Overproduction of mucus or viscid mucus may hinder ciliary action; viscid mucus may even become inspissated. Because their mucoid secretions are characteristically abnormal, children with cystic fibrosis are very susceptible to sinus infections.

Mucocillary Dysfunction

The cytotoxic effects of a viral infection can lead to temporary mucociliary dysfunction, as can cold air or some medications. Ciliary dysfunction may also occur secondary to inborn errors such as immotile cilia syndrome.

MEDICAL MANAGEMENT OF SINUSITIS IN CHILDREN

The main objectives of treating sinusitis are: (1) reestablishment of normal sinus physiology, (2) rapid sterilization of secretions, and (3) prevention of chronic sinusitis or complications. The initial approach to treating sinusitis in a patient of any age should always be medical. Only after optimal medical therapy has failed should surgery be considered.

Medical therapy for children with acute sinusitis usually includes antibiotics, decongestants, agents to liquify secretions, and humidification of inspired air (Table 8–2); less often children may be given antihistamines, cromolyn sodium, and local steroids (Table 8–2). Such therapy is curative in more than 80% of children with acute sinusitis.[11,12]

Antibiotic Medications

Antibiotic medications are the cornerstone of any medical regimen to treat sinusitis. The antibiotic should be selected on the basis of its effectiveness against the probable offending organism, which for acute sinusitis in children is most often *Streptococcus pneumoniae*, nontypable *Haemophilus influenzae*, or *Moraxella (Branhamella) catarrhalis*.[13] Anaerobes are likely to be prevalent in cases of chronic sinusitis, which should be taken into consideration in the selection of antibiotic therapy for this condition.[14,15]

A wide variety of antimicrobials available currently are effective in treating sinusitis. In two independent studies, Wald et al[16,17] showed amoxicillin to be as effective as cefaclor and amoxicillin/clavulanate potassium for treatment of acute sinusitis. Thus, the primary antibiotic treatment for children with uncomplicated acute sinusitis and no known allergy to penicillin is ampicillin (100 mg/kg/day) or amoxicillin (40 mg/kg/day) for a minimum of 14 days. Alternatives for initial therapy in patients who are allergic to penicillin include erythromycin (50 mg/kg/day), erythromycin-sulfisoxazole (Pediazole), and trimethoprim-sulfamethoxazole, although the last may be ineffective against group A streptococci.

Failure of an initial treatment, which occurs in approximately 20% of pediatric cases, may be due to the presence of beta-lactamase-positive (amoxicillin-resistant) strains of bacteria.[13,14] Such organisms are becoming increasingly prevalent. When initial antibiotic therapy has failed, we prescribe amoxicillin (40 mg/kg/day) with clavulanate potassium, cefaclor (40 mg/kg/day), cefixime (8 mg/kg/day), or cefuroxime axetil (125 mg twice daily). These medications should be given for 21 to 30 days to avoid changes leading to chronic sinusitis. A recent study by Sydnor et al[18] evaluated cefuroxime axetil and cefaclor for the treatment of acute maxillary sinusitis in adults and found cefuroxime axetil to be superior in this situation.

Other Medical Modalities

Antihistamines, decongestants, steroids, cromolyn sodium, systemically administered medications to liquify secretions, and humidification of inspired air may be used in conjunction with antibiotics to treat sinusitis in children. Although these modalities can help decrease edema and improve mucociliary clearance, their role in treating sinus disease has not been well established. Topical nasal decongestants should be used in children for 3 to 5 days only, and these agents can inhibit ciliary action. By drying secretions, antihistamines may make drainage more difficult. Despite these effects, topical decongestants and antihistamines can be beneficial in children with allergies.[19]

To prevent or manage sinusitis in children with allergies, the allergic disease must be controlled by altering the environment, pharmacotherapy, and immunotherapy when

Table 8–2 Medical Treatment Protocol for Sinusitis in Children

MEDICAL TREATMENT	INITIAL REGIMEN	DURATION	SECONDARY REGIMEN	DURATION
Antibiotics	Ampicillin, amoxicillin *Erythromycin, trimethoprim-sulfamethoxazole	14 days	Amoxicillin-clavulanate Cefaclor Cefuroxime axetil Cefixime	21–30 days
Decongestants	Pediatric nasal spray/drops	3–5 days	Pediatric nasal spray/drops Systemic	3–5 days 21–30 days
Antihistamines	—	—	Occasionally (late treatment)	7–14 days
Liquefying agents	+	14 days	+	21–30 days
Steroids (local spray) (systemic)	— —	— —	+ —	21 days —
Humidification of air	+	7–14 days	+	7–14 days

*Alternative treatment in children allergic to penicillin.

indicated.[20] Pharmacologic treatment for allergies in children includes cromolyn sodium, antihistamines (with or without decongestants), and, in resistant cases, topical steroids.[20]

ENDOSCOPIC SINUS SURGERY IN CHILDREN

When medical treatment has failed to promote adequate drainage of acutely infected sinuses or to prevent chronic or recurrent sinus disease, surgery may be indicated. Procedures used in the past for children whose sinusitis did not respond to medical therapy included antral lavage, creation of a nasoantral window, tonsillectomy, adenoidectomy, limited septoplasty, and partial turbinectomy. Indications for these procedures and their effectiveness are not well established, however, and currently the primary surgical treatment for chronic or recurrent sinusitis in children, as in adults, is ESS.

Preoperative Evaluation

Before ESS is undertaken, the extent of OMC disease must be documented reliably. In general, children will not tolerate office nasal endoscopy, and thus imaging studies are essential to diagnose OMC disease and plan surgical treatment.

Plain roentgenography of the paranasal sinuses in children may show some abnormalities (Fig. 8–3A), but computed tomography (CT) in the coronal plane is the most sensitive imaging modality and often the only way in which OMC disease and sinusitis can be diagnosed accurately (Figs. 8–3B and 8–4). For example, plain roentgenographs may demonstrate abnormalities in healthy children,[21] and in one study of 70 healthy children plain films either over- or underestimated the degree of sinus disease compared with CT.[11]

CT is not a perfect diagnostic tool, however. In reviewing CT findings in 300 patients who underwent ESS, we found that in almost 20% the extent of disease discovered at surgery was greater than had been indicated by preoperative CT, and 7% of children with normal preoperative CT scans were found to have significant sinus disease at the time of surgery.[19]

Endoscopic Sinus Surgery Technique in Children

The surgeon who is accustomed to performing ESS in adults and who undertakes this operation in children needs to remember that paranasal sinus structures are smaller in children, the depth of field is less, and relationships of structures to one another are different than in adults. Planning surgery carefully and handling tissues very gently will markedly reduce the amount of trauma caused by the procedure and will therefore decrease postoperative edema and possibly the formation of adhesions or granulation tissue so that morbidity is lower and the outcome of surgery is better.

The coronal CT scans obtained preoperatively should be displayed in the operating room for reference during ESS.

Children are given general anesthesia for ESS. The selection of anesthetic gas should be made in consultation with a pediatric anesthesiologist; in particular, the type of gas used may affect the concentration of epinephrine used for vasoconstriction.

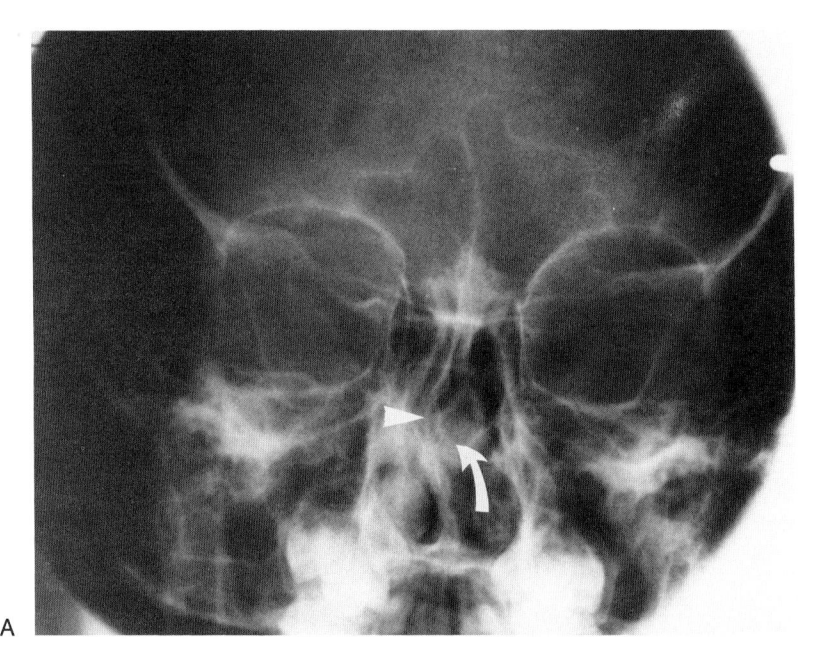

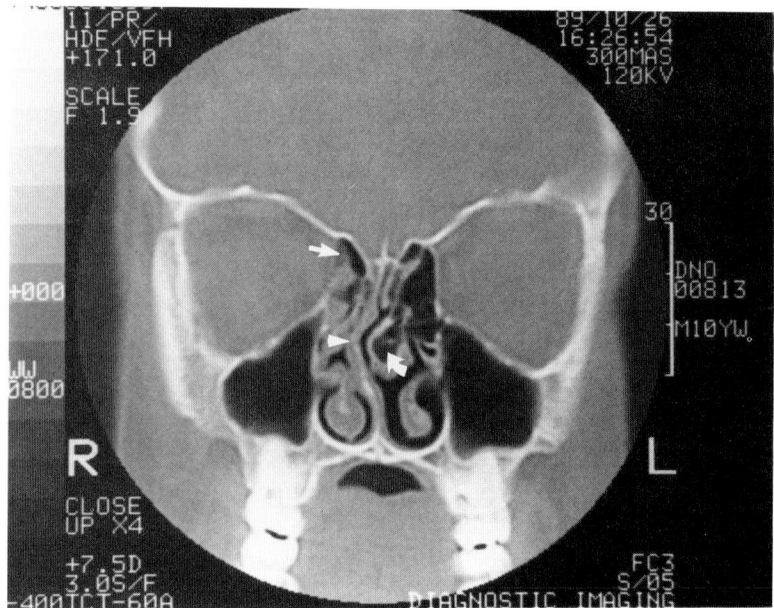

Figure 8–3. **A**: Plain x-ray of sinuses (Caldwell view) showing right septal deviation (arrowhead) and left concha bullosa (curved arrow) but no apparent sinus disease. **B**: Coronal CT of sinuses in same patient shows right ethmoid mucosal thickening (arrow), right septal deviation (arrowhead), and left concha bullosa (curved arrow).

Endoscopic Sinus Surgery in Children 253

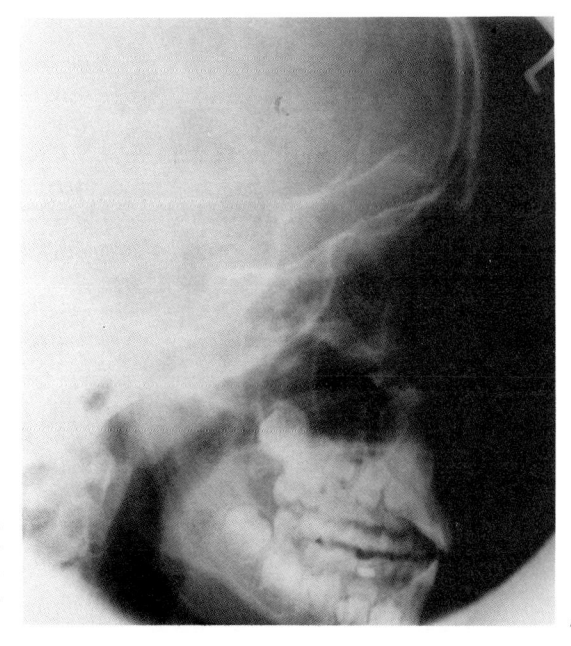

Figure 8–4. **A**: Plain x-ray of sinuses (lateral view) showing no apparent sphenoid disease. **B**: Coronal CT of sinuses of same patient shows a large right sphenoid mucous retention cyst (arrow).

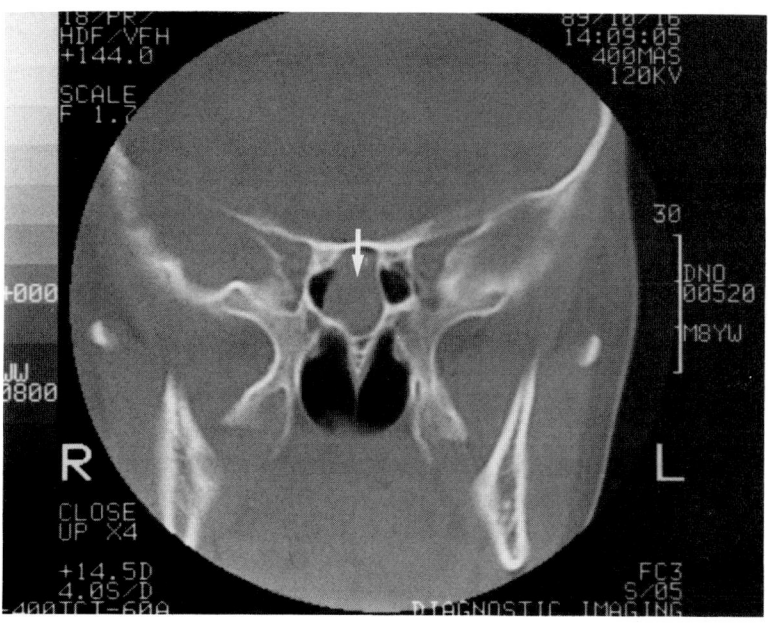

Vasoconstriction

On call to the operating room, the child's nose is sprayed with a topical decongestant such as phenylephrine or oxymetazoline.

After administration of the anesthesia a dental carpule syringe with a 27 gauge, 1.5 inch needle is used to inject the surgical site with 1 or 2% lidocaine with 1/50,000 epinephrine.

Next, the child's nose is packed with cotton pledgets dampened in phenylephrine or oxymetazoline. As in adults, pledgets should be left in the nose for a minimum of 10 minutes for maximal decongestion and hemostasis.

Procedure

Our procedure for ESS, based on the Messerklinger approach as described by Kennedy et al[22,23] and Stammberger[24], is essentially the same in children as in adults. The goal of surgery is to reestablish normal mucociliary clearance of the sinuses by opening the narrowed OMC, removing ethmoid sinus disease, and opening, when indicated, the natural ostia of the frontal, maxillary, and sphenoid sinuses. For visualization during ESS, we use the 0°, 4 mm rigid nasal endoscope in almost all children, even those as young as 14 months. In rare cases when this endoscope is too large, we use the 0°, 2.7 mm endoscope.

Surgery begins with an assessment of the septum, size of the middle turbinate, posterior nasal airway, and adenoids (if present). Infundibulotomy is then performed with a sickle knife under visualization through the 0°, 4 mm endoscope. After the uncinate process and bulla ethmoidalis have been removed, the anterior ethmoid air cells are opened and evacuated. Next the basal lamella is opened, and if any disease is present in posterior ethmoid cells, this is exenterated. We usually do not open the sphenoid sinus, unless there is evidence on CT scans of disease in this cavity.

The nasofrontal recess is inspected using a 30°, 4 mm endoscope. Any diseased mucous membrane is removed using upbiting instruments.

The natural ostium of the maxillary sinus is identified and enlarged by three to five times using Gruenwald forceps and backbiting instruments. The maxillary sinus is lavaged with saline; in rare cases the 70° endoscope may be needed for this step.

When a deviated septum, large middle turbinate, or concha bullosa obstructs the surgical field, a limited septoplasty or partial middle turbinectomy may be performed to improve exposure and facilitate aeration of the sinuses. In most cases, however, care is taken to minimize trauma to the middle turbinate and the septum to discourage the formation of adhesions or synechiae.

At the end of the procedure an antibiotic-steroid ointment* is used on the surgical site, but packing is generally not needed. The procedure can usually be completed in 30 to 60 minutes, with blood losses between 10 and 50 ml, and children are most often discharged the same day.

---

*Editors' note: Using ointment containing petrolatum in the surgical site is not endorsed by the editors because petrolatum-containing ointment placed in the surgical site has caused myospherulosis (see Chapters 5 and 7).

Postoperative and Follow-up Care

The success of ESS rests as much on postoperative management and follow-up care as on adequate removal of disease at surgery. Postoperatively, patients are prescribed a steroid spray, nasal decongestant, saline by nasal mist, and a broad-spectrum antibiotic for 6 weeks. During the fifth and sixth weeks, the child is weaned from the steroid spray and other medications.

Children are seen weekly for the first several weeks after ESS and then at longer intervals as healing progresses. Nasal endoscopy, for which the child must be under general anesthesia, is an essential component of postoperative care and is performed 2 to 3 weeks after the initial surgery. Following removal of any clots, crusts, granulation tissue, or adhesions, the maxillary sinus is examined and, as during the initial procedure, lavaged with saline solution. After this examination, as after ESS, an antibiotic-steroid ointment is applied.

Very rarely, a child needs to undergo a third endoscopic evaluation and treatment.

Results of Endoscopic Sinus Surgery in Children

We evaluated the results of ESS performed between January 1986 and June 1989 on 210 children aged 14 months to 16 years.[21] Approximately 50% of the children had been treated for allergies, 22% had asthma, 44% had undergone tonsillectomy and adenoidectomy, 28% had had tympanostomy tubes inserted at one time, and 30% had undergone sinus surgery previously.

Almost 80% of these children with other conditions were improved after the procedure performed during the study period, including 66% of children who had undergone sinus surgery previously[25] and 80% of the 8% of patients who had previously undergone ESS.[26] More than 80% of children with asthma said that their asthma was markedly improved after the operative procedure.[25]

None of the children in this series had a serious complication of ESS (blindness, extraocular muscle injury, cerebrospinal fluid leak, meningitis, or severe bleeding).

The most often-noted problems on follow-up endoscopy in this group of children were adhesions and formation of granulation tissue. No significant recurrence of polyps or delayed healing was noted. Some children had minimal return of preoperative symptoms in the early postoperative period, probably due to edema and unhealed tissues. These symptoms usually resolve during the 6 weeks' postoperative follow-up period, although treatment for allergy due to inhalants should continue until the allergy is under control.[25]

Children whose sinusitis does not resolve with ESS should undergo evaluations for systemic disorders such as cystic fibrosis, immotile cilia syndrome, Kartagener's syndrome, and immunodeficiency. An allergy evaluation should be performed by a pediatric otolaryngologist/allergist, possibly in consultation with a pediatric pulmonologist.

SUMMARY

Diagnosis and treatment of sinusitis in a child is best managed by a team approach, including a pediatrician or family practitioner, allergist, pulmonologist, immunologist, and infectious disease specialist in addition to the pediatric otolaryngologist. When appropriate medical therapy has failed to resolve chronic or recurrent sinusitis in children, ESS has proved a safe and cost-effective alternative. This procedure in children is similar to that for adults except for some differences in the paranasal sinus anatomy. Serious complications of ESS in children are rare, and the success rate of ESS may be as high as 80%, even in children with asthma or other complicating factors.

REFERENCES

1. Wald ER: Diagnosis and management of acute sinusitis. Pediatr Ann 17:629–638, 1988.
2. Gross CW, Gurucharri MJ, Lazar RH, Long TE: Functional endonasal sinus surgery in the pediatric age group. Laryngoscope 92:272–275, 1989.
3. Rice DH, Schaefer SD: Anatomy of the Paranasal Sinuses: Endoscopic Paranasal Sinus Surgery. New York: Raven Press, 1988, pp 3–35.
4. Kasper KA: Nasofrontal connections. A study based on one hundred consecutive dissections. Arch Otolaryngol 23:322–343, 1936.
5. Graney DO: Anatomy: Otolaryngology Head and Neck Surgery. St. Louis: CV Mosby, 1986, pp 845–852.
6. Van Alyea OE: Nasal Sinuses: An Anatomic and Clinical Consideration, ed. 2. Baltimore: Williams & Wilkins, 1951.
7. Schaefer JP: The sinus maxillaris and its relation in the embryo, child, and adult man. Am J Anat 10:313–367, 1910.
8. Van Alyea OE: The ostium maxillare—anatomic study of its surgical accessibility. Arch Otolaryngol 24:553–569, 1936.
9. Gonzalez C, Kolmer JW: Developmental Anatomy and Physiology of the Nose and Sinuses: Clinical Pediatric Otolaryngology. St. Louis: CV Mosby, 1986, pp 269–279.
10. Kennedy DW, Zinreich SJ: Functional endoscopic surgery. Adv Otolaryngol Head Neck Surg 3:1–26, 1989.
11. Lusk RP, Lazar RH, Muntz HR: The diagnosis and treatment of recurrent and chronic sinusitis in children. Pediatr Clin North Am 36:1411–1421, 1989.
12. Wald ER: Medical management: A pediatrician's perspective. Pediatr Infect Dis 4:565–566, 1985.
13. Wald ER: Diagnosis and management of acute sinusitis. Pediatr Ann 17:629–638, 1988.
14. Wald ER: Epidemiology, pathophysiology, and etiology of sinusitis. Pediatr Infect Dis 4(Suppl 6):551–554, 1985.
15. Brook I: Bacteriologic features of chronic sinusitis in children. JAMA 246:967–969, 1981.
16. Wald ER, Reilly JS, Casselbrant M, et al: Treatment of acute maxillary sinusitis in childhood: A comparative study of amoxicillin and cefaclor. J Pediatr 104:297–307, 1984.
17. Wald ER, Chiponis D, Ledemsa-Medina J: Comparative effectiveness of amoxicillin and amoxicillin clavulanate potassium in acute paranasal sinus infections in children: A double-blinded, placebo controlled trial. Pediatrics 77:795–800, 1986.
18. Sydnor A Jr, Gwaltney JM, Cocchetto DM, Scheld MW: Comparative evaluation of cefuroxime axetil and cefaclor for treatment of acute bacterial maxillary sinusitis. Arch Otolaryngol Head Neck Surg 115:1430–1433, 1989.
19. Lazar RH, Younis RT, Gross CW, Gurucharri MJ: Functional endonasal sinus surgery in pediatrics: A review of 210 patients. Head Neck 14:92–98, 1992.
20. Rachelelfsky GS, Katz RM, Siegel SC: Chronic sinusitis in the allergic child. Pediatr Clin North Am 35:1091–1101, 1988.
21. Caffey J: Pediatric X-ray Diagnosis: A Textbook for Students and Practitioners of Pediatrics, Surgery, and Radiology. Chicago: Yearbook, 1978.
22. Kennedy EW, Zinreich SJ, Rosenbaum AE, et al: Functional endoscopic sinus surgery: Theory and diagnostic evaluation. Arch Otolaryngol 111:576–582, 1985.
23. Kennedy DW: Functional endoscopic sinus surgery, technique. Arch Otolaryngol 111:643–649, 1985.
24. Stammberger H: Endoscopic endonasal surgery—new concepts and treatment of recurring rhinosinusitis. I. Anatomic and pathophysiologic considerations. II. Surgical technique. Otolaryngol Head Neck Surg 94:143–156, 1986.
25. Lazar RH, Younis RT, Parvey LS: Comparison of plain radiographs, coronal CT, and intraoperative findings in children with chronic sinusitis. Otolaryngol Head Neck Surg 107(1):29–34, 1992.
26. Lazar RH, Younis RT, Long TE, Gross CW: Revision functional endonasal sinus surgery. Ear Nose Throat J 71(3):131–133, 1992.

Appendix

Shadyside Hospital
Sinus Surgery Center
Mark May, M.D., Director

ENDOSCOPIC SINUS SURGERY PROTOCOL

Date:　　　　　　Name:　　　　　　　　　　　　Age/Sex:

Chief Complaint:

Hx Present Illness (brief):

Medication Allergies:

Present Medications:　Steroids　　　Aspirin　　　　NSAIDS

Past Medical History:　Hypertension　　　　　Smoker (pk/yr)

　　　　　　　　　　　Stroke　　　　　　　　Myocardial Infarction

　　　　　　　　　　　Diabetes　　　　　　　Obesity

　　　　　　　　　　　Asthma　　　　　　　　Bleeding Disorder

Surgical (Nonsinus) History:

Sinus Condition History

Medication History (courses/yr):   Antibiotics   Antihistamines

                                                        Decongestants   Nasal Spray

                                                        Allergy Shots   Steroids

Inhalant or Food Allergies (list):

Family History of Allergy:

Surgical History (Nasal or Sinus) (procedures/dates):

Caldwell-Luc

ESS

Nasoantral Window

Other _____

Intranasal Ethmoidectomy

Poor Prognosis (circle if +):
  I. Reactive Airway Disease
  II. Samter's Syndrome (aspirin sensitivity, nasal polyps, asthma)
  III. Recurrent Polyposis
  IV. Cystic Fibrosis
  V. Kartagener's Syndrome
  VI. Previous Nasosinus Surgery
  VII. Fungus

Symptom History

Mark + next to each symptom if present preoperatively on a chronic or recurrent basis. Rate the most bothersome three symptoms in red. Rate symptoms for each postoperative visit:
W = Worse   I = Improved   S = Same   0 = Gone

	Date	Date	Date	Date	Date	Date	Date	Date	Date
Nasal Stuffiness									
Nasal Airway Obstruction									
Postnasal Drainage									
Runny Nose									
Bloody Nose									
Puffy Eyes									
Eye Pressure/Pain									
Ear Pressure/Popping									
Headaches									
Facial Pressure									
Hoarseness									
Sore Throat									
Bad Breath									
Aching Teeth									
Taste/Smell Changes									
General Fatigue									
Dizziness/Lightheadedness									
Chronic Cough									
Itchy Nose									
Watery Eyes									
Red Eyes									
Scratchy Throat									
Frequent Throat Clearing									
Sneezing									
Other									

Nasal Endoscopic Findings

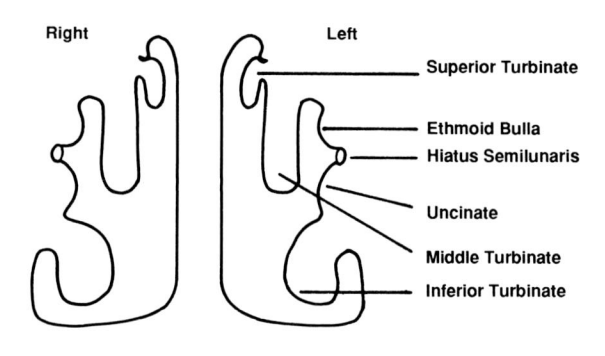

```
        Right        Left
                          ——— Superior Turbinate
                          ——— Ethmoid Bulla
                          ——— Hiatus Semilunaris
                          ——— Uncinate
                          ——— Middle Turbinate
                          ——— Inferior Turbinate
```

                                    Right   Left

Turbinoseptal (TS) Classification

Mucosa:

Septum:

Turbinates (Middle):

        (Inferior):

Uncinate Process:

Bulla Ethmoidalis:

Polyps:

Infection:

Other Findings on Head/Neck Exam:

Computed Tomographic Scan Findings

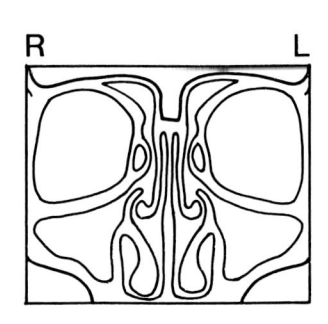

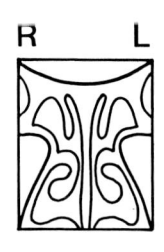

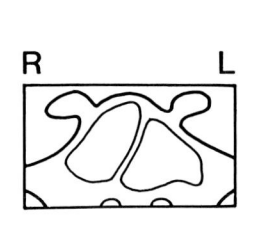

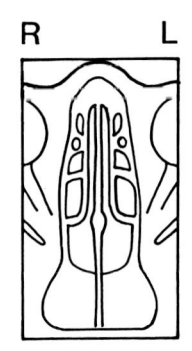

Classification of CT Findings—right, left, or both sides
- 0 = Normal—No Findings
- 1+ = Minimal—Disease limited to OMC
- 2+ = Moderate—Incomplete opacification of one or more major sinuses (frontal, maxillary, sphenoid)
- 3+ = Maximal—Complete opacification of one or more major sinuses, but not all
- 4+ = Most severe—Total opacification of all sinuses

Subclassification—CT plus endoscopy
- Anatomic Abnormality—Turbinoseptal or other deformities compromising OMC
- Hyperplasia—Thickened mucous membrane lining noted on CT scan
- Polyposis
- Suppurative Disease

Informed Consent

Reviewed:
- History and Indications
- Surgical Procedure
- Postoperative Course and Hospital Stay
- Necessity for Follow-up Visits
- Success Rate
- Alternative Measures

Reviewed possible intraoperative or postoperative complications:
- Bleeding
- Infection
- Dental, lip, or cheek sensory changes
- Possible need for additional surgery
- Visual loss or change
- CSF leak

**Are your symptoms troublesome enough to consider surgery?

Surgical Procedure Performed:

Right		Left
Septoplasty		
Turbinectomy	Bilateral	Turbinectomy
Anterior OMC	Bilateral	Anterior OMC
Maxillary Antrum Enlarged	Bilateral	Maxillary Antrum Enlarged
Maxillary Antrum Probed	Bilateral	Maxillary Antrum Probed
Agger Nasi	Bilateral	Agger Nasi
Ethmoidectomy (post. complete)	Bilateral	Ethmoidectomy
Sphenoidectomy	Bilateral	Sphenoidectomy
Maxillary Sinoscopy	Bilateral	Maxillary Endoscopy
Mini-Caldwell-Luc	Bilateral	Mini-Caldwell-Luc
Frontal Sinus Cannulation	Bilateral	Frontal Sinus Cannulation
Frontal Sinus Ostioplasty I, II, III		Frontal Sinus Ostioplasty I, II, III

DATE OF SURGERY: _____

Anesthesia: Local   General

Findings at Surgery

    Fungus
    Tumor
    Mucocele
    Antral Choanal Polyp

Operative Complications:

Minor	**Major**
Orbital Emphysema	Orbital Hematoma (treatment: _____)
Orbital Ecchymosis	Loss of Vision, including blindness
Dental/Lip Numbness	Diplopia (treatment: _____)
Asthma	Epiphora (treatment: _____)
Adhesions	Carotid Artery Violation (outcome: _____)
Epistaxis	Transfusion Needed (units _____)
Infection	CSF Leak (repaired? _____)
Permanent Pain/Numbness	Meningitis
Loss of Smell	Brain Abscess
	CNS Deficit (type: _____)
	Death (cause: _____)

Postoperative Results:

Time	Grade I	IIA	IIB	III	IVA	IVB	V	VI
6 months								
1 year								
2 years								
3 years								
4 years								
5 years								
6 years								
7 years								
8 years								
9 years								
10 years								

Revision Surgery

Time:
Due to: Ostium Stenosis   Adhesions
        Failure to Open Ostium   Failure to Open Sphenoid
        Failure to Open Ethmoid   Failure to Open Agger Nasi/Frontal Sinus
Procedure:
    Septoplasty   OMC   TE
    TES   Middle Turbinate Removed   Ostium Enlarged

Revision Surgery Operative Complications:

Minor	**Major**
Orbital Emphysema	Orbital Hematoma (treatment: _____)
Orbital Ecchymosis	Loss of Vision, including blindness
Dental/Lip Numbness	Diplopia (treatment: _____)
Asthma	Epiphora (treatment: _____)
Adhesions	Carotid Artery Violation (outcome: _____)
Epistaxis	Transfusion Needed (units _____)
Infection	CSF Leak (repaired? _____)
Permanent Pain/Numbness	Meningitis
Loss of Smell	Brain Abscess
	CNS deficit (type: _____)
	Death (cause: _____)

Reason for Revision Surgery Failure:
    Ostium Stenosis   Adhesions
    Failure to Open Ostium   Failure to Open Sphenoid Sinus
    Failure to Open Ethmoid Sinus   Failure to Open Agger Nasi/Frontal Sinus
    Mucosal Disease   Error in Diagnosis
        No Postoperative Follow-up
    Refused Revision Surgery

Time to Failure (months): _____

Index

(Italic page numbers indicate a figure or table.)

Adenocarcinoma, 38
Adenoid tissue, 69
Adenoidectomy, 255
Adhesions, 144, 150, *194*, 200, 201, 203, 230, 238, 255
   avoiding, 189–190
Agger nasi cells, 2–3, 4, *9*, 12, 13, *14*, 16, *17*, 34, 37, 74, *75*, *137*, 144, 147, *148*, 189
Air-fluid level, in maxillary antrum, *45*
Airway disease, 105, 106, 128, 170
Alfentanil, 94, 98, 99
Alkalol, 173
Allergy, 64, 65, 178, 239, 249, 254
   drug, 90
Amoxicillin, 66, 172, 249
Anatomy
   abnormalities, 72, 85, 185
   computed tomography, 29, *107*
   deformity, 64
   of ethmoid sinus, 32–34
      variants of normal, 34
   frontal sinus relationships, 157, *159*
   of lateral nasal wall, 2–15
   maxillary sinus
      variants of normal, 40
Anesthesia, 107, 165, 170
   bronchospasm and, 93, 98, 100
   care after, 101–102
   in children, 251
   emergence from, 100
   for endoscopic sinus surgery, 91–104
   evaluation, 91
   general, 97–100, 127, 203
      complications of, 100
      inhalation induction, 98
      intravenous induction, 98
   local, 93–97, 128–129
   maintenance of, 98–99
      inhalation agents, 98–99
      muscle relaxants, 98
   monitored care, 93–97, 126–127
      medications for, 94–95
   narcotic, 99–100
      advantages of, 100
      initiating, 99
      maintaining, 99–100
      side effects of, 100
   patient oxygenation during, 94
   surgeon's choice of, 126–129

Anosmia, *194*, 204, 238
Antacid, 93
Antibiotics, 66, 107, 172, 202, 249
Anticholinergic medications, 92
Antiemetics, 94–95
Antihistamines, 63, 172, 249
Antrocasal canal, *135*
Anxiety, 92, 93
Anxiolytic medications, 92
Appendix, 257–264
Artery
   cardiac, 229
   carotid, 15, 20, *21*, 45, *48*, 142, *143*, 194, 229
   ethmoid, 12, 16, *17*, *19*, *20*, *23*, 24–25, 26, *27*, 134, 137, *139*, *142*, 169, 202, 210, *219*, *220*
   nasofrotal, *27*
   ophthalmic, 12, *25*
   splenopalatine, *21*, 26, *28*, *143*, 144, 169–170
ASA triad, 62–63, 64, 128, 173, 187–188
Aspergillosis, *43*, 56
Aspiration, from oversedation, 97
Aspiration pneumonitis, 93
Aspirin, 63
   See also Samter's syndrome
Astemizole, 172
Asthma, 63, 92, 93, 98, 100, 128, 178, 187–188, 203–204, 237, 255
   patients with, 101
   See also Samter's syndrome
Atelectasis, 40, 42
Atracurium, 98
Azithromycin, 172

Basal lamella (third lamella), 4–6, *9*, 18, 20, *27*, 32, *33*, *41*, 134, 137, *138*, 202, 242
Beclomethasone, 173
Beta blockers, 63
Blade, tongue, *116*
Bleeding, 203
   of cardiac artery, 229
   drugs and, 63
   instruments to control, *115*
   postoperative, 229
   prevention and management of, 169–170
   prolonged, 106, 170
   tests for, 63
   See also Hemorrhage
Blindness, 24, 25, 26, 47, 90, *194*, 210
Brain, 142, *228*

265

complications in, 46, 140, 194, 223
Bronchospasm, 93, 98, 100, *194*
  from anesthesia with sedation, 97
Bulla ethmoidalis (second lamella), 3, 4, *5*, 6, *8*, 9, *10*, 12, *14*, 16, 18, *20*, 24, 32, *33*, 51, 72, 81, *83*, *84*, 85, 126, 130, 134, *135*, *136*, 137, 142, 241, 247

Calcifications, 42
Caldwell-Luc procedure, *39*, 42, *122*, 127, 164, 165, 167, *252*
Camera, 69, *70*, *71*, 72
Cancer
  See Carcinoma, Malignancies, Tumors
Canine fossa, 165, 204
  puncture technique, 165
Cannulas, *112*, *113*, 114, 134, *136*, 144, 150, *152*, 154, 157, *166*
Cantholysis, 202, 210, 221–222
Canthotomy, 202, 210, 221–222
Carcinoma
  of maxillary sinus, 46
  squamous cell, 38, *57*
Cardiovascular disease, 170
Carotid artery, 15, 20, *21*, 45, *48*, 142, *143*, *194*, 228
Carotid canal, *47*, *48*
Catecholamines, 96, 99
Catheters, *114*, 150, *157*
  balloon, 120, *124–125*, 170
  Hudson, *115*
Cautery, 170
Cavernous sinus, 24, 25
Cerebrospinal fluid leak, 16, 18, *19*, 20, 22, 24, *36*, 46, 81, 90, 129, 141, 142, *194*, 202, 223, 224, *225–227*
Children, 127, 181
  anesthesia in, 251
  endoscopic sinus surgery in, 244–256
  pathophysiology of sinusitis, 246–248
  surgery in, 244–256
Choana, 142, 169–170
  obstruction of, 126
Chordoma, of clivus, *48*
Clarithromycin, 172
Cleft palate, *38*
Clinoid process, 15, 44, *47*
Coagulator, suction, *115*
Cocaine, 63, 95, 128
  absorption of, 96
  and catecholamines, 96
  dose of, 96
  toxicity of, 96
Compartments, anterior and posterior, *5*
Complications, 193–242
  additional surgery, 90
  adhesions, 144, 150, *194*, 203, 238
  anosmia, *194*, 204, 238
  blindness, 24, 25, 26, 47, 90, *194*, 210
  brain, 46, 142, *194*
  bronchospasm, *194*
  carotid artery, 142, *194*, 229
  central nervous system deficit, *194*

cerebrospinal fluid leak, 16, 18, *19*, 20, 22, 24, *36*, 46, 81, 90, 129, 141, 142, *194*, 202, 223, 224, *225–227*
death, *194*
dental pain, *194*, 204, 238
diplopia, 24, 47, *194*
ecchymosis, *194*
emphysema, *194*
of endoscopic sinus surgery, 193–244
  reporting system, 193–195
    classification, 193–194
    incidence, 194–195
  reported, 195–201
    categorization, 199–200
      adhesions, 200
      bleeding, 200
      orbital hematoma, 203
    differences in enumeration, 195–198
      full disclosure, 195
      incidence, 195, *196–197*
      patients versus complications, 198
      versus traditional, *196–197*, *199*
      types reported, 195, 198
    for nonendoscopic surgery, 198
    position of surgeon during operation, 200
    surgeon's learning curve, 198–199
    versus traditional, 200–201
      adhesions, 201
      orbital, 200–201
      vascular, 201
    type of procedure, 199
epiphora, *194*
of general anesthesia, 100
hematoma
  orbital, *194*
  retrobulbar, 25
hemorrhage, 20, 25, 26, 45, 47, *48*, 90, *194*, 203
incidences of Levine and May, 201–204
  adhesions, 203
  anosmia, *194*, 204
  asthma, 203–204
  bleeding, 203
  dental or lip pain, 204
  dural, 202–203
  numbness, 204
  orbital, 203, 204
  technique differences, 201
infection, 90, *194*, 238
intracranial, 193
lacrimal, 193
meningitis, *194*
during monitored anesthesia care, 96–97
mortality, 20
of narcotic anesthesia, 100
numbness, *194*, 204, 238
optic nerve, 142
orbital, 7, 22, 24, 25, 26, 47, 193
prevention of, 142, 144, 204–223, 239–240
sensory changes, 90
vascular, 193
Computed tomography, *79*, 82, 85–87, 141, 142, 178, 179, *209*, *223*, *228*, 251, *252*, *253*, 261

Index

abnormal findings, *89*
anatomy on scans, *107*
axial plane, 85
of concha bullosa, 80
frontal sinus, 30, *31*, *158–164*
nasolacrimal duct, 31, *32*
objectives of, 29
of paranasal sinuses, 29–48
preoperative, 105, 184
screening, 49–51
  advantages of, 51
  technique for, 49
for suppurative sinusitis, 66, 74, *122–123*
technical aspects, 20
Concha bullosa, *23*, 24, 34, 35, 36, 78–81, *252*
ossified, *80*
Confusion, from anesthesia with sedation, 96
Congenital deformity, 34
Contrast agent, 56, 58
Cough, 64, 190
Cranial fossa, anterior, *13*, 16, *21*, *22*, 144
Cranial nerve
  II, *21*
  III, 24
  IV, 24
  V, 15
  VI, 24
Cribriform plate, 12, *13*, *14*, *17*, 18, *23*, 24, 32, *33*, *36*, *41*, 81, *82*, 129, *147*
Crista galli, 12, *18*, *24*, *41*
Cromolyn sodium, 249
Culture, aspirate for, 65
Cyst, retention, *34*, 42, *43*, *44*

Dacryocystorhinostomy, 230, *235*
Decongestants, 63, 66, 72, 107, 169, 172, 249, 254
Dental pain, 64, 204, 238
Diabetes, 170
Diagnosis, differential, 42, 52
Diclofenac, *63*
Diflunisal, *63*
Diplopia, 210, 223
Disease
  persistant, 189
  treatment-resistant, 189
Draf procedures, 157, *158–159*, *163–164*
Drainage
  frontal sinus, 11, 12
  nasolacrimal, 3–4
  sinus, 3–4, 6
Dressings, *116–117*, 203, 239
  postoperative, 170, 229
Drills, 157, *161*, *163*, *235*
Droperidol, 95
Drugs
  allergies, 91
  See also individual drugs, Medications
Dysplasia, fibrous, 30, 31

Ear pressure, 85
Ecchymosis, *194*, 203, 204, *205–206*, 208, *212–213*
Edema, 203, *209*

Emphysema, *194*, 203, 204, *206*, *207*, 208
Endonasal surgery, 67, 78, 165
Endoscopes, 69–71, 120
Endoscopic examination, 66–67, 69–85, *86*, 120–126, *127*, *152*, *156*, *160*, *164*
  equipment, 69–71
  middle turbinates and septum, 72–78
  technique, 71–72
Endoscopic sinus surgery, 60–90, 91–104, 105–175, 222
  in children, 244–256
    preoperative evaluation, 251
    results of surgery, 255
    technique of, 251
  choice of anesthesia, 127–128
  complications, 193–242
  functional, 105
  equipment for video, *111*
  results of surgery, 176–192
  revision, 188–190
    reasons for, 188–190
    treatment-resistant disease, 190
Endoscopic sinus surgery protocol, 61, 64, 85
Enflurane, 98
Epinephrine, 95, 99, *127*, 128, 169, *235*
  risk of, 95
Epiphora, 229
Ethmoid, 208, 210
  air cells, *19*, *38*, 137
  anterior, 4, *14*
  artery, 12, 16, *17*, *19*, *20*, *23*, 24–25, 26, 27, *134*, *137*, *139*, *142*, 169, 202, 210, *219*, *220*
  bleeding, 25
  box, 9, 15–21, *205*
  bulla, *See* Bulla ethmoidalis
  cells, *9*, *14*, *20*, *23*, 24, *25*, 26, 27, 28, 126
  foramen, anterior, 12
  infundibulum, 6, 11
  nerve, *26*, 128
Ethmoid sinus, 10, *38*, *40*, 239
  in children, 244
  computed tomography of, 32–38
  roof of, 3, 12, *14*, 15, 16, *17*, *19*, 20, *23*, 24, *26*, 32, *36*, 46, *87*, *106*, 137–141, 202, *219*, *228*
  surgical exposure of, 137
Exophthalmos, *216*

Facial pressure, *62*
Fentanyl, 92, 94, 98
Fluorescein, 154
Fluoroscopy, 144, 154, 157, *160*, 202
Fontanelle, 6, 8, 9, *43*, *135*, 165, 190, 237
Forceps, *112*, *113*, *114*, *119*, 129, 130, 133, 134, *137*, 141, *142*, 144, *145*, *146*, *148*, 157, *162*, *163*, 165, 169, 230, *231*, *236*
Frontal bone, *23*, *27*, 202
Frontal lobe, *16*
Frontal sinus, 10–13, *14*, *17*, 26, 27, 76, 87, *114*, *149*, *152*, *153*, 241
  in children, 246
  computed tomography of, 30, 31, *158–164*
  drainage, *155–156*

floor of, 13
osteoplasty, 157, *158–164*
polyps and, 190
Frontoethmoid cell, *22, 23*
Functional endoscopic surgery, 105
Fungus, 30, 42, *68*, 144, 164, 165
  aspergillosis, *43*, 56
  disease from, 66, 87

Gadolinium, 56, *58*
Glycopyrrolate, 92
Grafting, 223
Greater wing, of sphenoid, 13, 44
Ground lamella, *See* Basal lamella
Guaifenesin, 172
Gyri recti, 46

Haller cells, 34, 35, 37
Halothane, 98–99
Haemophilus influenzae, 66, 249
Headache, 62, 64, 78, 172, 190
Hematoma, 25, 194, 203
  retrobulbar, 210
Hemorrhage, 20, 25, 26, 45, *48*, 90, *194*, 203, 210, *217*, *220*, 222, 223, *228*
  See also Bleeding, Complications
Hemostasis, 169
Hiatus semilunaris, 3, 4, 5, 51, 72, 81, *130*, *135*
Hyperplastic disease, 180
Hypertension, 106, 107
  from anesthesia with sedation, 97
Hypoplasia, 40

Ibuprofen, *63*
Immunologic status, 182
Index procedure, 178
Indications for surgery, 184
Indomethacin, *63*
Infection, 90, 182, 185, *194*, 238
  chronic, 64 *See also* Fungus
Inferior meatus, 3
Inferior oblique muscle, 25
Inflammation, 35, 52, 53, *55*, 56, 182, 248
Informed consent, 90, 262
Informing patient, 87, 90
Infratermoral fossa, *45, 46*
Infundibulum, 3, 4, 5, *10*, 11, 16, *23*, 24, 27, 32, 34, *35*, 38, *39*, *41*, *137*, *231*
  ethmoid, 6, 11
  frontal, 6
Infusions, continuous, 99
Inhalation
  agents, 98–99
  induction, 98
Injection site, of anesthesia, *127*
Instruments for surgery, *112*, *140*
Internal carotid artery, 2
Internal maxillary os, 5
Intraorbital bleeding, 47
Irrigation
  surgery and, *119*, 165, *167–168*, 173
  of sinus, 66
Isoflurane, 98

Ketamine, 98
Knife, sickle, *112*, 130

Laboratory tests, 92
Lacrimal bone, 3, 34
Lacrimal duct, 22, 130, 230, *231–233*
Lacrimal sac, 3, 134, *137*, 144, *233–234*
Lacrimal fossa, *32*
Lacrimal system, 27
Lamella
  basal, 4, *5*, 9
  first, 3
  second, 3
  third, 4
Lamina papyracea, 3, *5*, 9, 11, *13*, *15*, 16, *20*, *21*, 22, *23*, 24, *27*, 32, *33*, *38*, *40*, *41*, 47, 137, *139*, 141, *149*, 204, 210
Latex, allergy to, 239
Lidocaine, 95, 98, 99, *127*, 128, 235
  toxicity of, 95
Ligament
  of eye, *22*
  of Zinn, *26*
Lymphoma, *45*
Lynch incision, 154, *155*

Magnetic resonance imaging, 52–58, 210, *228*
  limitations of, 56
  signal intensity, 53, 56
Malignancies, 37–38, 43, 46, *57*, 165
Marijuana, 63
Masses, 37
Maxilla
  antrum, *35*, *38*, *41*, 42, *43*, *45*
  orbital plate, 7
Maxillary os, *8*
Maxillary sinoscopy, instruments for, *113*
Maxillary sinus, 8, 22, 25, 28
  anatomy and variants, 40–42
    asymmetry, 40–41
    hypoplastic, 40
  carcinoma of, *46*
  in children, 245–246
  computed tomography of, 38–43
  disease, 164–165
    indications for, 165
  ostium, 7, 9, 16, *17*, 22, 24, *33*, 42, 74, 105, 120, *121*, *123*, *131*, *133*, 134, *135*, 150, 190, 202, 204, 230, 241, 245
    instrument for, 130, *131*, 134, *135*, *136*, 157, *204*, 208
  membranous, *6*
  surgery for, 134
  pathology of, 42–43
  roof of, *8*
  sinusitis, *39*, 42
Maxillary wall, *23*
Measurements
  angles of, 85, *88*, 89, *106*, *141*, 142
  preoperative, 85
Meatus
  antrostomy, *124*
  inferior, *24*

middle, 33, *38*
superior, *5*
Medications, 62–63, 91
  anticholinergic, 92
  anxiolytic, 92
  local, 95–96
  for minimal anesthesia care, 94–95
  postoperative, 172–173
    antibiotics, 172
    antihistamines, 172
    decongestants, 172
    mucolytics, 172
    steroids, 173
  preoperative, 92–93, 107
  during surgery, *110*
  See also Antibiotics, Antihistamines, Decongestants, Steroids
Merocel sponge, 170
Messerklinger procedure, 254
Metoclopramide, 93, 95
Microscope
  binocular, 120
  operating, 120–126, 157
Midfovia, measurement with, *89*
Midazolam, 92, 94
Monitored anesthesia care, 127
  with asthma patients, 93
  complications of, 96–97
  disadvantages, 93
  risk, 93
Moraxella (Branhamella) catarrhalis, 249
Mortality, 20
Mucocele, 30, 36, *40*, 42, 44, 53, 56, *57*
Mucociliary dysfunction, 248
Mucociliary flow, *5*, 7, 9, 13, 64, 105, 120, *121*, *123*, 181, 246, 248, 254
Mucolytics, 172
Mucopus, site of, 65
Mucosa, hyperplastic, 184
Mucus
  change in, 248
  inspissated, 56
Mupirocin, 170
Muscles, *22*, *23*, *214*
  extraocular, 24, *25*
  inferior oblique, *25*
  optic, 24
  rectus, 22, *23*, *24*, *25*, *26*, 223
  relaxants, 98
  superior oblique, 223
Mycosis, 44
Myospherulosis, 170, 239

Naproxen, *63*
Narcotics, 94
  anesthesia, 99–100
    advantages of, 100
    initiating, 99
    maintaining, 99–100
    side effects of, 100
  See also individual drugs
Nasal antrum surgery, *122–123*
Nasal cavity, *76*, *78*, *82*, *83*, *84*

Nasal examination, 68–85, 260
  endoscopy, 69–85
  external inspection, 68
  facial landmarks, 68
  internal examination, 68
  posterior rhinoscopy, 69
Nasal polyps, 62, 64
Nasal septum, *22*, *23*, *25*, 84, *150*, 241
  deviated, 34, *35*, *36*, *38*, 68, *79*, 207, 247, 252
  evaluation of, 72–78
  medial wall, 2
  right, 2
  surgery of, 129
Nasal specula, *110*
Nasal spine, 85, *88*
Nasal wall
  lateral, 1–28, *79*, 81, 85, 137
    anatomy of, 2–15
Nasoantral canal, *5*, *136*
Nasofrontal artery, 27
Nasofrontal "beak," 157, *160–162*
Nasofrontal isthmus, 9, 10, *13*, *14*, 27, 150, *153–154*, 157, *160*, *163–164*
Nasofrontal recess, 4, *5*, 6, 9, 10, 11, 12, 13, *14*, 16, *17*, *26*, *76*, *114*, 134, 144, *147*, 150, *152*, 157, *160*, *163*, 219
Nasolacrimal duct, 3, *4*, 12, *17*, 18, 22, 51, *53*, 134, *147*
  computed tomography of, 31, 32
Nasolacrimal sac, *14*, *17*, *147*
Nasomaxillary channel, 24
Nasopharynx, 72, 85, *125*
Nasosinus disorders, office evaluation of, 60–90
Nausea and vomiting, 170
Needle, *115*
Neoplasms, 43, 52, 56
Nerve hook, 144
Nitrous oxide, 98, 99
Nonsteroidal anti-inflammatory drugs, 63, 107
Nose
  polyposis, 62, 63
  symptoms in, 62
  See also Nasal examination
Numbness, 204, 237

Obstructions, 64, 66, 190, *233*
  middle turbinate, 150
  ostial, 246, 248
Odontogenic cyst, *39*
Office evaluation, of nasosinus disorders, 60–90
Olfactory area, 204
Olfactory groove, *23*, *36*
Olfactory nerve, *24*
Onodi cell, 24, 26, 27, 210, *211*
Opacification, *39*, *40*
  of concha bullosa, *36*
  of ethmoid air cells, *38*
  of middle turbinate, 34
  of sphenoid sinus, 44
Operating microscope technique
  binocular microscope, 120
  See also Microscope

Operating room
　anesthesia preparations in, 93
　on call to, 107
　during operation, 108
　set-up of, *109*
Operation, time of, 170
Ophthalmic artery, 12, *25*
Optic canal, 15
Optic muscles, 24
Optic nerve, 2, 15, 20, 24, 26, *47*, 137, 142, *143*, *212*, *217*
　pathology of, 36, 210
Orbit, *18*, 144, *148*
　decompression of, *221–222*
　fat, 22, *23*, 141, 203, 205, 208, 209
　structures, 22, *26*
Orbital apex, 24, *26*, *28*
Orbital apex syndrome, 24
Orbital cone, 24, *25*
Orbital contents, 47
Orbital penetration, 203, *212–217*
Orbital plate
　of maxilla, 7
Orbital structures, *23*
Orbital tone, *216*
Orbital zones, *205*
Orbital wall, 22
Osteoma, 30
Ostiomeatal complex (OMC), 4–6, 34, 35, *38*, 61, 66, 68, 78, 81, 87, 104, 129, 134, *136*, 150, 182, 184, 189, 246, *247*, 248, 251
　anterior, 4, 16–18
　posterior, 4
Ostioplasty, of frontal sinus
　candidates for, 157
　contraindications for, 157
　indications for, 157
　procedure, *158–164*
　technique, 157
Ostium
　accessory, 7, 9, 72, 120, *121*, *123*
　maxillary, *6*, 7, 74, 105
Outpatient treatment, 91
Oversedation, 96
Oxygenation, 94
Oxymetazoline, 66, 95, 107, 128, 169, 170, 229, 254

Pain, 172
　dental, 64, 204
Palatine bone, 9
Papilloma, inverted, 37, 43, *45*
Paranasal sinus, 22–26
　computed tomography of, 29–48
　developmental anatomy of, 243–245
　magnetic resonance imaging of, 52–56
　pathology of, 35–38
　radiology of, 29–59
　screening computed tomography of, 49–51
　three-dimensional reconstruction of, 51–52
Patient care, postoperative
　in children, 255
　discharge instructions, 173
　　activity, 173
　　nasal irrigations, 173
　medications, 172–173
　　antibiotics, 172
　　antihistamines, 172
　　decongestants, 172
　　mycolytics, 172
　　steroids, 173
　office visits, 173–174
　outpatient versus inpatient, 170–171
　routine orders, 171–172
Patient history, 60–64, 256
　chief complaint, 61
　medications, 62–64
　past illness, 61
　present illness, 62
　symptoms, 64
Patient selection, for surgery, 60–90
Patients
　with asthma, 101
　care after anesthesia, 101–102
　discharge criteria, 102
　discharge instructions, 102
　preoperative care, 107, 108
Penicillin, 172, 249
Petrolatum, 170
Phenylephrine, 95–96, 254
Phenylpropanolamine, 172
Phenytoin, 197
Photocoagulation, laser, 72
Photography, 72
　intranasal, 71
Piroxicam, *63*
Pituitary gland, 2, 15, *21*
Polyps, 35, 42, *55*, 81, *83*, *123*, 150, 173, 178, 188, 247, 255
　antral choanal, *35*
　and frontal sinus, 190
　multiple, *44*, 62, 63, 106, 127, 178, 184, 185, 188, 229
　　See also Samter's syndrome
　recurrence of, 178
Postnasal discharge, 62, *62*, 64, 190
Postoperative care, *See* Patient care
Prednisone, 173
Pressure
　ear, 85
　intraorbital, 202, 210
Preseptal air collection, *209*
Pseudoephedrine, 172
Pterygoid process, 13, 44
Pterygopalatine fissure, *28*
Pulmonary therapy, 107
Punch, antrum, *112*, 130, *133*, 134
Pupils, dilation of, 239

Radiology, 142, 150, 154, 178, 251, *252–253*
　for paranasal sinus, 29–59, 87
　preoperative, 106
　of sinus, 66, 85
　for suppurative sinusitis, 66
Ranitidine, 93
Reactive airway disease, 62

Rectus muscle, 22, *23*, *24*, *25*, *26*, 223
Restlessness, during anesthesia with sedation, 96
Results reporting system
 classification, *183*, *184*
 proposed management, *184*
 results of Levine and May series, 185–188
  category, *186*
  effects of disease on, 185–187
  preoperative factors on, 187–188
  prognosis, 188
  symptom profile, *186*
Rhinoscopy
 anterior, 69
 posterior, 69
Rhinosinusitis, 179

Saline solution, 154, 173
Samter's syndrome, 62–63, 64, 164, 184, 187
Sarcoma, 38
Scars, 204
Scissors, *113*, *114*
Sclerosis, *43*
Screening
 computed tomography, 49–51
 roentgenography for, 85
Sedatives
 with monitored anesthesia care, 93–97
 oversedation, 96
Sella turcica, 15
Semilunar hiatus, *See* Hiatus semilunaris
Septoplasty, 129, 170
Sinus
 disease, symptoms of, *62*, 127
 external surgery, 165, 169
 frontal, *6*
 imaging of, 152, 185–187
 lateralis, 6, 18, *20*, 32, *136*
 maxillary, *6*, 7–9, 22, *33*
 ostia, 51
 paranasal, *87*
 radiology, 66, 85
 terminalis, 6, 11
Sinusitis
 bacterial, *31*
 fungal, 30, 42, *68*, 87
 maxillary, *39*, *122*
 medical management of, 65–67
  of children, 247–250
  trial of, 65
 obstructive, 30
 pediatric, *245*
  protocol for treatment, 250
 sphenoid, *47*
 suppurative, 62, 64, 106, 107, 127, 172
  diagnosis of, 66
  treatment of, 66–67
   endoscopic management, 66–67
   medical management, 66
   surgical management, 66
Smell, alteration in, *62*, 64, 81
Speculum, 130
Sphenoethmoidectomy, 184
Sphenoethmoid junction, measurement with, *89*

Sphenoethmoid recess, 4, 13, *25*, 72, 81, 85, *86*
Sphenoid, measurement with, *89*
Sphenoid bone, greater wing of, 13
Sphenoiditis, *86*
Sphenoidotomy, 142–144
 procedure for, 144
Sphenoid sinus, 2, 4, 15, *21*, *25*, *27*, *28*, *47*, 126, *142*, *143*, 190, 210, 253
 anatomy, 44
 in children, 246
 complications in, 20, 241
 computed tomography of, 43–44
 disease, 85
 face of, 16, *141*, *141*, *145*, 146, 169–170
 internal carotid artery, 44–45, *143*
 opacification of, 44
 optic nerve, *143*
 ostium, 4
 pathology, 44
 retained secretions in, *58*
 roof of, 15
Splenopalatine artery, *21*, 26, *28*, *143*, 144, 169–170
Sphenopalatine ganglion, 128
Splenopalatine vessel, *25*, *28*
Sponge, 170
Squamous cell carcinoma, 38, 57
Stankiewicz maneuver, 204
Staphylococcus aureus, 238
Stenosis, 141, 150, 230, 237, 247
 of nasofrontal recess or isthmus, 150–154
Stents, 150
Sterilization, of equipment, *118*
Steroids, 62, 107, 173, 249
Streptococcus pneumoniae, 249
Succinylcholine, 98
Suction tip, 154
 Yankower, *117*
Sulindac, 63
Superior oblique muscle, *23*, *24*, *25*, *26*, *27*, 223
Supraorbital cell, *22*
Surgeon
 anesthesia choice of, 126–128
 endoscopic sinus, 1–28
Surgery
 approaches to sinus
  choice of anesthesia, 127–128
  choice of technique, 126
  operating microscope, 120–126
  two-handed technique, 108–120
  Wigand technique, 126
 case selection, 87, 90
 endonasal, 67, 78, 85
 endoscopic sinus, 91–104, 105–175, *177*, 180–182
  evaluation of results, 180
  late failures, 182
  results reporting system, 182–188
  step by step, 129, 150
 external sinus, 165, 169
 failure of, 190
 findings at, 263
 informed consent for, 90

indications for, 184
landmarks for, 137, 141
monitoring during, 129
plan of, 85
postoperative evaluation of, 174
preparation for, 106–107
  special considerations, 106–107
results, 176–190
  evaluation of, 174
  reporting systems, 176–182
revision of, 263
for sinus disease, 6, 60–90
  goal of treatment, 60
special situations, 150–169
success of, 190
traditional sinus, 176–179
  outcome measures, 179
  preoperative factors, 176, 178–179
  revision procedures, 178–179
  timing of evaluation of results, 179
of turbinates, 72
Symptom history, 61, 259
Symptomatology, 180–181
Synechiae, 189
Syringe, *115*

Taste, alteration in, *62*, 64
Terfenadine, 172
Theophylline, 99
Thiopental sodium, 98
Three-dimensional reconstruction, 51–52
Tolmetin, *63*
Tonsillectomy, 254
Torus tubarius, 4, *5*, 65, 72, 85
Toxic shock syndrome, 237–238
Transcanine fossa, *8*
  approach to, *121*, *123*, 165
  instruments for surgery, *113*
Transfusion, 202
Trephination, 154, *156*
Trigeminal nerve, 25

Trimethoprim-sulfamethoxazole, 66, 172
Trocar, 165, *166*, *167*
Tumors, 44, 56
Turbinates, 2–3, 32, 33, 41, 68, 69, *207*
  inferior, 4, *24*, 31
  middle, 3, *5*, 11, *14*, *15*, 16, *17*, 18, *21*, 22, *23*, 24, *25*, *28*, 34, *35*, *36*, *80*, *83*, *84*, 126, *135*, 144, 150, *151*, 169–170, 189, 190, 203, 223, *225–227*, 230, 242
  evaluation of, 72–78
  paradoxical, 34, *36*, *37*, 74, 77, 78, *79*, 246
  superior, *4*, 13, *25*, *39*, 72, 81, *82*, *136*
Turbinectomy, instruments for, *113*
Turbinoseptal deformity, 72, *73*
Two-handed technique, *See* Video endoscopic sinus surgery
Tympanostomy tube, 255

Uncinate process (first lamella), 3, *4*, *5*, 7, *8*, *10*, 11, 16, 22, 24, 27, 31, 32, *33*, 34, 35, *41*, 42, 51, 72, 81, *83*, *84*, 126, 130, *131*, *133*, *135*, *137*, *140*, 203, 204, *207*, 241
  structures lateral to, 6

Vasoconstrictors, 128
Vecuronium, 98
Vibrations, 208
Video camera, 70, 71, 72
Video endoscopic sinus surgery
  equipment, 108–120
    handling of, *118*
    sterilization of, *118*
Vision, *215*, *217*
Vomer, *41*

Washout sign, *224*
Wigand technique, 126

Zone A, 16–18, 147, 204, 208, *212*
Zone B, 18–20, 210
Zone C, 20–21, 210, 229